Cancer and Rheumatic Diseases

Editor

JOHN MANLEY DAVIS III

RHEUMATIC DISEASE CLINICS OF NORTH AMERICA

www.rheumatic.theclinics.com

Consulting Editor
MICHAEL H. WEISMAN

August 2020 • Volume 46 • Number 3

ELSEVIER

1600 John F. Kennedy Boulevard ● Suite 1800 ● Philadelphia, Pennsylvania, 19103-2899
http://www.theclinics.com

RHEUMATIC DISEASE CLINICS OF NORTH AMERICA Volume 46, Number 3
August 2020 ISSN 0889-857X, ISBN 13: 978-0-323-76126-0

Editor: Lauren Boyle
Developmental Editor: Nicole Congleton

Rheumatic Disease Clinics of North America (ISSN 0889-857X) is published quarterly by Elsevier Inc., 360 Park Avenue South, New York, NY 10010-1710. Months of issue are February, May, August, and November. Business and editorial offices: 1600 John F. Kennedy Boulevard, Suite 1800, Philadelphia, PA 19103-2899. Periodicals postage paid at New York, NY and additional mailing offices. Subscription prices are USD 362.00 per year for US individuals, USD 777.00 per year for US institutions, USD 100.00 per year for US students and residents, USD 427.00 per year for Canadian individuals, USD 971.00 per year for Canadian institutions, USD 100.00 per year for Canadian students/residents, USD 465.00 per year for international individuals, USD 971.00 per year for international institutions, and USD 230.00 per year for foreign students/residents. To receive student/resident rate, orders must be accompanied by name of affiliated institution, date of term, and the *signature* of program/ residency coordinator on institution letterhead. Orders will be billed at individual rate until proof of status received. Foreign air speed delivery is included in all *Clinics* subscription prices. All prices are subject to change without notice. **POSTMASTER:** Send address changes to *Rheumatic Disease Clinics of North America*, Elsevier Health Sciences Division, Subscription Customer Service, 3251 Riverport Lane, Maryland Heights, MO 63043. **Customer Service: 1-800-654-2452 (US and Canada). From outside of the US and Canada: 314-447-8871. Fax: 314-447-8029. For print support, e-mail: JournalsCustomerService-usa@elsevier.com. For online support, e-mail: JournalsOnlineSupport-usa@elsevier.com.**

Reprints. For copies of 100 or more of articles in this publication, please contact the Commercial Reprints Department, Elsevier Inc., 360 Park Avenue South, New York, New York, 10010-1710; Tel.: +1-212-633-3874, Fax: +1-212-633-3820, and E-mail: reprints@elsevier.com.

Rheumatic Disease Clinics of North America is covered in *MEDLINE/PubMed (Index Medicus), Current Contents/Clinical Medicine, Science Citation Index, ISI/BIOMED,* and *EMBASE/Excerpta Medica.*

Contributors

CONSULTING EDITOR

MICHAEL H. WEISMAN, MD
Professor of Medicine, Emeritus, Division of Rheumatology, Cedars-Sinai Medical Center, Distinguished Professor of Medicine, Emeritus, David Geffen School of Medicine, University of California, Los Angeles, Los Angeles, California, USA

EDITOR

JOHN MANLEY DAVIS III, MD, MS
Practice Chair and Vice Chair, Division of Rheumatology, Mayo Clinic, Associate Professor of Medicine, Mayo Clinic College of Medicine and Science, Rochester, Minnesota, USA

AUTHORS

NOHA ABDEL-WAHAB, MD, PhD
Assistant Professor, Division of Internal Medicine, Section of Rheumatology and Clinical Immunology, Lecturer, Department of Rheumatology and Rehabilitation, The University of Texas MD Anderson Cancer Center, Houston, Texas, USA; Faculty of Medicine, Assiut University Hospital, Assiut, Egypt

ROHIT AGGARWAL, MD, MSc
Division of Rheumatology and Clinical Immunology, Associate Professor, Department of Medicine, Myositis Center, University of Pittsburgh School of Medicine, UPMC Arthritis and Autoimmunity Center, Pittsburgh, Pennsylvania, USA

DANA P. ASCHERMAN, MD
Division of Rheumatology and Clinical Immunology, Department of Medicine, Myositis Center, University of Pittsburgh School of Medicine, Pittsburgh, Pennsylvania, USA

DELAMO I. BEKELE, MBBS
Instructor of Medicine and Fellow, Division of Rheumatology, Department of Internal Medicine, Mayo Clinic, Rochester, Minnesota, USA

SASHA BERNATSKY, MD, PhD
Professor, Department of Medicine, McGill University, Division of Clinical Epidemiology, Research Institute of McGill University Health Centre, Montreal, Quebec, Canada

LIVIA CASCIOLA-ROSEN, PhD
Professor of Medicine, Division of Rheumatology, Johns Hopkins School of Medicine, Baltimore, Maryland, USA

ANN E. CLARKE, MD, MSc
Professor of Medicine, Division of Rheumatology, University of Calgary, Calgary, Alberta, Canada

JOHN MANLEY DAVIS III, MD, MS
Practice Chair and Vice Chair, Division of Rheumatology, Mayo Clinic, Associate
Professor of Medicine, Mayo Clinic College of Medicine and Science, Rochester,
Minnesota, USA

CAROLINE GORDON, MD
Professor of Rheumatology, Institute of Inflammation and Ageing, College of Medical and
Dental Sciences, University of Birmingham, Edgbaston, United Kingdom

JAMES E. HANSEN, MD, MS
Associate Professor of Therapeutic Radiology, Department of Therapeutic Radiology,
Yale School of Medicine, New Haven, Connecticut, USA

ANN IGOE, MD
Arthritis and Clinical Immunology Program, Oklahoma Medical Research Foundation,
Departments of Medicine and Pathology, University of Oklahoma Health Sciences Center,
Oklahoma City, Oklahoma, USA

PARAS KARMACHARYA, MBBS
Rheumatology Fellow, Division of Rheumatology, Department of Medicine, Mayo Clinic,
Mayo Clinic College of Medicine, Rochester, Minnesota, USA

FAHAD KHAN, MD
Fellow, Division of Rheumatology and Immunology, Department of Internal Medicine,
Columbus, Ohio, USA

HILARY KLEPPEL, BS
Clinical Research Coordinator, Division of Rheumatology and Immunology, Department
of Internal Medicine, Columbus, Ohio, USA

ALEXANDRA LADOUCEUR, MD, PhD
Department of Medicine, McGill University, Montreal, Quebec, Canada

ALEXA MEARA, MD
Assistant Professor, Division of Rheumatology and Immunology, Department of Internal
Medicine, Columbus, Ohio, USA

SALI MERJANAH, MD
The MetroHealth System, Case Western Reserve University, Cleveland, Ohio, USA

SIAMAK MOGHADAM-KIA, MD, MPH
Division of Rheumatology and Clinical Immunology, Department of Medicine, Myositis
Center, University of Pittsburgh School of Medicine, VA Pittsburgh Healthcare System,
Pittsburgh, Pennsylvania, USA

CHESTER V. ODDIS, MD
Division of Rheumatology and Clinical Immunology, Department of Medicine, Myositis
Center, University of Pittsburgh School of Medicine, UPMC Arthritis and Autoimmunity
Center, Pittsburgh, Pennsylvania, USA

ALEXIS OGDIE, MD, MSCE
Associate Professor of Medicine and Epidemiology, Division of Rheumatology, Hospital
of the University of Pennsylvania, Perelman Center for Advanced Medicine, Philadelphia,
Pennsylvania, USA

MRINAL M. PATNAIK, MBBS, MD
Associate Professor of Medicine and Consultant, Division of Hematology, Department of Internal Medicine, Mayo Clinic, Rochester, Minnesota, USA

XERXES PUNDOLE, MD, PhD
Department of Health Services Research, The University of Texas MD Anderson Cancer Center, Houston, Texas, USA

ROSALIND RAMSEY-GOLDMAN, MD, DrPh
Professor of Medicine, Division of Rheumatology, Northwestern University Feinberg School of Medicine, Chicago, Illinois, USA

R. HAL SCOFIELD, MD
Arthritis and Clinical Immunology Program, Member, Oklahoma Medical Research Foundation, Professor, Departments of Medicine and Pathology, University of Oklahoma Health Sciences Center, US Department of Veterans Affairs, Oklahoma City, Oklahoma, USA

AMI A. SHAH, MD, MHS
Associate Professor of Medicine, Division of Rheumatology, Johns Hopkins School of Medicine, Baltimore, Maryland, USA

RAVI SHAHUKHAL, MD
Academic Hospitalist, Division of Internal Medicine, Lakes Regional General Hospital, Laconia, New Hampshire, USA

MARIA E. SUAREZ-ALMAZOR, MD, PhD
Department of Health Services Research, Department of General Internal Medicine, Section of Rheumatology and Clinical Immunology, The University of Texas MD Anderson Cancer Center, Houston, Texas, USA

BASILE TESSIER-CLOUTIER, MD
Postdoctoral Reseach Fellow, Department of Pathology and Laboratory Medicine, University of British Columbia, Vancouver, British Columbia, Canada

UMA THANARAJASINGAM, MD, PhD
Assistant Professor, Mayo Clinic, Rochester, Minnesota, USA

EMMA WEEDING, MD
Postdoctoral Fellow, Division of Rheumatology, Johns Hopkins School of Medicine, Baltimore, Maryland, USA

Contents

Foreword   **xi**

Michael H. Weisman

Preface: Timely Knowledge and Clinical Insights on Cancer and Rheumatic Disease   **xiii**

John Manley Davis III

Overview of the Associations Between Cancer and Rheumatic Disease   **417**

John Manley Davis III

People living with rheumatic diseases frequently encounter cancer, either as a potential harm of antirheumatic therapies or as a comorbidity that alters the conversation about management. This article provides a general overview of the issues related to cancer and rheumatic disease and serves as a springboard for the remaining chapters in this issue. Several topics are reviewed, including epidemiology, bidirectional causal pathways, and issues related to medications. Although uncertainties remain, the issue of cancer is of great importance to patients with rheumatic diseases, and an individualized, person-centered approach to assessment and management is necessary.

Autoimmunity, Clonal Hematopoiesis, and Myeloid Neoplasms   **429**

Delamo I. Bekele and Mrinal M. Patnaik

Clonal hematopoiesis has been linked with the development of hematologic malignancy and atherosclerotic cardiovascular disease; however, the association with autoimmune diseases remains to be defined. The link between autoimmune diseases and myeloid neoplasms (MNs) is complex, often multifactorial, and seems bidirectional. The limited data suggest an increased risk of MNs in rheumatoid arthritis and systemic lupus erythematosus. Paraneoplastic manifestations of MN include arthritis, vasculitis, and connective tissue disease. Treatment options for autoimmune disease such as cyclophosphamide and azathioprine have been associated with MNs, whereas the data for methotrexate and tumor necrosis factor inhibitors are equivocal.

Cancer and Rheumatoid Arthritis   **445**

Xerxes Pundole and Maria E. Suarez-Almazor

Management of rheumatoid arthritis (RA) in patients with cancer is complex and requires a multidisciplinary approach. A few studies have examined the risk for recurrence in patients with RA receiving disease-modifying antirheumatic drugs, primarily tumor necrosis factor-α inhibitors. Although these agents seem to be safe in patients with a history of cancer and no evidence of disease, additional information is needed to determine their potential effects in patients with RA and active cancer. Patients with RA undergoing cancer therapy, including surgery, radiation, chemotherapy, and immunotherapy, need to be carefully monitored because they are at increased risk for adverse events.

Risk of Malignancy in Spondyloarthritis: A Systematic Review   463

Paras Karmacharya, Ravi Shahukhal, and Alexis Ogdie

Systematic inflammatory diseases, including rheumatoid arthritis (RA), are associated with an increased risk of malignancies. However, the pathogenesis of spondyloarthritis (SpA), which includes both ankylosing spondylitis and psoriatic arthritis, is different from RA, and the risk of malignancy and sites involved may also be different. It is important to better understand associations of SpA with site-specific cancers to facilitate appropriate cancer screening. The goal of this review was to examine the association of SpA with malignancy and the potential impact of therapy for SpA on development of malignancy.

Sjögren Syndrome and Cancer   513

Ann Igoe, Sali Merjanah, and R. Hal Scofield

The association between malignancy and rheumatic diseases has been demonstrated in a multitude of studies. Little is understood regarding the pathogenesis of rheumatic and musculoskeletal diseases in association with malignancy. There is strong evidence regarding the association between Sjögren syndrome and lymphoma as well as risk factors for development of lymphoma in these patients. This article discusses the accumulating data on various malignancies described in primary Sjögren syndrome, highlighting non-Hodgkin lymphoma and thyroid, multiple myeloma, and skin cancers. These reported associations may have clinical implications in daily practice and contribute to understanding of both autoimmunity and cancer.

Cancer and Systemic Lupus Erythematosus   533

Alexandra Ladouceur, Basile Tessier-Cloutier, Ann E. Clarke, Rosalind Ramsey-Goldman, Caroline Gordon, James E. Hansen, and Sasha Bernatsky

Systemic lupus erythematosus is associated with a small overall increased cancer risk compared with the general population. This risk includes a 4-fold increased risk of non-Hodgkin lymphoma, but a decreased risk of other cancers (such as breast cancer). The pathophysiology underlying the increased risk of hematologic cancer is not fully understood, but many potential mechanisms have been proposed, including dysfunction of the tumor necrosis factor and other pathways. A decreased risk of breast, ovarian, and endometrial cancer might be driven by hormonal factors or lupus-related antibodies, but these links have not been proved.

Cancer and Scleroderma   551

Emma Weeding, Livia Casciola-Rosen, and Ami A. Shah

Individuals with scleroderma have an increased risk of cancer compared with the general population. This heightened risk may be from chronic inflammation and tissue damage, malignant transformation provoked by immunosuppressive therapies, or a common inciting factor. In unique subsets of patients with scleroderma, there is a close temporal relationship between the onset of cancer and scleroderma, suggesting cancer-induced autoimmunity. This article discusses the potential mechanistic links between cancer and scleroderma, the serologic and clinical risk factors associated with increased cancer risk in patients with scleroderma, and implications for cancer screening.

Risk Factors and Cancer Screening in Myositis 565

Siamak Moghadam-Kia, Chester V. Oddis, Dana P. Ascherman, and Rohit Aggarwal

The idiopathic inflammatory myopathies, particularly dermatomyositis, are associated with an increased risk of cancer. Lung, ovarian, breast, colon, prostate, and cervical cancers, and hematologic malignancies, are among the most common associated cancers. Risk stratification for cancer in patients with myositis is based on clinical risk factors/red flags, myositis clinical subtypes, and myositis-specific autoantibodies. Clinical risk factors include older age at disease onset, male gender, dysphagia, acute onset/refractory myositis, cutaneous ulceration, necrosis/vasculitis, and elevated inflammatory markers. Appropriate screening strategies are based on the risk level. Further studies are warranted to determine the role of advanced imaging and comprehensive cancer screening.

Paraneoplastic Musculoskeletal Syndromes 577

Fahad Khan, Hilary Kleppel, and Alexa Meara

Paraneoplastic syndromes are rare diseases caused by malignancies through means other than mass effect or metastasis. Paraneoplastic phenomena can be the first sign of cancer and can be fatal. Paraneoplastic rheumatic syndromes can occur with hematologic cancers, lymphoproliferative disease, and solid tumors. Diseases that feature an advanced age at onset, significant constitutional upset, inadequate response to treatment, and otherwise atypical characteristics should increase the index of suspicion for a paraneoplastic syndrome.

Immune Checkpoint Inhibition—Does It Cause Rheumatic Diseases? Mechanisms of Cancer-Associated Loss of Tolerance and Pathogenesis of Autoimmunity 587

Uma Thanarajasingam and Noha Abdel-Wahab

Mechanisms of immune checkpoints and their role in autoimmunity are discussed in the context of immune checkpoint inhibitor (ICI) therapy for cancer. The updated clinical spectrum of immune-related adverse events (irAEs), with an in-depth discussion of rheumatic irAEs, is presented. The relationship between ICI-induced loss of self-tolerance in cancer and the implications for understanding of irAEs, rheumatic irAEs in particular, is overviewed.

RHEUMATIC DISEASE CLINICS OF NORTH AMERICA

FORTHCOMING ISSUES

November 2020
**Health Disparities in Rheumatic Diseases:
Part I**
Candace H. Feldman, *Editor*

February 2021
**Health Disparities in Rheumatic Diseases:
Part II**
Candace H. Feldman, *Editor*

RECENT ISSUES

May 2020
**Spondyloarthritis: The Changing Landscape
Today**
Xenofon Baraliakos and Michael
Weisman, *Editors*

February 2020
**Education and Professional Development in
Rheumatology**
Karina D. Torralba and James D. Katz,
Editors

THE CLINICS ARE AVAILABLE ONLINE!
Access your subscription at:
www.theclinics.com

Foreword

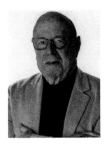

Michael H. Weisman, MD
Consulting Editor

John Davis has created a thoughtful and scholarly issue addressing the complex relationships between malignancy and chronic rheumatic diseases. The articles are practical in a clinical sense and support the concept of shared decision making when both the patient and his or her doctor face questions about options for further workup and management. As some wise clinicians used to say, it is not about treatment of a rheumatic disease (since we don't know the cause, how can we treat?), it is always about patient management, and malignancy potential fits directly into patient management. Now that we are regularly employing checkpoint inhibitors as part of cancer chemotherapy, the specificity of interruption of the immune system at certain targeted points with the subsequent display of rheumatic disease phenotypes of all kinds has eliminated the sharp distinctions between cancer and our rheumatic diseases. In his choice of articles and topics, John Davis has pointed out some areas of progress, but he has left open for further discussion the gaps in our understanding of why these events are taking place as our rheumatic diseases are becoming better controlled with drugs, or diagnosed earlier and managed efficiently before damage has occurred. Carefully done observational studies as well as basic science approaches in the research laboratory are reviewed in this issue; why some diseases are regularly associated with cancer (myositis, for example) and others are not (spondyloarthritis) are powerful incentives to keep these lines of research going. Much thanks to John for putting this important issue together.

Michael H. Weisman, MD
Division of Rheumatology
Cedars-Sinai Medical Center
David Geffen School of Medicine at University of California, Los Angeles
1545 Calmar Court
Los Angeles, CA 90024, USA

E-mail address:
michael.weisman@cshs.org

Rheum Dis Clin N Am 46 (2020) xi
https://doi.org/10.1016/j.rdc.2020.06.001
0889-857X/20/© 2020 Published by Elsevier Inc.

rheumatic.theclinics.com

Preface

Timely Knowledge and Clinical Insights on Cancer and Rheumatic Disease

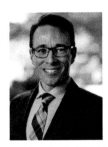

John Manley Davis III, MD, MS
Editor

Questions pertaining to cancer and rheumatic disease arise commonly in clinical practice. Clinicians commonly experience concern for the possibility that an atypical or undifferentiated inflammatory syndrome could be caused by an occult malignancy. Conversely, patients often raise justifiable concerns about the possibility a drug for their rheumatic disease may increase their lifetime risk of cancer. Estimates of the risk of cancer for a given rheumatic disease or related to a certain antirheumatic medication seem to vary from study to study. All parties to the care of patients with rheumatic diseases crave greater clarity on best practices for treatment and management. In this thematic issue on Cancer and Rheumatic Disease, experts in their fields provide their knowledge and clinical insights to address gaps in clinical practice and research. I am especially proud that all authors have taken a pragmatic and clinical approach by providing useful guidance on how to individualize patient assessment, with useful points on cancer screening as well as shared decision making about management. I am hopeful that the knowledge conveyed in this issue will provide an impetus for further clinical and translational studies on the interface between cancer and rheumatic diseases, which can be expected to provide new treatment options for people living with these conditions in the future. It has certainly been an honor and a privilege to work with my outstanding colleagues and with Elsevier to produce this thematic issue, and I am sincerely thankful to all for their great efforts. I hope

Rheum Dis Clin N Am 46 (2020) xiii–xiv
https://doi.org/10.1016/j.rdc.2020.05.001
0889-857X/20/© 2020 Published by Elsevier Inc.

rheumatic.theclinics.com

the readership of *Rheumatic Disease Clinics* finds the content of this issue valuable and useful in both the clinical and research settings.

John Manley Davis III, MD, MS
Mayo Clinic Rochester
200 1st Street Southwest
Rochester, MN 55905, USA

E-mail address:
davis.john4@mayo.edu

Overview of the Associations Between Cancer and Rheumatic Disease

John Manley Davis III, MD, MS

KEYWORDS

- Cancer • Malignancy • Rheumatic disease • Prognosis
- Immune checkpoint inhibitors • Immune-related adverse events • Treatment
- Biologic therapies

KEY POINTS

- People with rheumatic diseases in general experience a higher risk of cancer compared with their peers in the general population; the types of cancer and the magnitude of risk differ across the rheumatic diseases.
- Chronic immune activation and inflammation caused by rheumatic diseases seem to be central to the increased risk of malignancies experienced by patients.
- Bidirectional relationships exist between cancer and rheumatic diseases; this is best exemplified by emerging data in myositis and systemic sclerosis.
- Rheumatic immune-related adverse effects of immune checkpoint inhibitors for the treatment of various cancers highlight a delicate balance between malignancy and inflammatory rheumatic syndromes and are an emerging clinical challenge for management.
- When facing patients with an underlying rheumatic disease, it is crucial to appraise the individuals' knowledge, preferences, and values and engage them in shared decision making about options for management.

INTRODUCTION

Cancer is a vexing issue that frequently confronts patients with rheumatic diseases and their physicians. Many different types of cancer have been associated with rheumatic diseases, including hematologic and nonhematologic malignancies. In contrast, many different rheumatic diseases have known associations with malignancy. These points inform a variety of considerations regarding potential causality. First, inflammation is central to both cancer and rheumatic disease, which may explain in part the overlap in risk factors. Second, there are many examples of rheumatic diseases being associated with heightened risk of cancer, and there are examples of cancers potentially causing rheumatic diseases such as paraneoplastic syndromes, showing the

Division of Rheumatology, Mayo Clinic, 200 1st St SW, Rochester, MN 55905, USA
E-mail address: davis.john4@mayo.edu
Twitter: @JohnDavisIII (J.M.D.)

Rheum Dis Clin N Am 46 (2020) 417–427
https://doi.org/10.1016/j.rdc.2020.05.002
0889-857X/20/© 2020 Elsevier Inc. All rights reserved.

rheumatic.theclinics.com

bidirectional relationships between these neoplastic and inflammatory disease states. Third, medications may mediate the relationship between cancer and rheumatic disease. Although concerns have arisen that immunosuppressive, disease-modifying antirheumatic therapies may increase the cancer risk, long-term extensions of clinical trials as well as population-based trials increasingly provide reassurance that these agents can be used overall with safety with regard to cancer risk. More recently, an epidemic of rheumatic immune-related adverse events of checkpoint inhibitor therapy is transforming understanding of the interactions between immunity and oncogenesis. In this issue of *Rheumatic Disease Clinics of North America*, experts review the complex interrelationships between cancer, rheumatic disease, and treatment of these conditions in depth. They address key points to consider regarding cancer screening for patients with rheumatic diseases. Ultimately, this issue is expected to provide state-of-the-art information to guide clinicians and their patients.

OVERVIEW OF THE ASSOCIATIONS BETWEEN CANCER AND RHEUMATIC DISEASE

For the past several decades, knowledge of the relationship between cancer and rheumatic disease has been in existence. Historically, this knowledge has been classified according to hematologic and nonhematologic (ie, solid or visceral) malignancies. With respect to the hematologic category, higher rates of both lymphoid (eg, Hodgkin and non-Hodgkin lymphoma) and myeloid (eg, acute myeloid leukemia) neoplasms have been reported among patients with several rheumatic diseases; for example, rheumatoid arthritis (RA),[1–3] systemic lupus erythematosus,[4–7] and Sjögren syndrome.[8–10] More recently, as reviewed in this issue by Bekele and Patnaik,[11] an emerging relationship between rheumatic disease and clonal hematopoiesis provides new insights into the relationships between chronic inflammation and malignant cell transformation.[12]

With regard to the nonhematologic category, differential risk has been observed for various types of solid/visceral malignancies among patients with rheumatic diseases, including melanoma and nonmelanoma skin cancers, and breast, lung, liver, pancreas, bladder, prostate, uterine, and cervical cancers.[1,4,13–16] Associations vary in terms of cancer types and even direction of effect across the rheumatic diseases, which presumably may be related to basic demographics, risk factors, levels and sites of systemic inflammation, or degree of immune suppression associated with the antirheumatic therapies used. In this issue, Igoe and colleagues[17] highlight not only the hematologic but also the nonhematologic malignancies that associate with Sjögren syndrome, including the salivary glands, nasopharynx, thymus, and lung. As highlighted by Pundole and Suarez-Almazor[18] in this issue, preexisting interstitial lung disease in patients with RA is a risk factor for the development of lung cancer, which may relate to smoking as a shared risk factor or to chronic inflammation and activation of fibrogenic pathways. In an example of different associations by cancer type, the risks of lung cancer and melanoma are increased for patients with RA but decreased for breast and colorectal cancer.[19] Recently, it has been shown that the reduced risk of breast cancer in patients with RA cannot be explained by traditional risk factors.[20] The incidence rates for high-grade cervical dysplasia and cancer are higher for patients with systemic lupus erythematosus (SLE) than for patients with rheumatoid arthritis or psoriasis.[16] Further research is necessary to elucidate the underpinnings of these differential associations between cancer and rheumatic diseases.

OVERVIEW OF SHARED RISK FACTORS

In reviewing the most important risk factors for both cancer and rheumatic disease, it is likely that many of these are shared between the two disease categories. Previous studies have attempted to address the extent to which genetic risk factors overlap between cancer and rheumatic diseases. If genetic overlap plays an important role in the risk of these two conditions, the familial risk associations would be expected to be bidirectional. However, in the example of the association between RA and lymphoma, a personal history of cancer, including lymphoma, does not increase the risk of subsequent RA development. Similarly, having a family history of Sjögren syndrome does not associate with a higher risk of non-Hodgkin lymphoma, and vice versa.[21] A confirmed example of genetic overlap between cancer and rheumatic disease has been reported for Sjögren syndrome, in which genetic variation in tumor necrosis factor alpha–induced protein 3 (TNFAIP3), the gene that encodes the A20 protein and that is associated with several autoimmune diseases, has been found to be present in 77% of these patients who develop mucosa-associated lymphoid tissue lymphoma.[22] A recent large genome-wide association study has shown sparse overlap between genetic variants associated with RA, SLE, and non-Hodgkin lymphoma subtypes; however, only a few weakly associated loci were identified in common, explaining little overall risk.[23] Hence, it seems likely that other factors are more important in the risk of cancer in patients with rheumatic diseases.

One such factor that is central to both cancer and rheumatic disease is chronic inflammation, with numerous examples in the literature. In particular, this would partially explain why so many cancers follow the onset of autoimmune rheumatic diseases, such as in the cases of rheumatoid arthritis, lupus, and Sjögren syndrome.[24] For example, the incidence of lymphoma increases in the decade following the onset of RA.[24] The risk is highest among patients in the upper decile of cumulative disease activity and tends to decrease with use of disease-modifying medications to control disease activity.[25,26] In the case of Sjögren syndrome, the presence of rheumatoid factor and measures of disease activity (eg, low C4 level; cryoglobulinemia; lymphopenia; and the European League Against Rheumatism Sjögren's Syndrome Disease Activity Index, excluding the lymphoma domain) were found to be predictive of lymphoma.[27] The concept that chronic activation of the immune system, either by infection or autoimmune disease, mediates cancer development also holds for acute and chronic myeloid leukemias.[28,29] Using the Veterans Affairs Rheumatoid Arthritis cohort, Bryant and colleagues[30] showed that increased levels of cytokines and chemokines in the peripheral blood at baseline of men with RA was associated during longitudinal follow-up with overall cancer mortality. Furthermore, there was an interaction between tobacco smoking and the summary cytokine score, such that cancer mortality was much higher among men who were current smokers and had a high cytokine score than for either risk factor alone. With regard to gout, a disease that has been of great interest in recent years, there is increasing evidence that chronic gouty inflammation is associated with an increased risk of malignancies,[31–33] which may be attenuated by colchicine or urate level–lowering therapy.[34–36] In addition, aspirin and nonsteroidal antiinflammatory drugs in a recent meta-analysis were shown to decrease the risk of recurrent colorectal adenomas, a precursor to adenocarcinoma.[37] Hence, ongoing efforts to abrogate inflammation in patients with rheumatic diseases will be crucial to effectively mitigate risk of future malignancy.

Environmental risk factors are also shared between cancer and rheumatic diseases. Tobacco smoking is a well-known risk factor for both rheumatic diseases (eg, RA, SLE, and Sjögren) and a myriad of cancers, especially lung cancer.[38–42] Excess body fat and obesity are also established risk factors for several rheumatic diseases and cancers, the effects of which in these diseases may be mediated by the issue of chronic inflammation, mentioned earlier.[43–45] Dietary patterns, particularly those with inflammation-promoting foods, are associated with a higher risk of both RA and certain cancers.[46–52] The molecular mechanisms of these associations remain to be defined, but there is great interest in the role of the gut microbiome in mediating the effects of inflammatory dietary patterns on the host immune system, ultimately driving adaptive immune responses and chronic inflammation.[53–57] There may also be a role for the gut microbiome in driving cell growth and proliferation, altering food and drug metabolism, and modulating immune surveillance for malignant cells via the effects of circulating microbial metabolites.[54] It is also possible that live gut bacteria translocate across a dysfunctional gut barrier to interact with and instigate T-cell and B-cell activation and inflammatory responses that could play a role in both cancer and rheumatic diseases.[53,55,56] In addition, Epstein-Barr virus is an example of a viral pathogen that has been associated with lymphoproliferative disease in patients treated with immunosuppressive therapies, both in the cancer and rheumatic setting, and is also associated with the pathogenesis of RA, SLE, and Sjögren syndrome.[58,59]

POTENTIAL CAUSAL PATHWAYS FROM CANCER TO RHEUMATIC DISEASE

It has been known for decades that rheumatic conditions can represent paraneoplastic syndromes. As reviewed comprehensively in this issue by Khan and colleagues,[60] classical paraneoplastic rheumatic syndromes include carcinomatous polyarthritis, remitting symmetric seronegative synovitis with pitting edema (RS3PE), polymyalgia rheumatica–like syndromes, and palmar fasciitis with polyarthritis.[61–64] Recently, the spectrum of autoimmune and autoinflammatory syndromes associated with chronic myelomonocytic leukemia has become apparent.[65] Great progress has been made in understanding the nature of the associations between visceral malignancies and various subtypes of myositis and scleroderma. Moghadam and colleagues[66,67] in this issue review the relationships, both positive and negative, between myositis syndromes defined not only by their clinical manifestations but also by autoantibody specificities, particularly transcriptional intermediary factor-1-gamma (TIF-1-γ) and nuclear matrix protein-2 (NXP-2) autoantibodies. Also herein, Weeding and colleagues[68–71] elegantly summarize the novel associations linking cancer to the pathophysiology of certain subtypes of systemic sclerosis, particularly the diseases associated with anti-RNA polymerase I/III and anti–RNPC-3. These insights provide an opportunity to dissect the mechanistic links between oncogenesis and the loss of tolerance to tumor-associated antigens and the development of autoimmunity, culminating in these systemic rheumatic diseases.[72] Further, this information provides clinicians with the beginning of a basis to rationally identify patients at high risk for concomitant malignancy for comprehensive cancer screening.[73]

DRUG EFFECTS, CANCER, AND RHEUMATIC DISEASE

Since the initial use of immunosuppressive, disease-modifying medications for RA, there has been concern for the potential adverse effect of cancer. Over the years, many studies and meta-analyses have been undertaken,[3,74–82] a full review of which goes beyond the scope of this overview and is covered elsewhere in this issue. In recent years, the authors have gained confidence that the overall safety of targeted, biologic therapies for RA is excellent with only minimal excess risk of primary or recurrent malignancy.[83] Exceptions remain, of course, and perhaps lymphoma and other hematologic malignancies are the forms of cancer that remain as relative contraindications to certain antirheumatic therapies, particularly tumor necrosis factor (TNF) biologics more so than non-TNF biologics, JAK inhibitors, or conventional synthetic agents. Among patients with lymphoma, B-cell depletion therapy with rituximab maintains its role as the preferred therapeutic option.[84] However, because power is limited even with large, nationwide register–based studies to detect sparse adverse effects of biologic or targeted therapies, such as malignancies, shared decision making with patients about the potential benefits in relation to the potential harms, including malignancies, is very important. In their thoughtful review of this issue, Pundole and Suarez-Almazor[18] provide a clinically useful summary of available guidelines and commentary about individualizing decision making about antirheumatic therapies and other relevant management strategies in patients with cancer.

The advent and now widespread use of immune checkpoint inhibitor therapy for various cancers heralded an array of rheumatic syndromes, termed rheumatic immune-related adverse effects (rh-irAE), including inflammatory arthritis, polymyalgia, sicca syndrome, myositis, and sclerodermalike syndromes, that occur in 5% to 10% of patients with cancer treated with these agents.[85–89] In some cases, these syndromes have seemed to represent genuine drug-induced rheumatic diseases, fulfilling classification criteria, but other cases have presented atypical features.[90] These syndromes are often severe and can be life threatening. Uma Thanarajasingam and Noha Abdel-Wahab's article, "Immune Checkpoint Inhibition–Does It Cause Rheumatic Diseases? Mechanisms of Cancer-Associated Loss of Tolerance and Pathogenesis of Autoimmunity," in this issue review the literature on this topic in detail, including the pharmacology of immune checkpoint inhibitors, clinical features of rh-irAE, pathophysiology, and clinical management guidelines. rh-irAE seems to result from disinhibiting T-cell regulation, leading to unchecked activation of T-helper (Th) 1 and Th17 cells as well as B cells, driving autoimmunity and tissue inflammation. Many uncertainties remain, particularly the full spectrum of rh-irAE syndromes, similarities and differences of these from idiopathic rheumatic diseases, the underlying molecular mechanisms, ability to identify patients at risk of rh-irAE before immune checkpoint inhibitor therapy, best practices for use of steroids and antirheumatic disease-modifying therapies, and the long-term prognosis, both for the cancer and the rheumatic syndrome.

SUMMARY

When patients present with rheumatic syndromes, it is important to consider the possibility of an underlying or associated malignancy. Age-appropriate and sex-appropriate cancer screening is important for all patients with rheumatic diseases, and more comprehensive screening should be undertaken with consideration of diagnosis, clinical characteristics and serologic findings, disease activity and progression, cancer risk factors, and medication exposures. Elsewhere in this issue, more detailed guidance is presented on cancer screening, such as the risk stratification proposals of Moghadam-Kia and colleagues[91] and Weeding and colleagues.[92] With respect to making decisions with patients about treatment of their rheumatic disease, in general, the evidence is reassuring that the absolute probability of primary or recurrent malignancy is very low (typically, 2–5 per 1000 patients treated for 1 year); in patients with a prior cancer, the risk is especially low when the cancer is inactive and more than 5 years old. The complexity and, sometimes, the uncertainty of the relationship of an individual patient's cancer to the rheumatic disease warrant caution and deliberation by the patient's multidisciplinary team. Several important clinical questions still remain pertaining to cancer and rheumatic disease that require further clinical and translational research.

CLINICS CARE POINTS

- All adult patients with rheumatic diseases should undergo age- and sex-appropriate cancer screening at diagnosis.

- Comprehensive, disease-specific cancer screening is indicated in several higher risk rheumatic diseases, including myositis and systemic sclerosis.
- Effective control of systemic inflammation with disease-modifying antirheumatic drugs is important to mitigate the risk of future cancer in patients with rheumatic diseases.
- Collaborative decision-making between the patient, rheumatologist, and oncologist is crucial when considering treatment of a patient with active malignancy with immunosuppressive therapies.

DISCLOSURE

Dr J.M. Davis has received research grants from Pfizer and has served on advisory boards for Abbvie and Sanofi-Genzyme.

REFERENCES

1. Simon TA, Thompson A, Gandhi KK, et al. Incidence of malignancy in adult patients with rheumatoid arthritis: a meta-analysis. Arthritis Res Ther 2015;17:212.
2. Lim XR, Xiang W, Tan JWL, et al. Incidence and patterns of malignancies in a multi-ethnic cohort of rheumatoid arthritis patients. Int J Rheum Dis 2019;22(9):1679–85.
3. Askling J, Fored CM, Baecklund E, et al. Haematopoietic malignancies in rheumatoid arthritis: lymphoma risk and characteristics after exposure to tumour necrosis factor antagonists. Ann Rheum Dis 2005;64(10):1414–20.
4. Song L, Wang Y, Zhang J, et al. The risks of cancer development in systemic lupus erythematosus (SLE) patients: a systematic review and meta-analysis. Arthritis Res Ther 2018;20(1):270.
5. Bernatsky S, Boivin JF, Joseph L, et al. An international cohort study of cancer in systemic lupus erythematosus. Arthritis Rheum 2005;52(5):1481–90.
6. Apor E, O'Brien J, Stephen M, et al. Systemic lupus erythematosus is associated with increased incidence of hematologic malignancies: a meta-analysis of prospective cohort studies. Leuk Res 2014;38(9):1067–71.
7. Lu M, Bernatsky S, Ramsey-Goldman R, et al. Non-lymphoma hematological malignancies in systemic lupus erythematosus. Oncology 2013;85(4):235–40.
8. Tsukamoto M, Suzuki K, Takeuchi T. Ten-year observation of patients with primary Sjogren's syndrome: Initial presenting characteristics and the associated outcomes. Int J Rheum Dis 2019;22(5):929–33.
9. Retamozo S, Brito-Zeron P, Ramos-Casals M. Prognostic markers of lymphoma development in primary Sjogren syndrome. Lupus 2019;28(8):923–36.
10. Liang Y, Yang Z, Qin B, et al. Primary Sjogren's syndrome and malignancy risk: a systematic review and meta-analysis. Ann Rheum Dis 2014;73(6):1151–6.
11. Bekele D, Patnaik MM. Autoimmunity, clonal hematopoiesis and myeloid neoplasms. Rheum Dis Clin North Am 2020;46(3).
12. Savola P, Lundgren S, Keranen MAI, et al. Clonal hematopoiesis in patients with rheumatoid arthritis. Blood Cancer J 2018;8(8):69.
13. Ni J, Qiu LJ, Hu LF, et al. Lung, liver, prostate, bladder malignancies risk in systemic lupus erythematosus: evidence from a meta-analysis. Lupus 2014;23(3):284–92.
14. Yang Z, Lin F, Qin B, et al. Polymyositis/dermatomyositis and malignancy risk: a metaanalysis study. J Rheumatol 2015;42(2):282–91.
15. Zhang JQ, Wan YN, Peng WJ, et al. The risk of cancer development in systemic sclerosis: a meta-analysis. Cancer Epidemiol 2013;37(5):523–7.

16. Kim SC, Glynn RJ, Giovannucci E, et al. Risk of high-grade cervical dysplasia and cervical cancer in women with systemic inflammatory diseases: a population-based cohort study. Ann Rheum Dis 2015;74(7):1360–7.

17. Igoe A, Merjanah S, Scofield RH. Sjögren's Syndrome and Cancer. Rheum Dis Clin North Am 2020;46(3).

18. Pundole X, Suarez-Almazor ME. Cancer and rheumatoid arthritis. Rheum Dis Clin North Am 2020;46(3).

19. Smitten AL, Simon TA, Hochberg MC, et al. A meta-analysis of the incidence of malignancy in adult patients with rheumatoid arthritis. Arthritis Res Ther 2008; 10(2):R45.

20. Wadstrom H, Pettersson A, Smedby KE, et al. Risk of breast cancer before and after rheumatoid arthritis, and the impact of hormonal factors. Ann Rheum Dis 2020;79(5):581–6.

21. Ben-Eli H, Aframian DJ, Ben-Chetrit E, et al. Shared medical and environmental risk factors in dry eye syndrome, Sjogren's Syndrome, and B-cell non-hodgkin lymphoma: a case-control study. J Immunol Res 2019;2019:9060842.

22. Nocturne G, Boudaoud S, Miceli-Richard C, et al. Germline and somatic genetic variations of TNFAIP3 in lymphoma complicating primary Sjogren's syndrome. Blood 2013;122(25):4068–76.

23. Din L, Sheikh M, Kosaraju N, et al. Genetic overlap between autoimmune diseases and non-Hodgkin lymphoma subtypes. Genet Epidemiol 2019;43(7): 844–63.

24. Hellgren K, Smedby KE, Feltelius N, et al. Do rheumatoid arthritis and lymphoma share risk factors?: a comparison of lymphoma and cancer risks before and after diagnosis of rheumatoid arthritis. Arthritis Rheum 2010;62(5):1252–8.

25. Baecklund E, Iliadou A, Askling J, et al. Association of chronic inflammation, not its treatment, with increased lymphoma risk in rheumatoid arthritis. Arthritis Rheum 2006;54(3):692–701.

26. Baecklund E, Smedby KE, Sutton LA, et al. Lymphoma development in patients with autoimmune and inflammatory disorders–what are the driving forces? Semin Cancer Biol 2014;24:61–70.

27. Nocturne G, Virone A, Ng WF, et al. Rheumatoid factor and disease activity are independent predictors of lymphoma in primary sjogren's syndrome. Arthritis Rheumatol 2016;68(4):977–85.

28. Kristinsson SY, Bjorkholm M, Hultcrantz M, et al. Chronic immune stimulation might act as a trigger for the development of acute myeloid leukemia or myelodysplastic syndromes. J Clin Oncol 2011;29(21):2897–903.

29. Elbaek MV, Sorensen AL, Hasselbalch HC. Chronic inflammation and autoimmunity as risk factors for the development of chronic myelomonocytic leukemia? Leuk Lymphoma 2016;57(8):1793–9.

30. England BR, Sokolove J, Robinson WH, et al. Associations of circulating cytokines and chemokines with cancer mortality in men with rheumatoid arthritis. Arthritis Rheumatol 2016;68(10):2394–402.

31. Tu H, Wen CP, Tsai SP, et al. Cancer risk associated with chronic diseases and disease markers: prospective cohort study. BMJ 2018;360:k134.

32. Wang W, Xu D, Wang B, et al. Increased risk of cancer in relation to gout: a review of three prospective cohort studies with 50,358 subjects. Mediators Inflamm 2015;2015:680853.

33. Wandell P, Carlsson AC, Ljunggren G. Gout and its comorbidities in the total population of Stockholm. Prev Med 2015;81:387–91.

34. Shih HJ, Kao MC, Tsai PS, et al. Long-term allopurinol use decreases the risk of prostate cancer in patients with gout: a population-based study. Prostate Cancer Prostatic Dis 2017;20(3):328–33.

35. Chen CJ, Hsieh MC, Liao WT, et al. Allopurinol and the incidence of bladder cancer: a Taiwan national retrospective cohort study. Eur J Cancer Prev 2016;25(3): 216–23.

36. Kuo MC, Chang SJ, Hsieh MC. Colchicine significantly reduces incident cancer in gout male patients: a 12-year cohort study. Medicine (Baltimore) 2015;94(50): e1570.

37. Veettil SK, Lim KG, Ching SM, et al. Effects of aspirin and non-aspirin nonsteroidal anti-inflammatory drugs on the incidence of recurrent colorectal adenomas: a systematic review with meta-analysis and trial sequential analysis of randomized clinical trials. BMC Cancer 2017;17(1):763.

38. Bernatsky S, Ramsey-Goldman R, Petri M, et al. Smoking is the most significant modifiable lung cancer risk factor in systemic lupus erythematosus. J Rheumatol 2018;45(3):393–6.

39. Stone DU, Fife D, Brown M, et al. Effect of tobacco smoking on the clinical, histopathological, and serological manifestations of sjogren's syndrome. PLoS One 2017;12(2):e0170249.

40. Joseph RM, Movahedi M, Dixon WG, et al. Smoking-related mortality in patients with early rheumatoid arthritis: a retrospective cohort study using the clinical practice research datalink. Arthritis Care Res (Hoboken) 2016;68(11):1598–606.

41. Warren GW, Cummings KM. Tobacco and lung cancer: risks, trends, and outcomes in patients with cancer. Am Soc Clin Oncol Educ Book 2013;359–64. https://doi.org/10.1200/EdBook_AM.2013.33.359.

42. Sugiyama D, Nishimura K, Tamaki K, et al. Impact of smoking as a risk factor for developing rheumatoid arthritis: a meta-analysis of observational studies. Ann Rheum Dis 2010;69(1):70–81.

43. Nikiphorou E, Fragoulis GE. Inflammation, obesity and rheumatic disease: common mechanistic links. A narrative review. Ther Adv Musculoskelet Dis 2018; 10(8):157–67.

44. Liu Y, Hazlewood GS, Kaplan GG, et al. Impact of obesity on remission and disease activity in rheumatoid arthritis: a systematic review and meta-analysis. Arthritis Care Res (Hoboken) 2017;69(2):157–65.

45. Kolb R, Sutterwala FS, Zhang W. Obesity and cancer: inflammation bridges the two. Curr Opin Pharmacol 2016;29:77–89.

46. Sparks JA, Barbhaiya M, Tedeschi SK, et al. Inflammatory dietary pattern and risk of developing rheumatoid arthritis in women. Clin Rheumatol 2019;38(1):243–50.

47. Petersson S, Philippou E, Rodomar C, et al. The Mediterranean diet, fish oil supplements and Rheumatoid arthritis outcomes: evidence from clinical trials. Autoimmun Rev 2018;17(11):1105–14.

48. Namazi N, Larijani B, Azadbakht L. Association between the dietary inflammatory index and the incidence of cancer: a systematic review and meta-analysis of prospective studies. Public Health 2018;164:148–56.

49. Moradi S, Issah A, Mohammadi H, et al. Associations between dietary inflammatory index and incidence of breast and prostate cancer: a systematic review and meta-analysis. Nutrition 2018;55-56:168–78.

50. Johansson K, Askling J, Alfredsson L, et al. Mediterranean diet and risk of rheumatoid arthritis: a population-based case-control study. Arthritis Res Ther 2018; 20(1):175.

51. Jayedi A, Emadi A, Shab-Bidar S. Dietary inflammatory index and site-specific cancer risk: a systematic review and dose-response meta-analysis. Adv Nutr 2018;9(4):388–403.
52. Forsyth C, Kouvari M, D'Cunha NM, et al. The effects of the Mediterranean diet on rheumatoid arthritis prevention and treatment: a systematic review of human prospective studies. Rheumatol Int 2018;38(5):737–47.
53. Konig MF. The microbiome in autoimmune rheumatic disease. Best Pract Res Clin Rheumatol 2020;101473. https://doi.org/10.1016/j.berh.2019.101473.
54. Baffy G. Gut microbiota and cancer of the host: colliding interests. Adv Exp Med Biol 2020;1219:93–107.
55. Dehner C, Fine R, Kriegel MA. The microbiome in systemic autoimmune disease: mechanistic insights from recent studies. Curr Opin Rheumatol 2019;31(2): 201–7.
56. Gopalakrishnan V, Helmink BA, Spencer CN, et al. The influence of the gut microbiome on cancer, immunity, and cancer immunotherapy. Cancer Cell 2018;33(4): 570–80.
57. Rajagopala SV, Vashee S, Oldfield LM, et al. The human microbiome and cancer. Cancer Prev Res (Phila) 2017;10(4):226–34.
58. Draborg AH, Duus K, Houen G. Epstein-Barr virus in systemic autoimmune diseases. Clin Dev Immunol 2013;2013:535738.
59. Pattle SB, Farrell PJ. The role of Epstein-Barr virus in cancer. Expert Opin Biol Ther 2006;6(11):1193–205.
60. Khan F, Kleppel H, Meara AS. Paraneoplastic rheumatic and musculoskeletal syndromes. Rheum Dis Clin North Am 2020;46(3).
61. Muller S, Hider S, Helliwell T, et al. The real evidence for polymyalgia rheumatica as a paraneoplastic syndrome. Reumatismo 2018;70(1):23–34.
62. Manger B, Schett G. Palmar fasciitis and polyarthritis syndrome-systematic literature review of 100 cases. Semin Arthritis Rheum 2014;44(1):105–11.
63. Zupancic M, Annamalai A, Brenneman J, et al. Migratory polyarthritis as a paraneoplastic syndrome. J Gen Intern Med 2008;23(12):2136–9.
64. Karmacharya P, Donato AA, Aryal MR, et al. RS3PE revisited: a systematic review and meta-analysis of 331 cases. Clin Exp Rheumatol 2016;34(3):404–15.
65. Zahid MF, Barraco D, Lasho TL, et al. Spectrum of autoimmune diseases and systemic inflammatory syndromes in patients with chronic myelomonocytic leukemia. Leuk Lymphoma 2017;58(6):1488–93.
66. Best M, Molinari N, Chasset F, et al. Use of anti-transcriptional intermediary factor-1 gamma autoantibody in identifying adult dermatomyositis patients with cancer: a systematic review and meta-analysis. Acta Derm Venereol 2019;99(3):256–62.
67. Fiorentino DF, Chung LS, Christopher-Stine L, et al. Most patients with cancer-associated dermatomyositis have antibodies to nuclear matrix protein NXP-2 or transcription intermediary factor 1gamma. Arthritis Rheum 2013;65(11):2954–62.
68. Shah AA, Laiho M, Rosen A, et al. Protective effect against cancer of antibodies to the large subunits of both RNA polymerases I and III in scleroderma. Arthritis Rheumatol 2019;71(9):1571–9.
69. Shah AA, Xu G, Rosen A, et al. Brief report: anti-RNPC-3 antibodies as a marker of cancer-associated scleroderma. Arthritis Rheumatol 2017;69(6):1306–12.
70. Shah AA, Hummers LK, Casciola-Rosen L, et al. Examination of autoantibody status and clinical features associated with cancer risk and cancer-associated scleroderma. Arthritis Rheumatol 2015;67(4):1053–61.

71. Shah AA, Rosen A, Hummers L, et al. Close temporal relationship between onset of cancer and scleroderma in patients with RNA polymerase I/III antibodies. Arthritis Rheum 2010;62(9):2787–95.

72. Shah AA, Casciola-Rosen L. Mechanistic and clinical insights at the scleroderma-cancer interface. J Scleroderma Relat Disord 2017;2(3):153–9.

73. Igusa T, Hummers LK, Visvanathan K, et al. Autoantibodies and scleroderma phenotype define subgroups at high-risk and low-risk for cancer. Ann Rheum Dis 2018;77(8):1179–86.

74. Raaschou P, Soderling J, Turesson C, et al. Tumor necrosis factor inhibitors and cancer recurrence in Swedish patients with rheumatoid arthritis: a nationwide population-based cohort study. Ann Intern Med 2018;169(5):291–9.

75. Chen Y, Friedman M, Liu G, et al. Do tumor necrosis factor inhibitors increase cancer risk in patients with chronic immune-mediated inflammatory disorders? Cytokine 2018;101:78–88.

76. Wadstrom H, Frisell T, Sparen P, et al. Do RA or TNF inhibitors increase the risk of cervical neoplasia or of recurrence of previous neoplasia? A nationwide study from Sweden. Ann Rheum Dis 2016;75(7):1272–8.

77. Scott FI, Mamtani R, Brensinger CM, et al. Risk of nonmelanoma skin cancer associated with the use of immunosuppressant and biologic agents in patients with a history of autoimmune disease and nonmelanoma skin cancer. JAMA Dermatol 2016;152(2):164–72.

78. Bae SH, Ahn SM, Lim DH, et al. Safety of tumor necrosis factor inhibitor therapy in patients with a prior malignancy. Int J Rheum Dis 2016;19(10):961–7.

79. Nocturne G, Mariette X. Sjogren Syndrome-associated lymphomas: an update on pathogenesis and management. Br J Haematol 2015;168(3):317–27.

80. Mercer LK, Lunt M, Low AL, et al. Risk of solid cancer in patients exposed to anti-tumour necrosis factor therapy: results from the British Society for Rheumatology Biologics Register for Rheumatoid Arthritis. Ann Rheum Dis 2015;74(6):1087–93.

81. Wu CY, Chen DY, Shen JL, et al. The risk of cancer in patients with rheumatoid arthritis taking tumor necrosis factor antagonists: a nationwide cohort study. Arthritis Res Ther 2014;16(5):449.

82. Le Blay P, Mouterde G, Barnetche T, et al. Risk of malignancy including non-melanoma skin cancers with anti-tumor necrosis factor therapy in patients with rheumatoid arthritis: meta-analysis of registries and systematic review of long-term extension studies. Clin Exp Rheumatol 2012;30(5):756–64.

83. Xie W, Xiao S, Huang Y, et al. A meta-analysis of biologic therapies on risk of new or recurrent cancer in patients with rheumatoid arthritis and a prior malignancy. Rheumatology (Oxford) 2020;59(5):930–9.

84. Singh JA, Saag KG, Bridges SL Jr, et al. 2015 American College of rheumatology guideline for the treatment of rheumatoid arthritis. Arthritis Rheumatol 2016;68(1):1–26.

85. Richter MD, Crowson C, Kottschade LA, et al. Rheumatic syndromes associated with immune checkpoint inhibitors: a single-center cohort of sixty-one patients. Arthritis Rheumatol 2019;71(3):468–75.

86. Cappelli LC, Gutierrez AK, Baer AN, et al. Inflammatory arthritis and sicca syndrome induced by nivolumab and ipilimumab. Ann Rheum Dis 2017;76(1):43–50.

87. Calabrese C, Kirchner E, Kontzias A, et al. Rheumatic immune-related adverse events of checkpoint therapy for cancer: case series of a new nosological entity. RMD Open 2017;3(1):e000412.

88. Belkhir R, Burel SL, Dunogeant L, et al. Rheumatoid arthritis and polymyalgia rheumatica occurring after immune checkpoint inhibitor treatment. Ann Rheum Dis 2017;76(10):1747–50.
89. Cappelli LC, Gutierrez AK, Bingham CO 3rd, et al. Rheumatic and musculoskeletal immune-related adverse events due to immune checkpoint inhibitors: a systematic review of the literature. Arthritis Care Res (Hoboken) 2017;69(11): 1751–63.
90. Kostine M, Truchetet ME, Schaeverbeke T. Clinical characteristics of rheumatic syndromes associated with checkpoint inhibitors therapy. Rheumatology (Oxford) 2019;58(Suppl 7):vii68–74.
91. Moghadam-Kia S, Oddis CV, Ascherman DP, et al. Risk factors and cancer screening in myositis. Rheum Dis Clin North Am 2020;46(3).
92. Weeding EA, Casciola-Rosen L, Shah AA. Cancer and Scleroderma. Rheum Dis Clin North Am 2020;46(3).

Autoimmunity, Clonal Hematopoiesis, and Myeloid Neoplasms

Delamo I. Bekele, MBBS[a], Mrinal M. Patnaik, MBBS, MD[b],*

KEYWORDS

- Autoimmune disease • Myeloid neoplasms • Clonal hematopoiesis • DMARDs

KEY POINTS

- Clonal hematopoiesis is associated with chronic inflammation, endothelial dysfunction, and increased all-cause mortality, and may be linked to autoimmune disease.
- Autoimmune diseases, including rheumatoid arthritis and systemic lupus erythematosus, have been associated with an increased risk of myeloid neoplasms.
- Myeloid neoplasms have also been associated with autoimmune diseases and systemic inflammatory syndromes.
- Treatment of autoimmune diseases can give rise to therapy-associated myeloid neoplasms.

INTRODUCTION

The associations between rheumatologic disorders and malignancy have been well described in the literature. The causes vary from rheumatic comorbidity, unchecked chronic inflammation, to adverse effects of immunosuppressive agents. Certain rheumatologic disorders, including dermatomyositis, systemic sclerosis (SSc), rheumatoid arthritis (RA), systemic lupus erythematosus (SLE), and Sjögren syndrome (SS), have strongly been linked with malignancy.[1] Enhanced screening is usually undertaken, supported by other clinical manifestations, additional risk factors for malignancy (family history, cigarette smoking, and so forth), and disease-specific autoantibodies (anti-transcriptional intermediary factor 1 antibody/TIF1-Ab positivity in dermatomyositis[2] and RNA polymerase 3 positivity in SSc).[3] There is a lack of consensus for specific algorithms and the debate continues while further studies are conducted.

[a] Division of Rheumatology, Department of Internal Medicine, Mayo Clinic, Mayo Building, East 15-94, 200 First Street Southwest, Rochester, MN 55905, USA; [b] Division of Hematology, Department of Internal Medicine, Mayo Clinic, Mayo Building, East 10, 200 First Street Southwest, Rochester, MN 55905, USA
* Corresponding author.
E-mail address: Patnaik.Mrinal@mayo.edu

Rheum Dis Clin N Am 46 (2020) 429–444
https://doi.org/10.1016/j.rdc.2020.03.001
0889-857X/20/© 2020 Elsevier Inc. All rights reserved.

rheumatic.theclinics.com

The expanding use of immunotherapy (immune checkpoint inhibitors) for treatment of malignancy has led to multiple adverse effects, among which rheumatic manifestations are common, including severe manifestations such as myositis and vasculitis.[4] Rheumatic manifestations can be a precursor or can accompany precursor states associated with myeloid neoplasms (MNs).

This complex interplay affects survival, quality of life, and therapeutic management. Although several of these associations have been researched in detail and hypothesis proved, the interaction between autoimmunity and hematologic malignancy has been less well defined. One major challenge is the overall rarity in incidence of most MNs and rheumatic autoimmune diseases, RA being the main exception. The lack of large randomized studies can provide challenges in clinical care of these patients (management, screening, and prognosis). This article explores what is currently known of these associations in detail, namely the links of MNs with rheumatic diseases, along with the impact of therapeutic interventions for autoimmune disease; that is, disease-modifying antirheumatic drugs (DMARDs) and biologic agents with MNs.

RHEUMATOLOGIC ASSOCIATION WITH MYELOID NEOPLASMS
Disease Subsets

Clonal hematopoiesis

Before exploring MNs, this article covers novel premalignant hematologic conditions (ie, clonal hematopoiesis [CH]) and its association with autoimmune disorders. CH is defined as the acquisition and propagation of somatic mutations in hematopoietic stem cells in people with normal blood counts.[5,6] When these mutations are putative driver mutations, involving leukemia-associated genes, with a variant allele frequency greater than or equal to 2%, this is termed CH with a putative driver or CH of indeterminate potential (CHIP).[5] When CH can be detected in the context of low blood counts and the absence of a defining bone marrow disease state, this is called clonal cytopenia of undetermined significance. CHIP is an age-dependent phenomenon, with the incidence being less than 1% before the age of 40 years and greater than 30% beyond age 80 years.

Several genetic studies in apparently healthy individuals (from a hematological perspective) have identified somatic clonal mutations that predate the development of clinical manifestations. These CHIP states are associated with a low risk of evolution to MNs (dependent on the driver oncogene) but are associated with an increased risk of cardiovascular disease and all-cause mortality.[6,7] Importantly, the risk of cardiovascular disease in individuals with CHIP is maintained when traditional risk factors (smoking and a family history of atherosclerotic cardiovascular disease) are excluded. The hypothesis behind this phenomenon is that CHIP commonly involves mutations in epigenetic regulator genes, *DNMT3A*, *TET2*, and *ASXL1*. These mutations affect monocytes/macrophages, leading to an inflammatory phenotype with associated cytokine release and endothelial dysfunction.[6] Given an increased cardiovascular risk in most rheumatic diseases compared with the general population, it is speculated that this risk is in part caused by coexistent CH.

The impact of CHIP in RA has been evaluated in 1 single-center study comparing patients with RA (median age, 58.5 years), healthy controls, and patients with aplastic anemia. A prevalence of 17% was detected in patients with RA (n = 59), which increased with age, unsurprisingly.[8] No associations were identified with other prognostic factors in RA, such as smoking status or seropositivity. More studies are needed to confirm these findings and to explore the potential role of CH in other systemic rheumatic disorders. Given the inflammatory cytokines and chemokines that have been associated with CHIP, it could be hypothesized that these could result in autoimmune inflammatory syndromes, and further work in this area is much needed.

Autoimmune disorders and myeloid neoplasms

Autoimmune disorders are more commonly associated with myelodysplastic syndrome (MDS) and/or acute myeloid leukemia (AML). Most data regarding MNs in autoimmune disorders relate to RA and SLE. One large study in Sweden identified 42,262 hospitalized patients with RA followed over 24 years.[9] Of these, 52 patients developed AML over the course of the study period, with an overall increased risk ratio of 2.4 (95% confidence interval [CI], 1.79–3.15). Another large study using the Swedish Cancer registry stratifying patients into early RA (within 1 year of symptom onset) and advanced RA found 4 cases of AML in the former and 68 cases of AML in the latter group.[10] The standardized incidence ratio (SIR) was markedly increased in both groups (4.3 and 2.4 respectively). No cases of chronic myelogenous leukemia (CML) were noted in the early RA group, whereas 13 cases were seen in the advanced RA group with an SIR of 2.4 (95% CI, 1.3–4.1).

The associations between solid organ malignancies such as breast, cervical cancer, and non-Hodgkin lymphoma have been well described in the SLE literature. In contrast, the association of SLE with MNs has been assessed infrequently; the studies are limited and mostly observational. As such, it is hard to draw definitive conclusions regarding the cause of increased risks (underlying autoimmune disease, therapy, or unrelated contributors). A meta-analysis of 8 prospective lupus cohorts revealed an increased SIR of non-Hodgkin lymphoma, Hodgkin lymphoma, and leukemias (SIR of 2.3). There was no change after adjusting for age, sex, or location.[11] Two of these studies reported SIR of myeloid leukemia in patients with SLE of 3.4 (95% CI, 2.2–5.1). One group observed a large number of patients with SLE in California (n = 30,478); 29 cases of myeloid leukemia were noted, with an SIR of 2.96 (95% CI, 1.99–4.26).[12] A limitation of these studies is that they did not specify whether the leukemias were acute or chronic and sometimes did not differentiate between myeloid and lymphoid leukemias.

Although visceral malignancies have been clearly linked with SSc, there is little description of the interplay with MNs. A literature review (60-year duration) revealed 130 cases of hematologic malignancies, including leukemia (28 total, 2 cases of AML) and myeloproliferative disorders (11 cases of CML, 4 cases of myelofibrosis, and 1 case of polycythemia rubra vera).[13] However, these studies are difficult to interpret given the use of immunosuppressive agents and disease-modifying biologic therapies, which inherently increase the risk of neoplasms.

Autoimmune disorders occurring concurrently or after diagnosis of myeloid neoplasms

One of the most intriguing questions for hematologists and rheumatologists alike is the chicken-or-egg causality dilemma regarding the development of autoimmune disorders in patients with MNs: does autoimmune disorder predispose to MNs, do autoimmune disorders develop in these patients secondary to the neoplasm, or is the relationship bidirectional?

It has been well described in the literature that patients with MNs can present with concurrent or subsequent rheumatic manifestations. A wide range of rheumatic manifestations have been described in association with MDS, including inflammatory arthritis (eg, monoarthritis, polyarthritis, remitting seronegative symmetric synovitis with pitting edema syndrome), vasculitis (eg, polymyalgia rheumatica, relapsing polychondritis, and cutaneous vasculitis), and connective tissue disorders, including SS.

Approximately 10% to 25% of MDS cases are usually associated with rheumatic manifestations.[14,15]

The development of systemic vasculitis is limited to case reports and case series. One case series included a literature review that identified 55 cases in association with MDS, the most common of which was polyarteritis nodosa (PAN) (>25% of cases).[16] Absolute neutrophil count–associated vasculitis was rare in this series, which has been replicated in other small observational studies.

A nested case-control study using data from the United Kingdom (General Practice Research Database) identified 849 cases of MDS (either likely or possible) with approximately 4 times the number of matched controls. There was a marginally increased risk of MDS in patients with autoimmune disease (adjusted odds ratio [OR], 1.5; 95% CI, 1.1–2.0).[17] When stratifying by autoimmune disorder duration, a significantly increased adjusted OR of 2.1 (95% CI, 1.4–3.2) was noted for patients with long-standing autoimmune disease of greater than 10 years. This finding suggests that long-standing immune dysregulation has a major role in the pathogenesis of MNs.

Chronic myelomonocytic leukemia is an overlapping stem cell disorder with features of MDS and myeloproliferative neoplasms (MPNs); it also has a significant risk of transforming into acute leukemia. Definite autoimmune disease and systemic syndromes have been reported in this overlapping MN. A large study of 377 patients revealed that 20% had an autoimmune disorder.[18] Interestingly, in 58% of cases, these occurred before the diagnosis of chronic myelomonocytic leukemia (CMML) (a minority of autoimmune disorders were nonrheumatic: Hashimoto thyroiditis, myasthenia gravis, and granuloma annulare). Most responded to immunosuppression (77%) despite the heterogeneity of autoimmune disorder manifestations. Durable remissions were often seen with disease-specific interventions such as hypomethylating agents and allogenic stem cell transplant.

Autoimmune manifestations of CML include leukemic arthritis and bone pain. Leukemic arthritis can be symmetric or migratory polyarthritis and tends to be a manifestation of advanced disease.[19] It is less commonly seen in adult patients than in cases of pediatric leukemia; however, it can be challenging to manage and unresponsive to the usual immunosuppressants used to treat inflammatory arthritis/RA. The treatment of choice should be appropriate for the underlying leukemia.

In summary, there is a bidirectional association with several MNs and autoimmune disorders (**Table 1**). Given the temporal associations of MNs and autoimmune disorders and numerous confounding factors, large, well-designed, prospective studies are required to confirm these associations and guide therapeutic options.

Mechanisms of myeloid neoplasm in autoimmune disorders (pathogenesis and potential causes)

The pathogenesis of the development of MNs in autoimmune disorders remains convoluted and unclear. The heterogeneous nature of both groups contributes to this, along with difficulties establishing temporality. Understanding the mechanisms that drive these processes and the interplay between them is critical to determine the standard of care for screening, evaluation, and treatment of both disorders. **Fig. 1** provides a conceptual diagram.

Chronic immune stimulation Chronic inflammation as a risk factor for malignancy was first described in the nineteenth century by Virchow. More recent epidemiology studies have identified that chronic immune activation related to infections increases the risks of AML and MDS.[20]

Table 1
Summary of major autoimmune diseases that have been associated with myeloid neoplasms

Disease	Associations	Clinical Risks/Pearls
Autoimmune Disease		
Rheumatoid arthritis	AML, CML	—
SLE	AML, all MN	Lymphopenia increases risk: OR 14 (95% CI, 1.4–141)
MN		
MDS	Inflammatory arthritis, relapsing polychondritis, PMR, lupuslike syndrome, cutaneous vasculitis	—
CML	Carcinomatous polyarthritis	—
CMML	Rheumatoid arthritis, psoriasis, polymyalgia rheumatica, systemic vasculitis including PAN	—

Abbreviation: PMR, polymyalgia rheumatica.

A large project using data from the Surveillance, Epidemiology, and End Results (SEER) Medicare Assessment of Hematopoietic Malignancy Risk Traits (SMAHRT) study identified 13,486 cases of MNs, in which the presence of any autoimmune disorder was associated with an increased risk of AML with OR of 1.29 (95% CI,1.20–1.39). Statistically significant associations were detected for RA, SS, SLE, polymyalgia rheumatica, and PAN with MDS.[21]

Immune dysfunction has been implicated in the pathogenesis of many autoimmune disorders. One potential mediator is nuclear factor kB (NF-kB), which has been identified in MNs and autoimmune disorders. NF-kB regulates various aspects of the normal function of the innate and adaptive immune system.[22] It has been implicated in the pathogenesis of RA, inflammatory bowel disease (IBD), and atherosclerotic cardiovascular disease. Given the potential interplay between systemic autoimmune diseases and MNs, a potential role for NF-kB needs further exploration.

Genetic contributors The role of cytogenetic and molecular factors predisposing patients with autoimmune disorder to MN is still under investigation. Given common abnormalities between the 2 classes of disorders, some hypotheses can be made. These hypotheses include the role of *TP53* tumor suppressor genes (discussed later), the mammalian target of rapamycin pathway, and the role of human leukocyte antigen (HLA).

Data from the 1950s to 1980s highlight an increased risk of leukemia in patients with ankylosing spondylitis (AS). This increased risk was attributed at the time to radium exposure, which was used for management of AS in the prebiologic era.[23] The role of HLA-B27 in AS and other spondyloarthropathies, through interaction of the major histocompatibility complex with malignancy and spondyloarthritis, has not been well defined. It was investigated in a large study in Hong Kong: 59 carriers of HLA-B27 were identified to have a malignant hematologic disorder, 4 of whom had lymphoid malignancy. No case of MN was found.[24]

In mouse models, HLA class II genes have been associated with hematologic malignancy.[25] Although HLA-B27 has been established to be important in the heritability of AS,[26] a larger multicenter and multiethnic study by the Prospective Study of Outcomes in Ankylosing Spondylitis (PSOAS) cohort group highlighted potential roles of

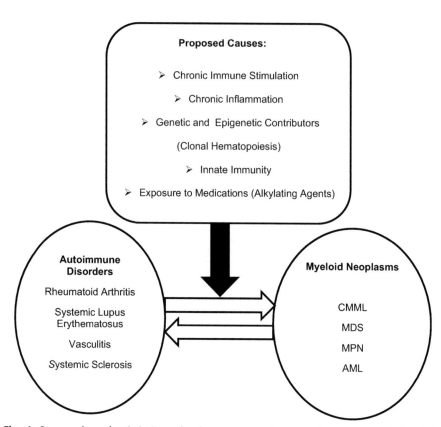

Fig. 1. Proposed mechanistic interplay between autoimmune disorders and MNs. AML, acute myeloid leukemia; CMML, chronic myelomonocytic leukemia; MDS, myelodysplastic syndrome; MPN, myeloproliferative neoplasms. (*Adapted from* Boddu PC, Zeidan AM. Myeloid disorders after autoimmune disease. *Ther-Relat Acute Leuk.* 2019;32(1):74-88; with permission.)

non-B27 class I HLA and also class II HLA in AS.[27] A study of HLA class 2 in patients with AS with malignancies has not been performed to the best of our knowledge and may be of benefit.

Innate immune system The role of interleukin (IL)-1 and *NLRP3* (nucleotide-binding domain–like receptor protein 3) in autoinflammatory disorders such as periodic fever syndromes is well established. Increased IL-1 levels have also been found in tissues of patients with autoimmune disorders inclusive of RA.[28] IL-1 has also been shown to play a role in the development of hematologic malignancy, including MNs.

The NLRP3 inflammasome (after upregulation by the *NF-kB* pathway) acts by downstream activation of IL-1 beta and IL-18, both of which are proinflammatory cytokines. Mouse models have identified a role of the inflammasome in RA, SLE, and even spondyloarthropathies (eg, AS).[29] The role of NLRP3 in the pathophysiology of malignancy and the role of other inflammasome complexes are still being determined. Note that activation of *NLRP3* has been associated with different cancer cell types, including melanoma and colon cancer. *NLRP3* has been proved to drive cell death through overexpression of proinflammatory pathways leading to increased apoptosis in

MDS.[30] Germline *MEFV1* mutations lead to the most common autoinflammatory/periodic fever syndrome, familial Mediterranean fever.[31] Interestingly, somatic mutations in the *MEFV* gene have been identified in a couple of patients with MDS who also presented with periodic fevers and cutaneous manifestations suggestive of Sweet syndrome.[32]

Therapy-associated myeloid neoplasms The medications used by rheumatologists to treat autoimmune disorders include antimetabolite medications (methotrexate, azathioprine, and mycophenolate mofetil), alkylating agents (cyclophosphamide), and biologic agents (tumor necrosis factor inhibitors [TNFi] and most recently non–tumor necrosis factor [TNF] biologics). Therapy-related MNs (t-MNs) have been well described with alkylating agents as well as DNA-topoisomerase agents (which are not commonly used in rheumatology practice). The risk of hematologic malignancy with antimetabolites has been considered lower historically, although there are newer data describing cases.[33]

Proposed causes for t-MNs include therapy-induced mutation to DNA damage sensing or repair genes (TP53), chromosome deletions with alkylating agents (chromosome 5 and 7 deletions),[34] and polymorphisms in genes that affect drug metabolism or transport.[35]

Somatic Mutations Associated with Myeloid Neoplasms and Autoimmune Disease

Common CHIP-associated mutations include *DNMT3A*, *TET2*, and *ASXL1*.[5] The *DNMT3A* gene is located at 2p23 and serves as one of the genes that encodes DNA methyltransferase enzymes, which play a role in methylation of CpG dinucleotides.[36] Mutations of this gene have been noted in a significant subset of patients with MDS and AML.[37]

TET2 encodes proteins that play a role in the control of DNA expression through demethylation.[38] *TET2* mutations are common in MNs, especially CMML.[39] *TET2* has also been reported to potentially participate in regulation of both the adaptive (T-helper [Th] 1 and Th17 cells) and innate immune systems.

The *ASXL1* (additional sex combs–like 1) gene regulates epigenetic marks and transcription through the polycomb repressor complex, with mutations being uniformly deleterious across MNs.[40–42]

Abnormal DNA methylation has been shown in several epigenetic studies of autoimmune disorders inclusive of RA, SLE, and SS.[31] A clear interaction between DNMT3A mutations and autoimmune disease has yet to be proved.

Other genes commonly associated with CHIP include *JAK2* and *TP53*. *JAK2* is a common driver mutation in MPNs and has been associated with leukocytosis, thrombocytosis, and thrombotic complications.[35] *TP53* somatic mutations are usually seen in the context of therapy-related MNs and are associated with very poor outcomes.[37]

The primary driver of progression from CHIP to an overt myeloid neoplasia is not completely understood, but the combination of inflammation and aging is thought to play a major role.[43]

Various reasons for the development of these somatic mutations have been identified, including environmental mutagens (radiation, cigarette smoke, air pollutants), mutagenic drugs (chemotherapeutic agents)[36] or impaired DNA repair, and altered telomere dynamics associated with aging.[31,41,44]

The data exploring these mutations in autoimmune and rheumatic disease are limited and the mechanisms are yet to be fully defined. However, *TP53* mutations have been extensively studied in mouse models; *TP53*-deficient mice are more likely to develop inflammatory arthritis.[45–47]

The 1 study that assessed CH in patients with RA along with aplastic anemia and healthy controls[8] identified *DNMT3A* mutations to be the most common (n = 4), followed by *TET2* (n = 3). None of these patients had MN or cancer. Interestingly, 1 patient with RA had a *TP53* mutation (17:g.7574003G>A), which was associated with cervical cancer requiring surgical intervention (unclear from data whether this was a somatic or germline mutation). Further studies are needed to assess whether chronic inflammation from autoimmunity favors the development of CHIP and subsequent MNs, or whether CHIP and MNs result in inflammation and autoimmunity.

Myeloid Sequelae of Rheumatologic Therapies/Medications

The determination and quantification of the risk of malignancy with DMARDs and biologic agents in rheumatic disease is extremely difficult. The overall burden of malignancy unrelated to rheumatic disease is high in the general population. Moreover, the risk of malignancy conferred by specific rheumatic diseases and the use of immunosuppressive agents, some of which are well known to have neoplastic potential, further complicates risk assessment. Given the broadness of this topic and matters discussed earlier, this article focuses on the myeloid sequelae of commonly used agents by rheumatologists. t-MNs comprise the spectrum of disorders that were discussed previously in the setting of chemotherapeutic, disease-modifying agents or other exposures such as radiation. This group can be divided into therapy-related AML, therapy-related MDS (t-MDS), and t-MDS/MPN. T-MNs are often characterized by specific cytogenetic changes, especially when they occur in the context of alkylator-based therapies.

Traditional immunosuppressive agents/disease-modifying antirheumatic drugs
The following commonly used immunosuppressive agents are discussed here: cyclophosphamide, azathioprine, methotrexate, and TNFi.

Cyclophosphamide Cyclophosphamide (CYC) has been long been attributed with significant risk of malignancy inclusive of lymphoma, leukemia, and visceral malignancies such as bladder cancer.[1] In light of these side effects and the development of multiple immunosuppressants within the last 2 decades, clinical use of CYC is now restricted to severe manifestations of rheumatic disease, such as diffuse alveolar hemorrhage, central nervous system vasculitis, and refractory renal involvement in SLE.[48–50] In addition, dose adjustments/reductions (eg, for the EuroLupus regimen for lupus nephritis) as well as intermittent intravenous administration rather than daily oral dosing of cyclophosphamide has become more common.[51] This trend is supported by noninferiority in clinical studies as well as reduction in adverse events.[52]

There have been clear links between cyclophosphamide usage and MNs (including MDS and CML). It typically takes 5 to 7 years after exposure to alkylating agents before t-MNs develop.[53,54] MDS is most common, with further clonal evolution to AML. Common karyotypic changes include deletions of chromosome 5 and/or 7 (7q/-7 and 7q/-5).[55]

There are some studies evaluating the role of CYC in t-MNs in specific autoimmune disorders. In patients with Granulomatosis with polyangiitis (GPA), approximately 8% of patients treated with CYC for remission induction and maintenance therapy developed MDS.[56] The rate was almost doubled with a high cumulative dose (>100 g). Multiple studies have identified an increased risk of both solid organ and hematologic malignancy in SLE, although this has been found to be independent of CYC use.[57,44]

The risk of hematologic malignancy is increased in patients with RA treated with cyclophosphamide[58] (**Table 2**). With the advent of many newer agents for RA in the last 10 to 20 years with favorable side effect profiles, cyclophosphamide has fallen out of use in the management of RA. In very rare and refractory cases (RA vasculitis or RA-associated large granular lymphocyte (LGL) leukemia), there may still be a role for cyclophosphamide. Clinicians deciding to initiate CYC in this subset of patients with RA should weigh this risk-benefit profile in addition to consideration of any alternate options.

Azathioprine Azathioprine is used to treat a wide spectrum of autoimmune disorders. Multiple studies have consistently shown an increased risk of lymphoproliferative disorders in patients with RA.[49] Although there was concern that this was related directly to the antimetabolite, a more recent systematic review revealed that the approximately 2-fold increase in lymphoma incidence in RA is related to the underlying disorder (severity and disease duration) and not the therapeutic agents (azathioprine and methotrexate).[33] This finding highlights the challenges in studying the complex multidirectional interplay between autoimmunity, malignancy, and immunosuppressive agents.

A Medline search in 2010 identified 56 cases of azathioprine-associated MDS and AML,[59] confirming the association of azathioprine with MNs. However, 52% of these cases were organ transplant recipients, and a markedly increased risk of solid organ, skin, and hematologic malignancies has been shown in organ transplant recipients. This increased risk may be related to higher doses of azathioprine in transplant patients in the setting of additional risk factors. The remainder of cases identified by Kwong[59] had autoimmune disorders; most of these were related to abnormalities in chromosome 7. In approximately 20% of the cases, recurrent cytopenias preceded t-MDS/AML, and this may be 1 indicator to follow for patients on azathioprine.

Focusing specifically on MNs, data were limited to case reports, and case series have been reported in RA, SLE, and IBD. However, a large case-control series[60] (see **Table 2**) identified a 7-fold increased risk of MN (AML or MDS) in patients with a primary autoimmune disease. Another case-control study found no association between azathioprine and MN, although the number of cases was small, which may have affected outcomes.[61]

Methotrexate Methotrexate is one of the most commonly used medications in rheumatology. It has been clearly shown to cause myelosuppression and lymphoproliferative disorders. The role of methotrexate in causing therapy-associated myeloid neoplasia is far from clear. The limited studies performed have found no association between methotrexate and myeloid neoplasia in RA.[62,63]

Biologic therapies (tumor necrosis factor inhibitors) TNFi are widely used for management of many rheumatic disorders, including RA, AS, and psoriatic arthritis. Safety data were initially accumulated during various clinical trials with subsequent population-based studies and through use of claims databases. Most of the studies have assessed the links of lymphomas and solid organ malignancies with TNFi.

The number of studies assessing MNs in patients with definite autoimmune disease is limited (**Table 3**). In a large Swedish cohort study of patients with RA divided into 3 groups (early RA/incident cohort, prevalent cohort/established RA and RA receiving TNFi), there was no significant increase in MPNs or hematologic malignancies in general in the group receiving a TNFi[10] (SIR 0 for AML and CML). Another large cohort study assessing TNFi use for RA in North America revealed a numerically significant hazard ratio of hematologic malignancy but the results were statistically insignificant.[64]

The large study by Ertz-Archambault and colleagues[60] identified 13 (15.1%) patients with MN who received a TNFi for autoimmune disease compared with 33 (19.2%)

Table 2
Selection of studies exploring the effects of select disease-modifying antirheumatic drug therapies and risk of myeloid neoplasms in autoimmune diseases

Medication	Author, Year	Study Design	Methods	Results	Conclusion
(1) Cyclophosphamide	Bernatsky et al,[62] 2008	Case control	Administrative database, 23,810 patients with RA	Adjusted rate ratio of hematologic malignancy: 1.84; 95% CI, 1.24–2.73	Increased risk of hematologic malignancy, cyclophosphamide exposure
	Baker et al,[67] 1987	Case control	Single-center US practice, patients with RA, 119 cyclophosphamide and 119 controls	37 malignancies in the CYC arm, only 2 leukemias noted (subtype not stated)	Although there is an increased risk of malignancy in CYC group, unable to conclude whether there is an increased risk of MN
(2) AZA	Bernatsky et al,[62] 2008	Case control	Administrative database, 23,810 patients with RA	Adjusted rate ratio of hematologic malignancy: 1.07; 95% CI, 0.74–1.54	No increased risk with Imuran exposure in this RA population
	Ertz-Archambault et al,[60] 2017	Case control	40,011 patients with a primary autoimmune disease, identified patients with concomitant MDS or AML and compared with controls (2 controls per case)	86 patients had either AML or MDS. OR of AZA: 7.05; 95% CI, 2.35–21.13	AZA exposure associated with a 7-fold risk of MN
	Lofstrom et al,[61] 2009	Nested case control	6438 SLE cases, 8 confirmed cases of SLE with myeloid leukemia	AZA: 0.8 (95% CI, 0.1–4.1)	AZA was not a cause of myeloid leukemia in SLE population
(3) Methotrexate	Bernatsky et al,[62] 2008	Case control	Administrative database, 23,810 patients with RA	Adjusted rate ratio of hematologic malignancy: 1.12; 95% CI, 0.93–1.34	MTX was not associated with an increased risk of MN

Abbreviations: AZA, azathioprine; MTX, methotrexate.
Data from Refs.[33,51,55,56]

Table 3
Studies exploring the effects of tumor necrosis factor inhibitors and risk of myeloid neoplasms in rheumatoid arthritis

Medication	Author, Year	Study Design	Methods	Results	Conclusion
TNFi	Setouguchi et al,[64] 2006	Cohort (using 3 health care databases)	Pooled cohort of patients with RA (2 US patients and 1 Canadian), 1152 received TNFi and 7306 MTX	11 hematologic malignancies, adjusted HR, 1.37; 95% CI, 0.71-2.65	No increased risk of hematologic malignancy in TNF-treated group compared with MTX
TNFi	Askling et al,[10] 2005	Population-based cohort study of RA	One prevalent cohort, 1 incident cohort, and 1 cohort of TNFi-treated patients (n = 4160)	11 hematopoietic malignancies (1999-2003), only 2 undefined leukemias. No cases of AML, CML, or PRV	No increased risk of MN in patients with RA treated with TNFi

Abbreviations: HR, hazard ratio; PRV, polycythemia rubra vera.
Data from Askling J, Fored CM, Baecklund E, et al. Haematopoietic malignancies in rheumatoid arthritis: lymphoma risk and characteristics after exposure to tumour necrosis factor antagonists. Ann Rheum Dis. 2005;64(10):1414-1420; and Tarr T, Gyorfy B, Szekanecz É, et al. Occurrence of Malignancies in Hungarian Patients with Systemic Lupus Erythematosus. Ann N Y Acad Sci. 2007;1108(1):76-82.

controls. An unadjusted OR of 0.71 (0.33–1.53) was detected; therefore, they concluded that there was no increased risk of MN with TNFi. Given that TNFi are recommended for patients with refractory inflammatory arthritides (RA, spondyloarthritis)[65,66] and are among the most frequently prescribed medications, these findings are reassuring, but they do need ongoing scrutiny.

SUMMARY

There is an increased risk of MNs in autoimmune disease. This risk is independent of other risk factors, such as smoking and immunosuppressive therapy. There are certain genetic predispositions, including somatic mutations, which may account for some of the risk and warrant further investigation. The strongest evidence for t-MN exist for cyclophosphamide, although recent studies have also identified azathioprine as a potential offending agent. Although larger studies are needed to reproduce these findings, these risks should be considered when deciding on immunosuppression for rheumatic disorders, especially in individuals with additional risk factors for malignancy.

CLINICS CARE POINTS

- Clonal hematopoiesis (CH) is associated with chronic inflammation, endothelial dysfunction and increased all-cause mortality. CH may be linked to autoimmune disease which warrants further exploration.
- Autoimmune diseases (AD) have been associated with an increased risk of myeloid neoplasms. The greatest risk is seen in RA and SLE patients though evidence of an association between MN and other AD's (vasculitis, sjogren's syndrome) has been identified in small observational studies.
- Myeloid neoplasms (MN) can present with features of concurrent or subsequent autoimmune diseases/systemic inflammatory syndromes.
- Therapy-associated myeloid neoplasms can develop as a delayed effect of treating an underlying autoimmune disorder. The strongest evidence exists for Cyclophosphamide and Azathioprine.
- More data evaluating the risks of MN with biologic agents is needed.

DISCLOSURE

D.I. Bekele: no disclosures. M.M. Patnaik: advisory board for Stem Line Pharmaceuticals.

REFERENCES

1. Turesson C, Matteson EL. Malignancy as a comorbidity in rheumatic diseases. Rheumatol Oxf Engl 2013;52(1):5–14.
2. Oldroyd A, Sergeant JC, New P, et al. The temporal relationship between cancer and adult onset anti-transcriptional intermediary factor 1 antibody–positive dermatomyositis. Rheumatol Oxf Engl 2019;58(4):650–5.
3. Shah AA, Rosen LC. Cancer and scleroderma: a paraneoplastic disease with implications for malignancy screening. Curr Opin Rheumatol 2015;27(6):563–70.
4. Shah AA, Casciola-Rosen L, Rosen A. Review: cancer-induced autoimmunity in the rheumatic diseases. Arthritis Rheumatol 2015;67(2):317–26.
5. Jaiswal S, Fontanillas P, Flannick J, et al. Age-related clonal hematopoiesis associated with adverse outcomes. N Engl J Med 2014;371(26):2488–98.

6. Jaiswal S, Natarajan P, Silver AJ, et al. Clonal hematopoiesis and risk of atherosclerotic cardiovascular disease. N Engl J Med 2017;377(2):111–21.
7. Libby P, Ebert Benjamin L. CHIP (clonal hematopoiesis of indeterminate potential). Circulation 2018;138(7):666–8.
8. Savola P, Lundgren S, Keränen MAI, et al. Clonal hematopoiesis in patients with rheumatoid arthritis. Blood Cancer J 2018;8(8). https://doi.org/10.1038/s41408-018-0107-2.
9. Hemminki K, Li X, Sundquist K, et al. Cancer risk in hospitalized rheumatoid arthritis patients. Rheumatology 2008;47(5):698–701.
10. Askling J, Fored CM, Baecklund E, et al. Haematopoietic malignancies in rheumatoid arthritis: lymphoma risk and characteristics after exposure to tumour necrosis factor antagonists. Ann Rheum Dis 2005;64(10):1414–20.
11. Apor E, O'Brien J, Stephen M, et al. Systemic lupus erythematosus is associated with increased incidence of hematologic malignancies: A meta-analysis of prospective cohort studies. Leuk Res 2014;38(9):1067–71.
12. Parikh-Patel A, Allen M, Cress R, et al. Cancer risk in a cohort of patients with systemic lupus erythematosus (SLE) in California. Cancer Causes Control 2008; 19(8):887–94.
13. Colaci M, Giuggioli D, Vacchi C, et al. Haematological malignancies in systemic sclerosis patients: case reports and review of the World Literature. Mikdashi J, ed. Case Rep Rheumatol 2017;2017:6230138.
14. Castro M, Conn D, Su W, et al. Rheumatic manifestations in myelodysplastic syndromes. J Rheumatol 1991;18(5):721–7.
15. Mekinian A, Braun T, Decaux O, et al. Inflammatory Arthritis in Patients With Myelodysplastic Syndromes. Medicine (Baltimore) 2014;93(1). https://doi.org/10.1097/MD.0000000000000011.
16. Oostvogels R, Petersen EJ, Chauffaille ML, et al. Systemic vasculitis in myelodysplastic syndromes. Neth J Med 2012;70(2):63–8.
17. Wilson AB, Neogi T, Prout M, et al. Relative risk of myelodysplastic syndromes in patients with autoimmune disorders in the General Practice Research Database. Cancer Epidemiol 2014;38(5):544–9.
18. Zahid MF, Barraco D, Lasho TL, et al. Spectrum of autoimmune diseases and systemic inflammatory syndromes in patients with chronic myelomonocytic leukemia. Leuk Lymphoma 2017;58(6):1488–93.
19. Ehrenfeld M, Gur H, Shoenfeld Y. Rheumatologic features of hematologic disorders. Curr Opin Rheumatol 1999;11(1):62–7.
20. Kristinsson SY, Björkholm M, Hultcrantz M, et al. Chronic immune stimulation might act as a trigger for the development of acute myeloid leukemia or myelodysplastic syndromes. J Clin Oncol 2011;29(21):2897–903.
21. Anderson LA, Pfeiffer RM, Landgren O, et al. Risks of myeloid malignancies in patients with autoimmune conditions. Br J Cancer 2009;100(5):822–8.
22. Liu T, Zhang L, Joo D, et al. NF-κB signaling in inflammation. Signal Transduct Target Ther 2017;2(1):17023.
23. Wick RR, Nekolla EA, Gaubitz M, et al. Increased risk of myeloid leukaemia in patients with ankylosing spondylitis following treatment with radium-224. Rheumatology 2008;47(6):855–9.
24. Au WY, Hawkins BR, Cheng N, et al. Risk of haematological malignancies in HLA-B27 carriers. Br J Haematol 2001;115(2):320–2.
25. Dorak MT, Chalmers EA, Gaffney D, et al. Human major histocompatibility complex contains several leukemia susceptibility genes. Leuk Lymphoma 1994; 12(3–4):211–22.

26. Chen B, Li J, He C, et al. Role of HLA-B27 in the pathogenesis of ankylosing spondylitis. Mol Med Rep 2017;15(4):1943–51.
27. Reveille JD, Zhou X, Lee M, et al. HLA class I and II alleles in susceptibility to ankylosing spondylitis. Ann Rheum Dis 2019;78(1):66–73.
28. Braddock M, Quinn A. Targeting IL-1 in inflammatory disease: new opportunities for therapeutic intervention. Nat Rev Drug Discov 2004;3(4):330–40.
29. Karan D. Inflammasomes: emerging central players in cancer immunology and immunotherapy. Front Immunol 2018;9:3028.
30. Basiorka AA, McGraw KL, Eksioglu EA, et al. The NLRP3 inflammasome functions as a driver of the myelodysplastic syndrome phenotype. Blood 2016;128(25): 2960–75.
31. Sönmez HE, Batu ED, Özen S. Familial Mediterranean fever: current perspectives. J Inflamm Res 2016;9:13–20.
32. Jo T, Horio K, Migita K. Sweet's syndrome in patients with MDS and MEFV mutations. N Engl J Med 2015;372:686–8.
33. Kaiser R. Incidence of lymphoma in patients with rheumatoid arthritis: a systematic review of the literature. Clin Lymphoma Myeloma 2008;8(2):87–93.
34. Boddu PC, Zeidan AM. Myeloid disorders after autoimmune disease. Ther Relat Acute Leuk 2019;32(1):74–88.
35. Churpek JE, Larson RA. The evolving challenge of therapy-related myeloid neoplasms. Best Pract Res Clin Haematol 2013;26(4):309–17.
36. Walter MJ, Ding L, Shen D, et al. Recurrent DNMT3A mutations in patients with myelodysplastic syndromes. Leukemia 2011;25(7):1153–8.
37. Roller A, Grossmann V, Bacher U, et al. Landmark analysis of DNMT3A mutations in hematological malignancies. Leukemia 2013;27(7):1573–8.
38. Ito S, D'Alessio AC, Taranova OV, et al. Role of Tet proteins in 5mC to 5hmC conversion, ES cell self-renewal, and ICM specification. Nature 2010;466(7310): 1129–33.
39. Coltro G, Mangaonkar AA, Lasho TL, et al. Clinical, molecular, and prognostic correlates of number, type, and functional localization of TET2 mutations in chronic myelomonocytic leukemia (CMML)—a study of 1084 patients. Leukemia 2019. https://doi.org/10.1038/s41375-019-0690-7.
40. Patnaik MM, Tefferi A. Chronic Myelomonocytic leukemia: 2020 update on diagnosis, risk stratification and management. Am J Hematol 2020;95(1):97–115.
41. Bejar R, Stevenson K, Abdel-Wahab O, et al. Clinical effect of point mutations in myelodysplastic syndromes. N Engl J Med 2011;364(26):2496–506.
42. Gelsi-Boyer V, Brecqueville M, Devillier R, et al. Mutations in ASXL1 are associated with poor prognosis across the spectrum of malignant myeloid diseases. J Hematol Oncol 2012;5(1):12.
43. SanMiguel JM, Loberg M, Heuer S, et al. Cell-extrinsic stressors from the aging Bone Marrow (BM) microenvironment promote Dnmt3a-mutant clonal hematopoiesis. Blood 2019;134(Supplement_1):5.
44. Wong TN, Miller CA, Jotte MRM, et al. Cellular stressors contribute to the expansion of hematopoietic clones of varying leukemic potential. Nat Commun 2018;9. https://doi.org/10.1038/s41467-018-02858-0.
45. Wu H, Chen Y, Zhu H, et al. The pathogenic role of dysregulated epigenetic modifications in autoimmune diseases. Front Immunol 2019;10. https://doi.org/10.3389/fimmu.2019.02305.
46. Nielsen C, Birgens HS, Nordestgaard BG, et al. The JAK2 V617F somatic mutation, mortality and cancer risk in the general population. Haematologica 2011; 96(3):450–3.

47. Olivier M, Hollstein M, Hainaut P. TP53 mutations in human cancers: origins, consequences, and clinical use. Cold Spring Harb Perspect Biol 2010;2(1). https://doi.org/10.1101/cshperspect.a001008.

48. Steinberg P, Discussant AD. The treatment of lupus nephritis. Kidney Int 1986;30(5):769–87.

49. Hoffman GS, Kerr GS, Leavitt RY, et al. Wegener granulomatosis: an analysis of 158 patients. Ann Intern Med 1992;116(6):488–98.

50. Berlit P. Diagnosis and treatment of cerebral vasculitis. Ther Adv Neurol Disord 2010;3(1):29–42.

51. Houssiau FA, Vasconcelos C, D'Cruz D, et al. Immunosuppressive therapy in lupus nephritis: the Euro-Lupus Nephritis Trial, a randomized trial of low-dose versus high-dose intravenous cyclophosphamide. Arthritis Rheum 2002;46(8):2121–31.

52. Tian M, Song X, Dong L, et al. Systematic evaluation of different doses of cyclophosphamide induction therapy for lupus nephritis. Medicine (Baltimore) 2017;96(51):e9408.

53. Kayser S, Döhner K, Krauter J, et al. The impact of therapy-related acute myeloid leukemia (AML) on outcome in 2853 adult patients with newly diagnosed AML. Blood 2011;117(7):2137–45.

54. Smith SM, Le Beau MM, Huo D, et al. Clinical-cytogenetic associations in 306 patients with therapy-related myelodysplasia and myeloid leukemia: the University of Chicago series. Blood 2003;102(1):43–52.

55. Godley LA, Larson RA. Therapy-related Myeloid Leukemia. Semin Oncol 2008;35(4):418–29.

56. Reinhold-Keller E, Beuge N, Latza U, et al. An interdisciplinary approach to the care of patients with Wegener's granulomatosis: long-term outcome in 155 patients. Arthritis Rheum 2000;43(5):1021–32.

57. Coombs CC, Zehir A, Devlin SM, et al. Therapy-related clonal hematopoiesis in patients with non-hematologic cancers is common and impacts clinical outcome. Cell Stem Cell 2017;21(3):374–82.e4.

58. Fierabracci A, Pellegrino M. The double role of p53 in cancer and autoimmunity and its potential as therapeutic target. Int J Mol Sci 2016;17(12). https://doi.org/10.3390/ijms17121975.

59. Kwong Y-L. Azathioprine: association with therapy-related myelodysplastic syndrome and acute myeloid leukemia. J Rheumatol 2010. https://doi.org/10.3899/jrheum.090834.

60. Ertz-Archambault N, Kosiorek H, Taylor GE, et al. Association of therapy for autoimmune disease with myelodysplastic syndromes and acute myeloid leukemia. JAMA Oncol 2017;3(7):936–43.

61. Löfström B, Backlin C, Sundström C, et al. Myeloid leukaemia in systemic lupus erythematosus—a nested case–control study based on Swedish registers. Rheumatology 2009;48(10):1222–6.

62. Bernatsky S, Clarke AE, Suissa S. Hematologic malignant neoplasms after drug exposure in rheumatoid arthritis. Arch Intern Med 2008;168(4):378–81.

63. Silman AJ, Petrie J, Hazleman B, et al. Lymphoproliferative cancer and other malignancy in patients with rheumatoid arthritis treated with azathioprine: a 20 year follow up study. Ann Rheum Dis 1988;47(12):988.

64. Setoguchi S, Solomon DH, Weinblatt ME, et al. Tumor necrosis factor α antagonist use and cancer in patients with rheumatoid arthritis. Arthritis Rheum 2006;54(9):2757–64.

65. Singh JA, Saag KG, Bridges SL Jr, et al. 2015 American College of Rheumatology guideline for the treatment of rheumatoid arthritis. Arthritis Care Res 2016; 68(1):1–25.

66. Ward MM, Deodhar A, Gensler LS, et al. 2019 Update of the American College of Rheumatology/Spondylitis Association of America/Spondyloarthritis Research and Treatment Network Recommendations for the treatment of ankylosing spondylitis and nonradiographic axial spondyloarthritis. Arthritis Rheumatol 2019; 71(10):1599–613.

67. Baker GL, Kahl LE, Zee BC, Stolzer BL, Agarwal AK, Medsger TA Jr. Malignancy following treatment of rheumatoid arthritis with cyclophosphamide: Long-term case-control follow-up study. Am J Med 1987;83(1):1–9. https://doi.org/10.1016/0002-9343(87)90490-6.

Cancer and Rheumatoid Arthritis

Xerxes Pundole, MD, PhD[a], Maria E. Suarez-Almazor, MD, PhD[a,b],*

KEYWORDS

- Cancer • Rheumatoid arthritis • Disease-modifying antirheumatic drugs
- Biologic therapy

KEY POINTS

- Patients with RA should undergo age- and sex-appropriate cancer screening. No additional screening is recommended for patients on DMARDs.
- Management of RA in patients with cancer requires a multidisciplinary approach that considers type of cancer, stage, prognosis, and life expectancy, and that takes into account patient values.
- Current evidence suggests that biologic and synthetic DMARDs can be used safely in patients with RA and a prior diagnosis of cancer with no evidence of disease for at least 5 years.
- There is a knowledge gap with respect to the effects of bDMARDs and tsDMARDs on cancer outcomes in patients with RA and active cancer.
- Patients with RA undergoing cancer therapy need to be carefully monitored because they are at increased risk of complications.

The link between cancer and rheumatoid arthritis (RA) is complex. With advances in the knowledge of the pathophysiology, long-term outcomes, and development of new agents for cancer and RA, the relationship between these diseases is becoming more evident, and also more challenging. Here we describe related clinically important issues: cancer risk in RA, cancer risk related to therapy to treat RA, treatment of RA in patients with cancer, and treating cancer in patients with RA.

RA is an inflammatory autoimmune condition that symmetrically affects the small joints of the hands and feet and eventually involves large joints. The global prevalence of RA is almost 20 million and the incidence and prevalence rates of RA are increasing.[1] If not treated RA progression results in damage of articular bone and

[a] Department of Health Services Research, The University of Texas MD Anderson Cancer Center, Unit 1444, 1515 Holcombe Boulevard, Houston, TX 77030, USA; [b] Department of General Internal Medicine, Section of Rheumatology and Clinical Immunology, The University of Texas MD Anderson Cancer Center, Houston, TX, USA
* Corresponding author. Department of Health Services Research, The University of Texas MD Anderson Cancer Center, Unit 1444, 1515 Holcombe Boulevard, Houston, TX 77030.
E-mail address: msalmazor@mdanderson.org

Rheum Dis Clin N Am 46 (2020) 445–462
https://doi.org/10.1016/j.rdc.2020.05.003
0889-857X/20/© 2020 Elsevier Inc. All rights reserved.

rheumatic.theclinics.com

cartilage. In the past two decades the development of several new agents has revolutionized the treatment of RA resulting in improved clinical outcomes.[2] However, there are uncertainties as to whether these newer agents used to treat RA can increase the risk of cancer or affect its progression. To determine this, it is essential to first understand the baseline risk of cancer in RA.

CANCER RISK IN RHEUMATOID ARTHRITIS

The association between cancer and RA was first reported in 1978 in a study that identified an increased risk of lymphoma in patients with RA.[3] Since then several observational studies have been conducted to evaluate the risk of cancer in patients with RA. A recent meta-analysis conducted by Simon and colleagues[4] included studies from 2008 to 2014, and in their analysis, they also included studies that were previously analyzed by Smitten and colleagues[5] from 1990 to 2007. The pooled results showed that the standardized incidence ratio (SIR) in patients with RA compared with the general population for any cancer (all sites) was 1.09 (95% confidence interval [CI], 1.06–1.13). However, the risk was not the same across all cancer sites.

In the meta-analysis by Simon and colleagues,[4] the overall pooled SIR for lymphoma was 2.46 (95% CI, 2.05–2.96) for malignant lymphoma, 3.21 (95% CI, 2.42–4.27) for Hodgkin disease, and 2.26 (95% CI, 1.82–2.81) for non-Hodgkin lymphoma. The risk of lung cancer (SIR 1.64; 95% CI, 1.51–1.79) and melanoma (SIR 1.23; 95% CI, 1.01–1.49) were also increased. In contrast, however, the risks of breast cancer and of colorectal cancer were decreased, with SIR of 0.86 (95% CI, 0.73–1.01) and 0.78 (95% CI, 0.71–0.86), respectively.

This differential risk of cancer across sites may be attributable to several reasons. First, it is well known that inflammation in general and inflammatory cells play a role in the development of neoplasms.[6] RA causes a chronic inflammatory state and thus, RA itself, by causing a persistent inflammatory status, could be responsible for the increased risk of lymphoma.[7–9] Sustained immune activation in patients with Sjögren syndrome and Hashimoto thyroiditis has been linked to mucosa-associated lymphoid tissue lymphomas.[10] Many other cancer types have also been associated with chronic inflammation,[6,11,12] providing further evidence that chronic inflammation may play a role in lymphoma development in patients with RA. Second, cancer and RA could have shared risk factors, as is seen with lung cancer and RA. Smoking is a risk factor for developing lung cancer in up to 85% of cases,[13] and is also a known risk factor for RA, increasing risk up to 40%.[14] Inflammation in the airways is common in RA, even at early stages, and it has been suggested that it triggers the production of pathogenic antibodies, especially against citrullinated antigens, causing RA.[15] In addition, patients with RA can develop interstitial lung disease over time. It has been suggested that preexisting interstitial lung disease is associated with lung cancer, because many patients present with parenchymal imaging findings at cancer diagnosis.[16,17] Again, it is unclear whether this represents the effects of a common risk factor, primarily smoking, or whether the inflammation and fibrogenetic pathways related to interstitial lung disease might result in carcinogenesis. This relationship has not been studied in patients with RA.

Patients with RA have a lower risk of colorectal cancer. The cyclooxygenase (COX)-2 enzyme pathway is responsible for prostaglandin E_2 production, a known regulator of key oncogenic processes.[18] It is known that selective COX-2 inhibition results in tumor regression,[19] and at a population level, the use of nonsteroidal anti-inflammatory drugs (NSAIDs), which are COX inhibitors, is associated with a decreased risk of colorectal cancer.[20,21] NSAIDs are commonly used for pain control in patients with RA, even before RA diagnosis, and perhaps a similar effect to that seen in the general population of reduced risk of colorectal cancer may be attributable to the common use of NSAIDs.

Patients with RA also have a decreased incidence of breast cancer.[22] The decreased risk is seen before and after patients develop RA. Because there is a female predominance for RA, it has been suggested that hormonal factors may play a role; however, women with breast cancer who have received antiestrogen therapy with tamoxifen or aromatase inhibitors do not seem to be at increased risk for RA compared with those who do not receive these therapies.[22]

Genetic predispositions and gene-environment interactions may also play a role in the differential risk of cancers in patients with RA, which needs further exploration.

CANCER RISK IN RHEUMATOID ARTHRITIS IN ASSOCIATION WITH USE OF ANTIRHEUMATIC DRUGS

The mainstay of RA treatment is disease-modifying antirheumatic drugs (DMARDs). These agents are categorized into conventional synthetic (cs) DMARDs, biologic (b) DMARDs, and targeted synthetic (ts) DMARDs. With the increasing use of DMARDs in the management of RA, there is a critical need to understand whether or not the risk of cancer is increased with these agents. Here we briefly describe the risk of de novo cancer specifically in patients with RA receiving csDMARDs, bDMARDs, and tsDMARDs.

Conventional Synthetic Disease-Modifying Antirheumatic Drugs

The most commonly used DMARDs in RA are csDMARDs and include methotrexate, sulfasalazine, hydroxychloroquine, cyclosporine, azathioprine, and leflunomide. These agents are used as single agent or in combination with other DMARDs. Methotrexate is considered to be a safe and effective therapy for RA.[23] Overall methotrexate does not seem to increase cancer risk at large.[24] However, an Australian study[25] showed an increased risk of melanoma, non-Hodgkin lymphoma, and lung cancer in patients with RA exposed to methotrexate. This study did not have a control group of untreated RA; hence, it is difficult to ascertain whether the increased risk was from methotrexate or from the disease itself, especially in an Australian population with a high baseline risk of melanoma. In Japanese patients with RA a higher dose of methotrexate was associated with an increased risk of lymphoproliferative diseases.[26] Conflicting results of cancer risk have also been reported with cyclosporine,[27–29] azathioprine,[30] and leflunomide use in RA.[31] Lastly, little evidence is available on the use of sulfasalazine and hydroxychloroquine and cancer risk; however, neither are thought to be significant immunosuppressants.

Biologic Disease-Modifying Antirheumatic Drugs

Since the late 1990s, bDMARDs have become the second commonest class of DMARDs used in RA management. They are broadly categorized into tumor necrosis factor-α inhibitors (TNFi) (etanercept, adalimumab, certolizumab pegol, golimumab, infliximab, and related biosimilars) and non-TNFi agents (tocilizumab, sarilumab, abatacept, anakinra, and rituximab). In patients with RA there is conflicting evidence if TNFi increases cancer risk. Some meta-analyses and registry data have shown no increased cancer risk in patients receiving TNFi,[32–35] but other studies have shown increased risk of nonmelanoma skin cancer.[36–38] Similarly conflicting results have been reported for lymphoma risk.[39,40] However, TNFi agents are used in patients with severe disease, and deciphering the effects of RA, which is associated with increased baseline lymphoma risk, especially in those with persistently active disease, from the potential effects of treatment with TNFi is challenging.

The non-TNFi are used typically following inadequate response to other DMARDs and/or TNFi. A claims-based study of three large US insurance companies[41] and a Swedish study[42] did not show increased risk for cancer with tocilizumab, an interleukin-6 receptor inhibitor; abatacept, a fusion protein composed of the Fc region of the immunoglobulin IgG1 and the extracellular domain of cytotoxic T-lymphocyte-associated protein 4; or rituximab, a chimeric monoclonal antibody against CD20. However, nonmelanoma skin cancers were excluded in evaluation of the primary outcome in both studies. In the Swedish study, an increased risk of squamous cell skin cancer was observed in the abatacept cohort versus csDMARDs (hazard ratio [HR], 2.15; 95% CI, 1.31–3.52). However, because of the limitations of the study, authors concluded that firm conclusions could not be made. Less information is available for anakinra, an interleukin-1 receptor antagonist, rarely used for RA. One challenge in assessing the risk of non-TNFi is that most patients with RA receive TNFi before non-TNFi agents, so disentangling the effects of continued risk from TNFi from the potential confounding by indication is problematic.

Targeted Synthetic Disease-Modifying Antirheumatic Drugs

The agents available for the treatment of RA are expanding. Currently there are three tsDMARDs approved for RA treatment. Tofacitinib, baricitinib, and upadacitinib are all janus kinase inhibitors. These agents are small molecules and available in oral formation. No signals of cancer risk were observed with tofacitinib in a meta-analysis of 4000 patients from clinical trials,[43] and in 3-year data of postmarketing surveillance from Pfizer.[44] Limited other information is available on the cancer risk with tofacitinib and the other janus kinase inhibitors. As such the limited evidence thus far stems from clinical trials, and well-controlled large observational studies are needed to clarify cancer risk with tsDMARDs.

CANCER SCREENING IN PATIENTS WITH CANCER

In patients with RA and no prior cancer, the nationally recommended age- and sex-specific cancer screening guidelines for breast, cervical, endometrial, colorectal, lung, and prostate should be followed.[45] In a recent systematic review of guidelines, we found agreement in most guidelines to screen for cancer before RA therapy initiation, but disagreements on the comprehensiveness of screening were noted.[46] In the same review, there was an overall agreement to be vigilant for symptoms or signs of cancer among patients with RA receiving DMARDs, but specific details were lacking. The benefits of screening for skin cancer have not been thoroughly evaluated; however, this may be considered, especially in patients receiving bDMARDs because some studies have shown increased risk of nonmelanoma skin cancer.

SAFETY OF DISEASE-MODIFYING ANTIRHEUMATIC DRUGS IN PATIENTS WITH RHEUMATOID ARTHRITIS AND PRIOR OR CONCOMITANT CANCER

In patients with a history of cancer or with active cancer, the use of DMARDs may confer a different risk profile as it relates to recurrences and development of a second new cancer. csDMARDs, including methotrexate, leflunomide, hydroxychloroquine, and sulfasalazine, do not have significant immunosuppressive properties and are often used in patients with RA and cancer, which is not considered a contraindication for their use, although well-controlled data are scarce.[46,47] However, clinical trials of bDMARDs and tsDMARDs have systematically excluded patients with prior cancer because of initial concerns of the possible adverse effects on tumor immunity. Hence, the available evidence arises from observational data, and recommendations are largely based on expert opinion. Most of these observational studies have evaluated bDMARDs, and no studies have evaluated tsDMARDs in patients with cancer.

We summarize the evidence from observational studies on the use of DMARDs in patients with RA and cancer in **Tables 1** and **2**. Four European registries have provided data: (1) the British Society for Rheumatology Biologics Register, a national prospective observational study established in the United Kingdom[48–51]; (2) the Swedish biologics register (Anti-Rheumatic Therapy in Sweden)[52–54]; (3) the nationwide Danish DANBIO Registry[55,56]; and (4) the nationwide German biologics register RABBIT.[9] In addition, three other studies have evaluated the effects of bDMARDs in patients with prior malignancy in the United States using the national Veterans' Affairs administrative databases and electronic medical records,[57] and the Medicare administrative database.[58,59]

Eleven studies evaluated new or recurrent cancer in patients with RA who received TNFi compared with those who received csDMARDs (see **Table 1**). Of these, six studies showed a numerical, but not statistically significant, increased risk of new or recurrent cancer.[9,52–54,56,58] One study using data from the Medicare registry showed increased risk of a second nonmelanoma skin cancer (adjusted HR, 1.49; 95% CI, 1.03–2.16) in patients with prior nonmelanoma skin cancer receiving TNFi.[59] Two studies evaluated TNFi in patients with cervical carcinoma in situ and none progressed to cancer.[50,55]

Three studies evaluated the effect of rituximab in patients with prior malignancy,[51,56,59] of which two showed a numerical but statistically nonsignificant increased risk of second malignancy (see **Table 2**).[56,59] One study evaluated the effects of anakinra (n = 11),[9] and another evaluated the effects of abatacept compared with methotrexate monotherapy on risk of second nonmelanoma skin cancer (HR, 1.40; 95% CI, 0.48–4.03)[59]; however, no firm conclusions could be drawn because of the limited sample sizes. Most studies did not show statistically significant differences among groups; however, clinically meaningful risk cannot be ruled out given the effect size of the estimates and that several of the 95% CIs had upper limits greater than 2.0. Furthermore, most studies analyzed data from European registries, had small sample sizes, evaluated TNFi alone, had primarily patients with a remote history of cancer, and were not able to account for all confounders, especially cancer site and/or stage. There is still an urgent need for data to evaluate (1) differential effects of bDMARDs by cancer stage, especially in patients with active cancer or in those with advanced stage at primary diagnosis; (2) potential differences according to cancer type and histology; (3) safety and cancer outcomes on patients receiving non-TNFi biologics or tsDMARDs; and (4) cumulative dose and time-varying effects of these agents on cancer outcomes.

RECOMMENDATIONS ON THE MANAGEMENT OF RHEUMATOID ARTHRITIS IN PATIENTS WITH CANCER

We recently summarized published recommendations on the use of DMARDs in patients with RA and cancer.[46] These guidelines were based primarily on expert opinion, given the lack of evidence for the use of specific RA therapies across various cancers, and differences were observed among recommendations. Guidelines evaluating development of de novo cancer in a patient with RA generally agreed that the treatment of RA should be re-evaluated and most recommended discontinuation of bDMARDs. For patients with preexisting cancer who develop RA, most

Table 1
Risk of recurrent or new primary cancer development in patients with RA and cancer receiving TNFi versus csDMARDs

Country (Registry)	Study	TNFi	csDMARDs	Measure	Point Estimate (95% CI) TNFi vs csDMARDs (Ref)	Prior Cancer	Outcome	Adjustment Factors
United Kingdom (BSRB)	Dixon et al,[48] 2010	177	117	IRR	0.45 (0.09–2.17)	Any cancer except CIS and NMSC	New primary, recurrence, metastases	Propensity adjusted
	Mercer et al,[49] 2012	177	106	HR	0.70 (0.26–1.94)	Skin cancer	BCC	Treatment weighting
	Mercer et al,[50] 2013	190	48	—	None in TNFi group	CIS	Female genital cancer	None
	Silva-Fernandez et al,[51] 2016	243	159	HR	0.56 (0.36–0.88)	Any cancer except NMSC	New or recurrent cancer except NMSC	Age, gender, and smoking status
Sweden (ARTIS)	Raaschou et al,[53] 2013	54	295	aHR	3.2 (0.80–13.1)	Invasive or in situ melanoma	New melanoma	Age and sex
	Raaschou et al,[52] 2015	120	120	aHR	1.10 (0.40–2.80)	Breast cancer	Recurrence	Breast cancer characteristics and comorbidities
	Raaschou et al,[54] 2018	467	2164	aHR	1.06 (0.73–1.54)	Solid organs	Recurrence	Sex, birth year, index cancer year of diagnosis, type and stage, education level, and comorbid conditions
Denmark (DANBIO)	Cordtz et al,[55] 2015	233	442	—	None in either group	CIS or CD	Progression	None
	Dreyer et al,[56] 2018	1326[a]		aHR	1.21 (0.73–2.03)	Any cancer except NMSC	Second malignancy	Age, gender, calendar time, cancer site, and extent of disease
				aHR	1.42 (0.91–2.20)		Death	

Country	Study	Total patients	Number of patients			Any cancer except NMSC	Recurrence	None
Germany (RABBIT)	Strangfeld et al,[9] 2010	72	43	IRR	1.40 (0.50–5.50)	Any cancer except NMSC	Recurrence	None
United States (Veterans Affairs)	Philips et al,[57] 2015	31	149	aHR	0.75 (0.31–1.85)	HNC	Recurrence or HNC-attributable death	Age, stage at diagnosis, years from RA to HNC diagnosis, modified Romano score, smoking, alcohol, radiation, chemotherapy, surgery
United States (Medicare)	Mamtani et al,[58] 2016	273	1092	HR	1.11 (0.64–1.95)	Breast cancer	Breast cancer	No covariates modified HR >10% hence not adjusted for
	Scott et al,[59] 2016[b]	109	335	aHR	1.49 (1.03–2.16)	NMSC	Second NMSC	Anti-TNF exposure before incident NMSC; no other covariates modified HR by >10%

Abbreviations: aHR, adjusted hazard ratio; BCC, basal cell carcinoma; CD, cervical dysplasia; CIS, carcinoma in situ; HNC, head and neck cancer; IRR, incidence rate ratio; NMSC, nonmelanoma skin cancer.
[a] Total patients with extent of disease recorded.
[b] Number of patients in each group unknown, number of events reported.
Data from Refs.[9,48–59]

Table 2
Risk of recurrent or new primary cancer development in patients with RA and cancer receiving rituximab versus csDMARDs

Country (Registry)	Study	RTX	csDMARDs	Adjusted HR (95% CI) RTX vs csDMARDs (Ref)	Prior Cancer	Outcome	Adjustment Factors
United Kingdom (BSRB)	Silva-Fernandez et al,[51] 2016	23	159	0.44 (0.11–1.82)	Any cancer except NMSC	New or recurrent cancer except NMSC	Age, gender, and smoking status
Denmark (DANBIO)	Dreyer et al,[56] 2018	1326[a]		1.05 (0.47–2.34) 1.11 (0.53–2.35)	Any cancer except NMSC	Second malignancy Death	Age, gender, calendar time, cancer site, and extent of disease
United States (Medicare)	Scott et al,[59] 2016	320[b]	—	1.44 (0.26–8.08)	NMSC	Second NMSC	RTX exposure before incident NMSC; no other covariates modified HR by >10%

Abbreviations: NMSC, nonmelanoma skin cancer; RTX, rituximab.
[a] Total patients with extent of disease recorded.
[b] RTX with methotrexate versus methotrexate. No of patients unknown; number of events are reported.
Data from Refs.[51,56,59]

recommendations suggested that bDMARDs should not be used in patients with active cancer and could be used primarily only in those with no evidence of disease. In general, use of csDMARDs was considered safe.

Several guidelines addressed their recommendations from the perspective of time from cancer diagnosis. For patients with a history of cancer of at least 5 years, most guidelines considered bDMARDs to be generally safe but recommended caution with use. Some guidelines did not recommend use of TNFi at all in patients with pre-existing cancer. For patients with a more recent history of cancer, of 5 years or less, most guidelines did not recommend treatment with TNFi. With respect to other non-TNF bDMARDs, most stated that these agents could be used with caution. Abatacept was not recommended by some. In general, rituximab was considered to be safe. Consultation with an oncologist was recommended before initiation of any bDMARDs. No clear guidance was provided on treatment with tsDMARDS because many of these recommendations were published before the approval of these agents, but those who considered it, stated that csDMARDs therapy was preferred.

In patients with a history of a hematologic cancer, csDMARDs were preferred over TNFi, based on the American College of Rheumatology guidelines, but the Canadian guidelines expressed caution against the use of leflunomide and methotrexate in patients with a history of lymphoma. The consensus of most guidelines was that rituximab can be used, and abatacept and tocilizumab should be used with caution, but were nevertheless preferred over TNFi.

Some guidelines considered patients with premalignant conditions. Treatment with bDMARDs or cyclosporine was not recommended, or caution was advised if used. Among bDMARDs an exception was rituximab, which in one guideline was suggested to be a consideration in patients with in situ cancer.

Most guidelines considered cancer as a class, and distinctions were only provided in some with respect to solid tumors, hematologic cancers, or skin cancers. Although duration from diagnosis of cancer was often considered, other important issues, such as stage of disease, prognosis, potential for cure, or life expectancy, were not addressed. These are issues that are fundamental for decision-making and that need to be considered at the individual level, taking into account patient preferences and values for quality of life and survival. Given the uncertainties on the potential effects of bDMARDS and tsDMARDS on recurrence and survival in patients with recently diagnosed cancer, patients may have different preferences, as exemplified next:

- Patient A is a 62-year-old woman with RA and recently diagnosed with estrogen-positive stage 1 breast cancer. She elects to continue therapy with TNFi because the 10-year probability of survival for this cancer after surgery, radiation, and hormonal therapy is high.
- Patient B is a 35-year-old man with RA and stage 3 melanoma. The survival rates for this cancer are not as good as for Patient A. Furthermore, melanoma is a highly immunogenic tumor, susceptible to immune attack. The patient wants to minimize the risk of a potential recurrence after treatment and decides to stop TNFi therapy.
- Patient C is a 68-year-old woman with RA, well controlled with TNFi, just diagnosed with metastatic adenocarcinoma of the pancreas. Given the poor prognosis of her cancer, the patient decides to continue treatment with TNFi to maintain her symptom control and maximize her quality of life for the remaining time she may survive.

For these three patients with RA and recently diagnosed cancer, there is no distinction in the recommendations about treatment with TNFi according to published guidelines. However, their age, type of cancer, stage, and prognosis, and patient values, are instrumental in informing the most appropriate therapeutic decision.

USE OF CORTICOSTEROIDS IN PATIENTS WITH RHEUMATOID ARTHRITIS AND CANCER

Corticosteroids are frequently used in patients with cancer and RA to treat flares or as bridge therapy before other DMARDs can be started. These drugs are also used in the treatment of certain cancers, such as lymphoma or myeloma, and in addition, they play an important role in supportive therapy.[60] Dexamethasone is often used concomitantly with chemotherapy infusions to reduce nausea and vomiting. For patients with advanced cancer, corticosteroids are often used to improve performance status, and in this situation, dosing is higher.

The effects of chronic steroid therapy on cancer recurrence or progression are largely unknown. Because corticosteroids are potent, wide-ranging, immunosuppressant drugs, they could conceivably impair tumor immunity. However, this issue remains controversial because some studies report tumor progression and others inhibition.[61] These effects may vary according to tumor type because corticosteroids are effective in the treatment of lymphoproliferative diseases. With the advent of immunotherapy, there is also limited evidence that suggests that patients with cancer who are treated with corticosteroids at a dose of greater than or equal to 10 mg prednisone equivalent at the initiation of immunotherapy may have worse cancer outcomes than those who do not.[62] Given this knowledge gap with respect to cancer outcomes, for patients requiring corticosteroids only for management of RA flares, and not as treatment of their cancer, low doses are recommended. High dosages can also increase the risk for infection, a common complication in the cancer population.

CANCER TREATMENT IN PATIENTS WITH RHEUMATOID ARTHRITIS

The treatment of cancer is often considered a priority compared with comorbidities, such as RA; hence, it is common that RA treatment is discontinued or withheld for a period of time. The consequences of such gaps in RA treatment on patients' outcomes and quality of life are unknown and have not been clearly documented.

Surgery

Surgery is one of the pillars of cancer therapy. Management of patients with RA in the perioperative setting can present unique challenges. Patients with RA frequently use NSAIDs, which inhibit COX-1 resulting in antiplatelet effects. Thus, patients being considered for surgery are at risk for bleeding, and in the preoperative period they should discontinue NSAIDs.[63] Glucocorticoids are also commonly used in patients with RA. Chronic use of glucocorticoids is associated with surgical site infections[64] and can result in poor healing of surgical site wounds.[65] It is thus advisable to taper glucocorticoids before surgery if feasible. Furthermore, in patients receiving long-term glucocorticoid therapy the hypothalamic-pituitary-adrenal axis is commonly suppressed. Patients taking greater than or equal to 20 mg of prednisone for 3 weeks or more may have adrenal suppression, which could result in hypotension and shock. In such circumstances patients should be given supplemental corticosteroids perioperatively to prevent adrenal insufficiency.[66]

Risk of infections after surgery is a major concern in patients with RA who are often immunosuppressed. For that reason, surgeons often request that RA therapies be discontinued before surgery. Most of the available data concern orthopedic surgery.[67,68] The use of hydroxychloroquine, methotrexate, and leflunomide is considered to be safe in the perioperative period because studies have failed to identify an increased risk of infections.[69–73] However, because these studies focused mainly on joint-replacement surgery, results may not be generalizable to all surgical procedures. As far as use of bDMARDs, a large retrospective cohort study using Medicare and Truven MarketScan administrative data showed that the risk of infection requiring hospitalization and prosthetic joint infection were similar across biologic agents in patients undergoing total hip or knee arthroplasty.[68] An analysis of the Danish DANBIO registry showed a slightly increased risk of infection following total hip or knee arthroplasty (HR, 1.35 [0.65–2.80]) albeit not statistically significant in patients receiving bDMARDs compared with those that did not receive biologics.[67] The joint guidelines between the American College of Rheumatology and the American Association of Hip and Knee Surgeons recommend stopping bDMARDs and planning the surgery at the end of the dosing cycle.[74] For restarting bDMARDs, they recommend waiting for a period of typically 14 days following surgery when there is evidence of wound healing. They also provided guidance on tsDMARD tofacitinib and recommended withholding tofacitinib for 7 days before elective arthroplasty. Few studies have provided information on the safety of RA treatments on nonorthopedic surgical outcomes, and to our knowledge, none have specifically addressed oncologic surgery.[75,76] Increased infections and delayed wound healing are to be expected. For this reason, recommendations for general oncologic surgery at this time should follow those proposed for joint replacement.

Radiation

There has been a concern with the use of radiation in patients with autoimmune rheumatic diseases, primarily in those with systemic sclerosis, and to a lesser degree, in patients with systemic lupus erythematosus.[77,78] In general, RA is not considered a contraindication for radiation therapy. In a review of medical records of 131 patients with RA that received a mean of 45 Gy of radiation, no differences were found in acute effects, such as mucositis, dysphagia, and skin changes, and late effects, such as cardiac toxicity, small-bowel obstruction, and tissue fibrosis or necrosis in patients with RA compared with patients with non-RA connective tissue diseases receiving radiation.[79] In another study patients with breast cancer with RA who received a median of 60 Gy of radiation did not show a significant difference in acute or late toxicity, compared with patients without RA with breast cancer who received radiation.[80] However, a few case reports have shown adverse toxicities from radiation in patients with RA.[81,82] We recommend a cautious approach to the use of radiation in patients with RA until further data are available.

Chemotherapy and Other Drug Therapies

Although there are guidelines for the management of RA in patients with a cancer history, the American College of Rheumatology does not have any current recommendations for the management of RA in patients with active cancer.[47] There have been theoretic concerns that some DMARDs may suppress the immune system, which may adversely affect cancer treatment. There is a general consensus in clinical practice that bDMARDs should be held in patients with active cancer receiving chemotherapy to avoid an increase in adverse events, especially infections. Anecdotally, patients with RA receiving chemotherapy often have improvement in their disease activity because the chemotherapy agents used are immunosuppressive, and also because corticosteroids are often given with the chemotherapy infusions. Finally, csDMARDs and tsDMARDs can interact with other drugs, and this should be taken into consideration, not just with chemotherapeutic agents, but also with targeted cancer therapies, which can present important drug interactions (eg, imatinib and cyclosporine).

Immune Checkpoint Inhibitors

In the last decade, improvement in the safety and efficacy of several cancers with the use of immune checkpoint inhibitors (ICI) has led to Food and Drug Administration approval of several ICI. These agents target the cytotoxic T-lymphocyte-associated protein-4, programmed cell death protein-1, or programmed death ligand-1 pathways. Activation of the immune system with ICI agents can also result in unwanted and off-target inflammatory or autoimmune effects, commonly referred to as immune-related adverse events (irAE).[83,84] Inflammatory arthritis is the most commonly reported rheumatologic irAE.[85–87] Most often patients present with seronegative polyarthritis or oligoarthritis, but occasionally develop well-defined seropositive RA.[83] Generally speaking, these irAE occur late, can have varying presentation affecting small and large joints, and lower and upper extremities.[83,88–90] Most patients receive corticosteroids to treat their arthritis irAE but some may develop chronic arthritis requiring DMARDs for disease control.[90] The effects of immunosuppressive therapies for arthritis on cancer outcomes in patients receiving ICI remain largely understudied. However, a recent study showed that patients with cancer receiving TNFi for the treatment of corticosteroid-refractory irAE had lower survival compared with patients who received only steroids.[91]

Patients with preexisting autoimmune disease including RA have been excluded from clinical trials of ICI and hence the available evidence stems from observational research. In patients with preexisting RA, the rate of arthritis irAE is estimated to be up to 44%[83]; however, most studies evaluating flares of RA following ICI therapy in patients with preexisting RA have had small sample sizes.[92–97] Further research is needed to evaluate the effects of flares and therapies to manage flares on cancer outcomes.

SUMMARY

One in three people, including patients with RA, develop cancer over their lifetime,[98] and patients and providers are thus frequently faced with making complex decisions related to RA and cancer therapy. Overall, the risk of cancer does not seem to be increased for most DMARDs, other than some small safety signals seen with TNFi and the development of lymphoma and skin cancer. Treatment of RA in patients with cancer is complex. Conventional DMARDs can generally be used even in patients with active cancer if they are not receiving chemotherapy and there are no drug interactions. In general, in patients with active cancer the use of bDMARDs and tsDMARDs is not recommended, especially when they are receiving concomitant cancer therapies. In patients with premalignant conditions these agents can be used with caution if required to control disease activity, with careful monitoring and repeated screening. Patients with cancer can receive csDMARDs if there are no contraindications related to concomitant therapies. bDMARDs, especially TNFi, and tsDMARDs should be avoided in patients with recently diagnosed cancer, at least until treatment is completed. An exception is rituximab, which has generally been considered safe in patients with cancer. Biologics and tsDMARDs can be considered in patients with a prior history of cancer and no evidence of disease for at least a few years. In patients with advanced metastatic disease, quality of life considerations are crucial, and use of effective RA therapy including biologics should be considered to improve patients' well-being at the end of life.

Cancer treatment in patients with RA also needs special attention. Patients with RA undergoing surgery, radiation, chemotherapy, or immunotherapy need careful monitoring because they are more susceptible to adverse events from these treatments than patients without RA.

Given the complexities in the clinical management of patients with RA and cancer, a multidisciplinary approach is encouraged to enhance patient well-being without detriment in cancer outcomes. Given the importance of balancing quality of life and survival, patient preferences should always be taken into consideration. Choices about therapy should be consensual, using principles of shared decision-making to ensure that patients understand potential harms and benefits, and that their preferences and values are considered in the management plan.

CLINICS CARE POINTS

- Biologic and tsDMARDs can be considered in patients with a remote history of cancer, and no recurrences.
- Patient preferences and values should be considered in treatment decision making in patients with RA and cancer, with appropriate discussions on quality of life and survival trade-offs.
- Patients with RA receiving cancer therapy including chemotherapy, radiation, and/or immunotherapy should be monitored closely for toxicities.

DISCLOSURE

M.E. Suarez-Almazor has received consultant fees from Agile Therapeutics, AMAG Pharmaceuticals, and Gilead. X. Pundole, none.

REFERENCES

1. Safiri S, Kolahi AA, Hoy D, et al. Global, regional and national burden of rheumatoid arthritis 1990-2017: a systematic analysis of the Global Burden of Disease study 2017. Ann Rheum Dis 2019;78(11):1463–71.
2. Burmester GR, Pope JE. Novel treatment strategies in rheumatoid arthritis. Lancet 2017;389(10086):2338–48.
3. Isomaki HA, Hakulinen T, Joutsenlahti U. Excess risk of lymphomas, leukemia and myeloma in patients with rheumatoid-arthritis. J Chronic Dis 1978;31(11):691–6.
4. Simon TA, Thompson A, Gandhi KK, et al. Incidence of malignancy in adult patients with rheumatoid arthritis: a meta-analysis. Arthritis Res Ther 2015;17:212.
5. Smitten AL, Simon TA, Hochberg MC, et al. A meta-analysis of the incidence of malignancy in adult patients with rheumatoid arthritis. Arthritis Res Ther 2008; 10(2):R45.
6. Coussens LM, Werb Z. Inflammation and cancer. Nature 2002;420(6917):860–7.
7. Baecklund E, Iliadou A, Askling J, et al. Association of chronic inflammation, not its treatment, with increased lymphoma risk in rheumatoid arthritis. Arthritis Rheum 2006;54(3):692–701.
8. Gridley G, Klippel JH, Hoover RN, et al. Incidence of cancer among men with the Felty syndrome. Ann Intern Med 1994;120(1):35–9.
9. Strangfeld A, Hierse F, Rau R, et al. Risk of incident or recurrent malignancies among patients with rheumatoid arthritis exposed to biologic therapy in the German biologics register RABBIT. Arthritis Res Ther 2010;12(1):R5.
10. Zucca E, Bertoni F. The spectrum of MALT lymphoma at different sites: biological and therapeutic relevance. Blood 2016;127(17):2082–92.
11. Karin M. Nuclear factor-kappaB in cancer development and progression. Nature 2006;441(7092):431–6.
12. Karin M, Greten FR. NF-kappaB: linking inflammation and immunity to cancer development and progression. Nat Rev Immunol 2005;5(10):749–59.

13. Warren GW, Cummings KM. Tobacco and lung cancer: risks, trends, and outcomes in patients with cancer. Am Soc Clin Oncol Educ Book 2013;359–64. https://doi.org/10.1200/EdBook_AM.2013.33.359.

14. Sugiyama D, Nishimura K, Tamaki K, et al. Impact of smoking as a risk factor for developing rheumatoid arthritis: a meta-analysis of observational studies. Ann Rheum Dis 2010;69(1):70–81.

15. Kelmenson LB, Demoruelle MK, Deane KD. The complex role of the lung in the pathogenesis and clinical outcomes of rheumatoid arthritis. Curr Rheumatol Rep 2016;18(11):69.

16. Gibiot Q, Monnet I, Levy P, et al. Interstitial lung disease associated with lung cancer: a case-control study. J Clin Med 2020;9(3) [pii:E700].

17. Naccache JM, Gibiot Q, Monnet I, et al. Lung cancer and interstitial lung disease: a literature review. J Thorac Dis 2018;10(6):3829–44.

18. Shao J, Jung C, Liu C, et al. Prostaglandin E2 Stimulates the beta-catenin/T cell factor-dependent transcription in colon cancer. J Biol Chem 2005;280(28): 26565–72.

19. Giardiello FM, Casero RA Jr, Hamilton SR, et al. Prostanoids, ornithine decarboxylase, and polyamines in primary chemoprevention of familial adenomatous polyposis. Gastroenterology 2004;126(2):425–31.

20. Din FV, Theodoratou E, Farrington SM, et al. Effect of aspirin and NSAIDs on risk and survival from colorectal cancer. Gut 2010;59(12):1670–9.

21. Ruder EH, Laiyemo AO, Graubard BI, et al. Non-steroidal anti-inflammatory drugs and colorectal cancer risk in a large, prospective cohort. Am J Gastroenterol 2011;106(7):1340–50.

22. Wadstrom H, Pettersson A, Smedby KE, et al. Risk of breast cancer before and after rheumatoid arthritis, and the impact of hormonal factors. Ann Rheum Dis 2020;79(5):581–6.

23. Lopez-Olivo MA, Siddhanamatha HR, Shea B, et al. Methotrexate for treating rheumatoid arthritis. Cochrane Database Syst Rev 2014;(6):CD000957.

24. Raheel S, Crowson CS, Wright K, et al. Risk of malignant neoplasm in patients with incident rheumatoid arthritis 1980-2007 in relation to a comparator cohort: a population-based study. Int J Rheumatol 2016;2016:4609486.

25. Buchbinder R, Barber M, Heuzenroeder L, et al. Incidence of melanoma and other malignancies among rheumatoid arthritis patients treated with methotrexate. Arthritis Rheum 2008;59(6):794–9.

26. Kameda T, Dobashi H, Miyatake N, et al. Association of higher methotrexate dose with lymphoproliferative disease onset in rheumatoid arthritis patients. Arthritis Care Res (Hoboken) 2014;66(9):1302–9.

27. Arellano F, Krupp P. Malignancies in rheumatoid arthritis patients treated with cyclosporin A. Br J Rheumatol 1993;32(Suppl 1):72–5.

28. van den Borne BE, Landewe RB, Houkes I, et al. No increased risk of malignancies and mortality in cyclosporin A-treated patients with rheumatoid arthritis. Arthritis Rheum 1998;41(11):1930–7.

29. Durnian JM, Stewart RM, Tatham R, et al. Cyclosporin-A associated malignancy. Clin Ophthalmol 2007;1(4):421–30.

30. Bernatsky S, Clarke AE, Suissa S. Hematologic malignant neoplasms after drug exposure in rheumatoid arthritis. Arch Intern Med 2008;168(4):378–81.

31. Strangfeld A, Hyrich K, Askling J, et al. Detection and evaluation of a drug safety signal concerning pancreatic cancer: lessons from a joint approach of three European biologics registers. Rheumatology (Oxford) 2011;50(1):146–51.

32. Dreyer L, Mellemkjaer L, Andersen AR, et al. Incidences of overall and site specific cancers in TNFalpha inhibitor treated patients with rheumatoid arthritis and other arthritides: a follow-up study from the DANBIO Registry. Ann Rheum Dis 2013;72(1):79–82.

33. Haynes K, Beukelman T, Curtis JR, et al. Tumor necrosis factor alpha inhibitor therapy and cancer risk in chronic immune-mediated diseases. Arthritis Rheum 2013;65(1):48–58.

34. Lopez-Olivo MA, Tayar JH, Martinez-Lopez JA, et al. Risk of malignancies in patients with rheumatoid arthritis treated with biologic therapy: a meta-analysis. JAMA 2012;308(9):898–908.

35. Thompson AE, Rieder SW, Pope JE. Tumor necrosis factor therapy and the risk of serious infection and malignancy in patients with early rheumatoid arthritis: a meta-analysis of randomized controlled trials. Arthritis Rheum 2011;63(6):1479–85.

36. Chakravarty EF, Michaud K, Wolfe F. Skin cancer, rheumatoid arthritis, and tumor necrosis factor inhibitors. J Rheumatol 2005;32(11):2130–5.

37. Tseng HW, Lu LY, Lam HC, et al. The influence of disease-modifying anti-rheumatic drugs and corticosteroids on the association between rheumatoid arthritis and skin cancer: a nationwide retrospective case-control study in Taiwan. Clin Exp Rheumatol 2018;36(3):471–8.

38. Wang JL, Yin WJ, Zhou LY, et al. Risk of non-melanoma skin cancer for rheumatoid arthritis patients receiving TNF antagonist: a systematic review and meta-analysis. Clin Rheumatol 2019;39(3):769–78.

39. Mariette X, Tubach F, Bagheri H, et al. Lymphoma in patients treated with anti-TNF: results of the 3-year prospective French RATIO registry. Ann Rheum Dis 2010;69(2):400–8.

40. Wolfe F, Michaud K. The effect of methotrexate and anti-tumor necrosis factor therapy on the risk of lymphoma in rheumatoid arthritis in 19,562 patients during 89,710 person-years of observation. Arthritis Rheum 2007;56(5):1433–9.

41. Kim SC, Pawar A, Desai RJ, et al. Risk of malignancy associated with use of tocilizumab versus other biologics in patients with rheumatoid arthritis: a multidatabase cohort study. Semin Arthritis Rheum 2019;49(2):222–8.

42. Wadstrom H, Frisell T, Askling J, Anti-Rheumatic Therapy in Sweden Study Group. Malignant neoplasms in patients with rheumatoid arthritis treated with tumor necrosis factor inhibitors, tocilizumab, abatacept, or rituximab in clinical practice: a nationwide cohort study from Sweden. JAMA Intern Med 2017;177(11):1605–12.

43. Curtis JR, Lee EB, Kaplan IV, et al. Tofacitinib, an oral Janus kinase inhibitor: analysis of malignancies across the rheumatoid arthritis clinical development programme. Ann Rheum Dis 2016;75(5):831–41.

44. Cohen S, Curtis JR, DeMasi R, et al. Worldwide, 3-year, post-marketing surveillance experience with tofacitinib in rheumatoid arthritis. Rheumatol Ther 2018;5(1):283–91.

45. Smith RA, Andrews KS, Brooks D, et al. Cancer screening in the United States, 2019: a review of current American Cancer Society guidelines and current issues in cancer screening. CA Cancer J Clin 2019;69(3):184–210.

46. Lopez-Olivo MA, Colmegna I, Karpes Matusevich AR, et al. Systematic review of recommendations on the use of disease-modifying antirheumatic drugs in patients with rheumatoid arthritis and cancer. Arthritis Care Res (Hoboken) 2020;72(3):309–18.

47. Singh JA, Saag KG, Bridges SL, et al. 2015 American College of Rheumatology guideline for the treatment of rheumatoid arthritis. Arthritis Rheumatol 2016; 68(1):1–26.

48. Dixon WG, Watson KD, Lunt M, et al. Influence of anti-tumor necrosis factor therapy on cancer incidence in patients with rheumatoid arthritis who have had a prior malignancy: results from the British Society for Rheumatology Biologics Register. Arthritis Care Res (Hoboken) 2010;62(6):755–63.

49. Mercer LK, Green AC, Galloway JB, et al. The influence of anti-TNF therapy upon incidence of keratinocyte skin cancer in patients with rheumatoid arthritis: longitudinal results from the British Society for Rheumatology Biologics Register. Ann Rheum Dis 2012;71(6):869–74.

50. Mercer LK, Low AS, Galloway JB, et al. Anti-TNF therapy in women with rheumatoid arthritis with a history of carcinoma in situ of the cervix. Ann Rheum Dis 2013; 72(1):143–4.

51. Silva-Fernandez L, Lunt M, Kearsley-Fleet L, et al. The incidence of cancer in patients with rheumatoid arthritis and a prior malignancy who receive TNF inhibitors or rituximab: results from the British Society for Rheumatology Biologics Register-Rheumatoid Arthritis. Rheumatology (Oxford) 2016;55(11):2033–9.

52. Raaschou P, Frisell T, Askling J, et al. TNF inhibitor therapy and risk of breast cancer recurrence in patients with rheumatoid arthritis: a nationwide cohort study. Ann Rheum Dis 2015;74(12):2137–43.

53. Raaschou P, Simard JF, Holmqvist M, et al. Rheumatoid arthritis, anti-tumour necrosis factor therapy, and risk of malignant melanoma: nationwide population based prospective cohort study from Sweden. BMJ 2013;346:f1939.

54. Raaschou P, Soderling J, Turesson C, et al. Tumor necrosis factor inhibitors and cancer recurrence in Swedish patients with rheumatoid arthritis: a nationwide population-based cohort study. Ann Intern Med 2018;169(5):291–9.

55. Cordtz R, Mellemkjaer L, Glintborg B, et al. Malignant progression of precancerous lesions of the uterine cervix following biological DMARD therapy in patients with arthritis. Ann Rheum Dis 2015;74(7):1479–80.

56. Dreyer L, Cordtz RL, Hansen IMJ, et al. Risk of second malignant neoplasm and mortality in patients with rheumatoid arthritis treated with biological DMARDs: a Danish population-based cohort study. Ann Rheum Dis 2018;77(4):510–4.

57. Phillips C, Zeringue AL, McDonald JR, et al. Tumor necrosis factor inhibition and head and neck cancer recurrence and death in rheumatoid arthritis. PLoS One 2015;10(11):e0143286.

58. Mamtani R, Clark AS, Scott FI, et al. Association between breast cancer recurrence and immunosuppression in rheumatoid arthritis and inflammatory bowel disease: a cohort study. Arthritis Rheumatol 2016;68(10):2403–11.

59. Scott FI, Mamtani R, Brensinger CM, et al. Risk of nonmelanoma skin cancer associated with the use of immunosuppressant and biologic agents in patients with a history of autoimmune disease and nonmelanoma skin cancer. JAMA Dermatol 2016;152(2):164–72.

60. Lossignol D. A little help from steroids in oncology. J Transl Int Med 2016; 4(1):52–4.

61. Lin KT, Wang LH. New dimension of glucocorticoids in cancer treatment. Steroids 2016;111:84–8.

62. Arbour KC, Mezquita L, Long N, et al. Impact of baseline steroids on efficacy of programmed cell death-1 and programmed death-ligand 1 blockade in patients with non-small-cell lung cancer. J Clin Oncol 2018;36(28):2872–8.

63. Franco AS, luamoto LR, Pereira RMR. Perioperative management of drugs commonly used in patients with rheumatic diseases: a review. Clinics 2017; 72(6):386–90.
64. Stuck AE, Minder CE, Frey FJ. Risk of infectious complications in patients taking glucocorticosteroids. Rev Infect Dis 1989;11(6):954–63.
65. Wang AS, Armstrong EJ, Armstrong AW. Corticosteroids and wound healing: clinical considerations in the perioperative period. Am J Surg 2013;206(3):410–7.
66. Nicholson G, Burrin J, Hall G. Peri-operative steroid supplementation. Anaesthesia 1998;53(11):1091–104.
67. Cordtz R, Odgaard A, Kristensen LE, et al. Risk of medical complications following total hip or knee arthroplasty in patients with rheumatoid arthritis: a register-based cohort study from Denmark. Semin Arthritis Rheum 2020; 50(1):30–5.
68. George MD, Baker JF, Winthrop K, et al. Risk of biologics and glucocorticoids in patients with rheumatoid arthritis undergoing arthroplasty: a cohort study. Ann Intern Med 2019;170(12):825–36.
69. Escalante A, Beardmore TD. Risk factors for early wound complications after orthopedic surgery for rheumatoid arthritis. J Rheumatol 1995;22(10):1844–51.
70. Bibbo C, Goldberg JW. Infectious and healing complications after elective orthopaedic foot and ankle surgery during tumor necrosis factor-alpha inhibition therapy. Foot Ankle Int 2004;25(5):331–5.
71. Grennan DM, Gray J, Loudon J, et al. Methotrexate and early postoperative complications in patients with rheumatoid arthritis undergoing elective orthopaedic surgery. Ann Rheum Dis 2001;60(3):214–7.
72. Perhala RS, Wilke WS, Clough JD, et al. Local infectious complications following large joint replacement in rheumatoid arthritis patients treated with methotrexate versus those not treated with methotrexate. Arthritis Rheum 1991;34(2):146–52.
73. Tanaka N, Sakahashi H, Sato E, et al. Examination of the risk of continuous leflunomide treatment on the incidence of infectious complications after joint arthroplasty in patients with rheumatoid arthritis. J Clin Rheumatol 2003;9(2):115–8.
74. Goodman SM, Springer B, Guyatt G, et al. 2017 American College of Rheumatology/American Association of Hip and Knee Surgeons guideline for the perioperative management of antirheumatic medication in patients with rheumatic diseases undergoing elective total hip or total knee arthroplasty. Arthritis Rheumatol 2017;69(8):1538–51.
75. Morel J, Locci M, Banal F, et al. Safety of surgery in patients with rheumatoid arthritis treated with tocilizumab: data from the French (REGistry -RoAcTEmra) Regate registry. Clin Exp Rheumatol 2020;38(3):405–10.
76. Latourte A, Gottenberg JE, Luxembourger C, et al. Safety of surgery in patients with rheumatoid arthritis treated by abatacept: data from the French Orencia in Rheumatoid Arthritis Registry. Rheumatology (Oxford) 2017;56(4):629–37.
77. Wo J, Taghian A. Radiotherapy in setting of collagen vascular disease. Int J Radiat Oncol Biol Phys 2007;69(5):1347–53.
78. Giaj-Levra N, Sciascia S, Fiorentino A, et al. Radiotherapy in patients with connective tissue diseases. Lancet Oncol 2016;17(3):e109–17.
79. Morris MM, Powell SN. Irradiation in the setting of collagen vascular disease: acute and late complications. J Clin Oncol 1997;15(7):2728–35.
80. Dong Y, Li T, Churilla TM, et al. Impact of rheumatoid arthritis on radiation-related toxicity and cosmesis in breast cancer patients: a contemporary matched-pair analysis. Breast Cancer Res Treat 2017;166(3):787–91.

81. Bliss P, Parsons C, Blake P. Incidence and possible aetiological factors in the development of pelvic insufficiency fractures following radical radiotherapy. Br J Radiol 1996;69(822):548–54.

82. Robertson JM, Clarke DH, Matter RC, et al. Breast conservation therapy. Severe breast fibrosis after radiation therapy in patients with collagen vascular disease. Cancer 1991;68(3):502–8.

83. Pundole X, Abdel-Wahab N, Suarez-Almazor ME. Arthritis risk with immune checkpoint inhibitor therapy for cancer. Curr Opin Rheumatol 2019;31(3):293–9.

84. Suarez-Almazor ME, Kim ST, Abdel-Wahab N, et al. Review: immune-related adverse events with use of checkpoint inhibitors for immunotherapy of cancer. Arthritis Rheumatol 2017;69(4):687–99.

85. Belkhir R, Burel SL, Dunogeant L, et al. Rheumatoid arthritis and polymyalgia rheumatica occurring after immune checkpoint inhibitor treatment. Ann Rheum Dis 2017;76(10):1747–50.

86. Kostine M, Rouxel L, Barnetche T, et al. Rheumatic disorders associated with immune checkpoint inhibitors in patients with cancer-clinical aspects and relationship with tumour response: a single-centre prospective cohort study. Ann Rheum Dis 2018;77(3):393–8.

87. Cappelli LC, Gutierrez AK, Baer AN, et al. Inflammatory arthritis and sicca syndrome induced by nivolumab and ipilimumab. Ann Rheum Dis 2017;76(1):43–50.

88. Lidar M, Giat E, Garelick D, et al. Rheumatic manifestations among cancer patients treated with immune checkpoint inhibitors. Autoimmun Rev 2018;17(3):284–9.

89. Smith MH, Bass AR. Arthritis after cancer immunotherapy: symptom duration and treatment response. Arthritis Care Res 2019;71(3):362–6.

90. Cappelli LC, Brahmer JR, Forde PM, et al. Clinical presentation of immune checkpoint inhibitor-induced inflammatory arthritis differs by immunotherapy regimen. Semin Arthritis Rheum 2018;48(3):553–7.

91. Verheijden RJ, May AM, Blank CU, et al. Association of anti-TNF with decreased survival in steroid refractory ipilimumab and anti-PD1 treated patients in the Dutch Melanoma Treatment Registry. Clin Cancer Res 2020;26(9):2268–74.

92. Puri A, Homsi J. The safety of pembrolizumab in metastatic melanoma and rheumatoid arthritis. Melanoma Res 2017;27(5):519–23.

93. Danlos FX, Voisin AL, Dyevre V, et al. Safety and efficacy of anti-programmed death 1 antibodies in patients with cancer and pre-existing autoimmune or inflammatory disease. Eur J Cancer 2018;91:21–9.

94. Kahler KC, Eigentler TK, Gesierich A, et al. Ipilimumab in metastatic melanoma patients with pre-existing autoimmune disorders. Cancer Immunol Immunother 2018;67(5):825–34.

95. Leonardi GC, Gainor JF, Altan M, et al. Safety of programmed death-1 pathway inhibitors among patients with non-small-cell lung cancer and preexisting autoimmune disorders. J Clin Oncol 2018;36(19):1905–12.

96. Richter MD, Pinkston O, Kottschade LA, et al. Brief report: cancer immunotherapy in patients with preexisting rheumatic disease: the Mayo Clinic experience. Arthritis Rheumatol 2018;70(3):356–60.

97. Abdel-Wahab N, Shah M, Lopez-Olivo MA, et al. Use of immune checkpoint inhibitors in the treatment of patients with cancer and preexisting autoimmune disease: a systematic review. Ann Intern Med 2018;168(2):121–30.

98. Siegel RL, Miller KD, Jemal A. Cancer statistics, 2019. CA Cancer J Clin 2019;69(1):7–34.

Risk of Malignancy in Spondyloarthritis
A Systematic Review

Paras Karmacharya, MBBS[a], Ravi Shahukhal, MD[b],
Alexis Ogdie, MD, MSCE[c],*

KEYWORDS

- Spondyloarthritis • Psoriatic arthritis • Ankylosing spondylitis • Malignancy • Cancer
- Tumor necrosis factor inhibitors

KEY POINTS

- There is conflicting evidence on the association between spondyloarthritis (SpA) and malignancies overall.
- There seems to be a higher incidence of nonmelanoma skin cancer in psoriatic arthritis (PsA) and both monoclonal gammopathy of unknown significance and multiple myeloma in ankylosing spondylitis (AS).
- A few studies have reported a higher incidence of lymphoma in both PsA and AS but the results were inconsistent.
- It is unclear if traditional immunosuppressive agents, tumor necrosis factor inhibitors, or nonsteroidal anti-inflammatory drugs modulate the risk of cancer in SpA. However, if there is an increased risk, it seems to be quite small.
- Although no specific screening recommendations for malignancy in SpA are available at present, it would be prudent to perform age-appropriate screening in all patients at minimum with a consideration for annual skin checks in patients with moderate-to-severe psoriasis.

INTRODUCTION

Spondyloarthritis (SpA) includes a group of chronic inflammatory diseases, such as ankylosing spondylitis (AS, or axial spondyloarthritis, AxSpA), psoriatic arthritis

[a] Division of Rheumatology, Department of Medicine, Mayo Clinic, Mayo Clinic College of Medicine, 200 First Street Southwest, Rochester, MN 55905, USA; [b] Division of Internal Medicine, Lakes Regional General Hospital, 80 Highland Street, Laconia, NH 03246, USA; [c] Division of Rheumatology, Hospital of the University of Pennsylvania, Perelman Center for Advanced Medicine, 3400 Civic Center Boulevard, South Pavilion, 1st Floor, Philadelphia, PA 19104, USA
* Corresponding author.
E-mail address: alogdie@pennmedicine.upenn.edu
Twitter: @paraskarmachary (P.K.)

Rheum Dis Clin N Am 46 (2020) 463–511
https://doi.org/10.1016/j.rdc.2020.04.001
0889-857X/20/© 2020 Elsevier Inc. All rights reserved.

rheumatic.theclinics.com

(PsA), inflammatory bowel disease–associated arthritis, and reactive arthritis. These diseases share a common tissue distribution and affect the axial and/or peripheral joints as well as entheses. In addition to the musculoskeletal involvement, they may have extra-articular manifestations, such as psoriasis, uveitis, and inflammatory bowel disease. Beyond extra-articular manifestation, these diseases also may be associated with other medical comorbidities, potentially including malignancies.

Systematic inflammatory diseases, including rheumatoid arthritis (RA), are associated with an increased risk of malignancies.[1] Chronic inflammation with high levels of elevated chemokines, cytokines (serum interleukin-1, 6, and tumor necrosis factor [TNF]-α) and growth factors can lead to DNA damage, chromosomal instability, and epigenetic alterations favoring malignant transformation in affected cells.[2,3] RA in particular is associated with an overall increased risk of malignancies, specifically lymphomas (standardized incidence ratios [SIR] up to 13 compared with the general population).[1] Similarly, the immunosuppressive agents used to treat inflammatory diseases have also been implicated in increasing the risk for cancer, although the degree of risk and difference among therapies remains unclear.

Malignancy, either related to an inflammatory disease or its treatments, is most often studied in the setting of RA; however, the pathogenesis of SpA is different from RA,[4] and the risk of malignancy and sites involved also may be different. It is important to better understand associations of SpA with site-specific cancers to facilitate proper screening. The goal of this review was to examine the association of the 2 most common types of SpA, PsA and AxSpA, with malignancy and the potential impact of therapy for SpA on development of malignancy.

METHODS

A comprehensive search of several databases from inception to January 11, 2020, was conducted. The databases included MEDLINE, EMBASE, Cochrane Central Register of Controlled Trials, and Scopus. ACR and EULAR abstracts published in the past 2 years were included as well. Search strategy included terms under 2 broad themes: (1) SpA (ie, spondylarthritis, spondyloarthritis, psoriatic arthritis, AS, spondylitis), and (2) malignancy (ie, cancer, neoplasms, malignancy). Studies reporting the relative association of malignancy with SpA or the prevalence/incidence of malignancy were included. Case reports, case series, nonhuman studies, and articles in language other than English were excluded. Two authors (PK and RS) screened abstracts for eligibility, retrieved full-texts, and excluded irrelevant articles. Disagreements were resolved by discussion about eligibility. Bibliographies belonging to included studies, reviews, and relevant articles were screened for additional studies. Relevant data were extracted by PK, and checked by RS.

RISK FOR MALIGNANCY IN PSORIATIC ARTHRITIS

Data on the risk of malignancy in PsA are conflicting, with most studies showing no significant association (**Table 1**). A recent systematic review and meta-analysis by Luo and colleagues[5] found a significantly higher risk of overall malignancy compared with the general population (relative risk [RR] 1.29; 95% confidence interval [CI] 1.04–1.60). However, none of the individual studies included in the meta-analysis, except Lange and colleagues,[6] showed a significantly higher overall risk of cancer. Although all included studies used cohort designs, there was significant heterogeneity ($I^2 = 71\%$) among them. This heterogeneity may have been in part related to the differing PsA populations (eg, different therapy exposures) and varied follow-up periods (3–15 years). Interestingly, in the subgroup analysis, only patients with

Table 1
Summary of studies examining the risk of malignancy among patients with spondyloarthritis (SpA)

Author, Year	Study Design	Study Period	No. of SpA Pts	SpA Definition	Relevant Study Questions	Comparison Group	Therapies	Follow-up Period, y	Types of Malignancies Reported	Estimate of Risk, Measure of Effect (95% CI)
SpA										
Bautista-Molano et al,[61] 2018	Cross-sectional, ASAS-COMOSPA study (from 3 Latin American countries-Argentina, Mexico, and Colombia)	NA (Cross-sectional study)	390	Pts ≥18 y fulfilling ASAS criteria (either axial or peripheral)	Overall prevalence of malignancy in SpA	GP	NSAIDs MTX SSZ TNFi	NA	Colon cancer, skin (melanoma and basocellular carcinoma), lymphoma (HL and NHL), breast, cervix, and prostate.	Prevalence of malignancies: Overall- 2.8% (95% CI 1.4–5.1) GP- 2.6% (NR) SRR for malignancies- 1.0
Fanto et al,[62] 2016	Retrospective, cohort study, single center (S. Andrea-Sapienza University, Rome, Italy)	2005–2011	197	SpA- AS or PsA- PsA- pts fulfilling Moll and Wright criteria AS pts fulfilling mNY criteria Previous history of malignancy excluded	Risk of malignancy in RA and SpA patients under immunosuppressive therapy	GP of Italy matched for age, sex, and area of residence	TNFi + DMARDs or DMARDs alone	Median - 5.03 (IQ range 3.7–6.9)	All cancers- solid cancers, hematologic malignancy and NHL	SIR of malignancy in SpA vs GP: Overall malignancy- 0.88 (0.29–2.05) Solid tumors SIR- 0.69 (0.19–1.77) Hematologic SIR 2.04 (0.05–11.37) NHL SIR- 4.35 (0.11–24.23) Age and sex adjusted HR for medications only calculated for RA

(continued on next page)

Table 1
(continued)

Author, Year	Study Design	Study Period	No. of SpA Pts	SpA Definition	Relevant Study Questions	Comparison Group	Therapies	Follow-up Period, y	Types of Malignancies Reported	Estimate of Risk, Measure of Effect (95% CI)
Hellgren et al,[15] 2017	Population-based, nationwide cohort study- ARTIS and DANBIO biologics registers, linked with the nationwide Swedish and Danish Cancer Registers	2001–2011	TNFi-17406 TNFi naïve-28,164	AS ICD-10 code (M45) PsA ICD-10 code (L40.5)	Cancer risk in SpA treated with TNFi compared with biologic naïve and GP	Swedish age-matched and sex-matched GP comparator cohort (n = 131,687)	TNFi treated TNFi naïve	Up to 10 y	Cancer overall Prostate Lung Colorectal Malignant lymphoma Breast Melanoma	TNFi naïve SpA vs GP (RR): 1.1 (1.0–1.2) 1.2 (1.1–1.4) 1.0 (0.7–1.2) 0.7 (0.5–0.8) 1.0 (0.7–1.3) 1.0 (0.8–1.2) 1.0 (0.7–1.3)

Study	Design	Year	N	Inclusion	Objective	Comparator	Exposure		Cancers	Results
Jiang et al,[47] 2018	Cross-sectional, single-center study from Third Affiliated Hospital of Sun Yat-sen University	2013–2015	346	Pts ≥18 y fulfilling ASAS criteria for SpA were recruited from the Third Affiliated Hospital of Sun Yat-sen University.	Prevalence of comorbidities and evaluation of screening in Chinese pts with SpA	None	NSAID use DMARDs use (ever): -MTX -SSZ -Biologic therapy	NA	Prostate cancer Breast cancer	160/280 (57.1%) male pts had screening for prostate cancer with PSA, while breast cancer was optimally screened in 21/66 (31.8%) female patients. 1/160 (0.6%) was confirmed with prostate cancer. None of the female pts ever did a cervical smear. 10 pts underwent colonoscopy or digital rectal examination. Only 4 pts once went to see a dermatologist in a recent year.
Molto et al,[46] 2016	ASAS-COMOSPA study Cross-sectional, multicentric and international study (from 22 countries from 4 continents- Africa, America, Asia, Europe)	NA	3984	Patients ≥18 y fulfilling ASAS criteria (either axial or peripheral)	Prevalence of malignancies in SpA	None	NSAID DMARDs (methotrexate, sulfasalazine, biologic therapies)	NA	Colon cancer Skin(melanoma and basocellular carcinoma) Breast and cervix Prostate for men Lymphoma	Prevalence of malignancies: Overall- 3.0% (2.46-3.52) Cervical cancer- 1.2% (0.3-1.7) Basocellular cancer- 0.8% (0.6-1.2) Melanoma- 0.7% (0.4-1.0) Most prevalent risk factors for cancer- family history of breast (15%) and colon cancer (8%)

(continued on next page)

Table 1
(continued)

Author, Year	Study Design	Study Period	No. of SpA Pts	SpA Definition	Relevant Study Questions	Comparison Group	Therapies	Follow-up Period, y	Types of Malignancies Reported	Estimate of Risk, Measure of Effect (95% CI)
PsA										
Eder et al,[24] 2012	Cross-sectional, single center (University of Toronto PsA clinic)	2008–2011	361	Pts fulfilling CASPAR criteria	Prevalence of monoclonal gammopathy in PsA	Case-MGUS, n = 35, control-no MGUS = 326	NR	NA	MGUS MM	35/361 (9.7%) had monoclonal gammopathy in at least 2 separate samples. 7/29 (24%) who were tested for Bence Jones protein tested positive. 1 patient diagnosed as MM. Longer disease duration (OR-1.04; 95% CI 1.01–1.07) and high ESR (OR-1.03; 95% CI 1.01–1.04) were associated with MGUS.
Edson-Heredia et al,[11] 2015	Retrospective study from CPRD	2006–2010	1952	Psoriasis (without PsA) and PsA as diagnosed by general practitioner or specialist	Incidence rates of malignancies in psoriasis and PsA	Cohort of pts with psoriasis (n = 27,672; mild, n = 22,174, severe, n = 5498)	NSAIDs (45.1%), Systemic therapies (mainly MTX and SSZ), and opiate and nonopiate analgesics	Mean = 3.0 (SD - 1.3)	Skin cancer (melanoma and NMSC)	HR (All psoriasis vs PsA): 0.33 (0.05–2.43) 1.14 (0.41–3.16) HR (PsA vs severe psoriasis)[a]: Melanoma - 0.12 (0.02–0.90) NMSC - 0.4 (0.14–1.16) HR adjusted for age, gender, smoking, and index year.

Study	Study type	Dates	N	Diagnosis	Objective	Comparator	Treatment	Person-years	Outcomes	Results
Gross et al,[7] 2014	Multicentered, longitudinal, prospective registry (CORRONA)	Aug 2003-Oct 2010	2970	Rheumatologist's diagnosis (at least 2 study visits during the time period)	Compare the incidence rates of malignancy among PsA and RA pts in CORRONA registry	RA pts in CORRONA (n = 19,260)	MTX Non-MTX DMARD TNFi Other biologics	PsA-7133 PY, RA-53864 PY	All malignancies NMSC All malignancies • NMSC • Non-NMSC (solid + hematologic) Solid • Breast • Prostate • Colorectal • Melanoma Hematologic • Lymphoma • MM • Leukemia	IR of cancer in PsA (per 100 PY): 0.56 (0.40-0.76) 0.21 (0.12-0.35) IRR of cancer in PsA vs RA: 1.18 (0.82-1.69) 1.05 (0.61-1.80) 0.97 (0.61-1.42) 0.90 (0.57-1.45) 1.54 (0.67-3.23) 0.56 (0.16-1.86) 1.33 (0.47-5.70) 1.33 (0.44-5.28) 1.17 (0.36-2.89) 1.00 (0.17-3.11) 7.78 (0.48-122.23) 1.00 (0.12-7.64)
Hagberg et al,[14] 2016	Retrospective cohort study from CPRD, UK	1988-2012.	8943	PsA as diagnosed by general practitioner or specialist	Incidence rate of cancers in patients with PsA vs without PsA	Pts without PsA (n = 82,601)	Systemic therapies DMARDs/biologics (eg, MTX, SSZ, and ADA), immunosuppressants (eg, AZT and leflunomide), and corticosteroids	Solid cancer-3139 PY, Hematological cancer-261 PY, NMSC-1561 PY	Solid, hematologic, and NMSC	IRR of malignancy in PsA vs no PsA: Solid cancer- 1.01 (0.90-1.13) Hematologic cancer- 1.52 (1.10-2.10) NMSC- 0.97 (0.82-1.14)

(continued on next page)

Table 1
(continued)

Author, Year	Study Design	Study Period	No. of SpA Pts	SpA Definition	Relevant Study Questions	Comparison Group	Therapies	Follow-up Period, y	Types of Malignancies Reported	Estimate of Risk, Measure of Effect (95% CI)
Hellgren et al,[22] 2014	Population-based, prospective cohort study from Swedish National Patient Register	2001–2010	19,283	ICD codes for AS, PsA	Risk of malignant lymphoma in AS, PsA	Randomly selected from Swedish Population Register (matched for age, sex, and county of residence)	TNFi MTX/ SSZ Oral GC	10,912 PY	Malignant lymphoma	HR of lymphoma in PsA vs GP: Overall- 1.2 (0.9–1.7)
Hellgren et al,[15] 2017	Population-based, nation-wide cohort study-ARTIS and DANBIO biologics registers, linked with the nation-wide Swedish and Danish Cancer Registers	2001–2011	TNFi-3833 TNFi naïve-15,908	ICD-10 code for PsA (L40.5)	Cancer risk in SpA treated with TNFi	Swedish age-matched and sex-matched GP comparator cohort (n = 74,010)	TNFi treated TNFi naïve	Up to 10 y	Cancer overall Prostate Lung Colorectal Malignant lymphoma Breast Melanoma	TNFi naïve PsA vs GP (RR): 1.0 (0.9–1.1) 1.1 (0.9–1.3) 1.0 (0.7–1.3) 0.8 (0.6–1.1) 1.0 (0.6–1.4) 0.9 (0.8–1.1) 0.9 (0.6–1.3)

							All pts ≥ 1 y follow-up	All cancers	
Kaine et al,[57] 2019	Retrospective, observational, cohort study using MarketScan Databases and Medicare Supplemental databases	Jan 2008–Sep 2015	14,898	≥1 inpatient or ≥2 outpatient diagnosis of PsA (ICD-9-CM 696.0) >30 d apart but within ≤365 d of each other	Incidence rates of comorbidities in pts with PsA compared with GP	Pts without AS (matched on age, geographic region, calendar year, and sex, n = 35,037)	NR	All pts ≥ 1 y follow-up	All cancers	IRR of malignancy in PsA vs GP: 1.09 (1.01–1.17)
Rohekar et al,[50] 2008	Prospective cohort study from University of Toronto Psoriatic Arthritis Clinic	1978–2004	665	Rheumatologist's diagnosis	Prevalence of malignancy in PsA	GP (Ontario)	NSAIDs DMARDs Immunosuppressants	NR	All cancers	SIR for malignancy PsA vs GP: All cancers - 0.98 (0.77–1.24) Hematologic - 0.69 (0.26–1.83) Lung- 0.88 (0.46–1.69) Breast-1.55 (0.92–2.62) Prostate —0.65 (0.29–1.44) ESR, cm/h was the only significant predictor of malignancy in Cox regression, HR-1.13 (1.02–1.25), TNFi and DMARDs were not.
Tan,[25] 2018 (abstract)	Population-based matched retrospective cohort	1997–2012	81,568 incident cases of PsO/PsA	Incident psoriasis/PsA defined as ≥ one of the	Risk of cancer in patients with psoriasis/PsA	Matched on age, sex, and calendar year	NR	623,843.5 PY 623,625.8 PY 623,818.6 PY 621,233.8 PY	Eye and orbit Female genitals other than cervix, uteri, corpus uteri, and ovary Other urinary	IRR of cancer in psoriasis/PsA vs matched controls: 4.25 (1.21–14.91) 2.57 (1.55–4.25) 1.90 (1.04–3.47) 1.82 (1.54–2.14)

(continued on next page)

Table 1
(continued)

Author, Year	Study Design	Study Period	No. of SpA Pts	SpA Definition	Relevant Study Questions	Comparison Group	Therapies	Follow-up Period, y	Types of Malignancies Reported	Estimate of Risk, Measure of Effect (95% CI)
	study from administrative health data (British Columbia, Canada)			following: 1 diagnostic code for psoriasis/ PsA by a rheumatologist/ dermatologist; ≥ 2 diagnostic codes for PsO/ PsA, ≥ 2 mo apart in a 2-year period by a nonrheumatologist/ dermatologist; or ≥1 hospitalization with diagnostic code for psoriasis/ PsA.		from the database.		PY 622,877.2 PY 620,065.8 PY 622,791 PY 622,845.1 PY 623,196.9 PY	NMSC Lung Prostate Melanoma Colon Rectum	1.17 (1.05–1.31) 1.12 (1.01–1.25) 1.07 (NR) 0.84 (0.72–0.99) 0.79 (0.64–0.98)
Wilton et al,[12] 2016	Retrospective. popu-	1970–2008	217	PsA meeting CASPAR	Cumulative incidence of	Age and sex-	NR	38	Any malignancy (including NMSC) Any malignancy	HR for incidence of malignancy in PsA vs those without PsA.

Author	Design	Years	N	Definition	Objective	Comparison	Follow-up	Cancer site	Result
	based (Olmsted County) cohort study				in PsA	patients from Olmsted County (n = 434)		Solid tumors	1.41 (0.96–2.07)
								Hematologic	**1.64 (1.03–2.61)**
								NMSC	1.48 (0.89–2.48)
								Breast (female only)	2.48 (0.75–8.13)
								Prostate	1.23 (0.72–2.09)
									3.59 (1.22–10.61)
									1.83 (0.75–4.46)

AxSpA

Author	Design	Years	N	Definition	Objective	Comparison	Follow-up	Cancer site	Result
Alehashemi,[36] 2018 (abstract)	Retrospective, cohort study (Medicare databases)	1999–2013	13,305	2 identical AS ICD-9 codes at least 30 d apart	Cancer risk in AS compared with those without AS in the US Medicare beneficiaries	Medicare without AS, matched on age and sex (n = 6,749,053)	NR Followed until 2015 (130841 PY)	Kidney	SIR in AS vs no AS in Medicare beneficiaries (statistical significant only): 1.57 (1.34–1.80)
								Melanoma	1.49 (1.27–1.71)
								Thyroid	1.43 (1.02–1.85)
								Leukemia	1.44 (1.24–1.65)
								NHL	1.36 (1.19–1.53)
								MM	1.32 (1.01–1.64)
								Prostate	1.34 (1.25–1.42)
								Esophagus	**0.58 (0.36–0.81)**
								Stomach	**0.55 (0.32–0.79)**
								Colorectal	**0.81 (0.71–0.91)**
								Lung	**0.72 (0.64–0.81)**
									SIR of cancer of upper airways, small intestine, liver/gallbladder, pancreas, female breast, uterus, bladder, connective tissue/bone, brain/eye/nervous system, HL were not statistically significant.
Anderson et al,[37] 2009	Population-based, case-control study using SEER	Lymphoid malignancies diagnosed between	44,350 lymphoid malignancy cases	ICD codes (hospital, physician, and outpatient Medicare claims)	Risk of specific lymphoid malignancies in autoimmune conditions	Medicare beneficiaries (matched on calendar year of dx,	NR NA	NHL	OR for prevalence of AS in pts with lymphoid malignancies vs controls:
								Diffuse large B cell lymphoma	1.1 (0.7–1.5)
								T-cell NHL	0.9 (0.5–1.7)
								Marginal zone lymphoma	0.9 (0.2–3.4)
								Follicular lymphoma	2.2 (0.9–5.4)

(continued on next page)

Table 1
(continued)

Author, Year	Study Design	Study Period	No. of SpA Pts	SpA Definition	Relevant Study Questions	Comparison Group	Therapies	Follow-up Period, y	Types of Malignancies Reported	Estimate of Risk, Measure of Effect (95% CI)
	database (SMAHRT study)	1993–2002,			Outcome: Malignancy Exposure: AS	age category and sex, n = 122,531			Chronic lymphocytic leukemia	0.80 (0.3–2.3) 1.1 (0.6–2.0)
Askling et al,[63] 2006	Nation-wide, popu-lation-based case-control study from the Swedish Inpatient Register	1964–2000	50,615 cases of lymp-homa	ICD codes	Association between AS and malignant lymphomas Outcome: Malignancy Exposure: AS	GP (92,928 matched controls)	NR	NA	Malignant lymphomas -NHL -HL -Chronic lymphocytic leukemia	OR of AS in malignant lymphoma vs controls: 1.0 (0.6–1.7) 0.8 (0.4–1.5) 1.7 (0.2–12) 1.9 (0.6–5.9)
Becker et al,[38] 2005	Popu-lation-based, case-control study from Germany	1999–2002	710	Self-report of physician-diagnosed AS	Association between history of AS and lymphoma Outcome: Malignancy Exposure: AS	GP (matched on age, sex and study region, n = 710)	NR	NA	All lymphomas	OR of AS in pts with lymphoma vs controls: 0.79 (0.59–1.05)
Brown et al,[32] 2008	Retros-pective cohort study	from July 1, 1969,	4641 (MM) and	ICD codes	Risk of MM, MGUS among	Men without AS	None	1 y after the date	MM MGUS	RR of malignancy among men with AS vs no AS: Overall- 2.29 (1.55–3.40)

Study	Design	Period	N	Population	Objective	Comparator	Drug	Follow-up	Outcomes	Results
	from US VA hospitals	to September 30, 1996,	2046 (MGUS)	US male veterans with prior AS				or the first hospital discharge to the end of observation period		Whites- 1.82 (1.12–2.98) Blacks- 4.23 (2.20–8.16) Overall- 2.02 (1.14–3.56)
Burmester et al,[13] 2013	Pooled data from clinical trials (Europe, North America, South America, Asia, Australia, New Zealand, and South Africa)	Through Nov 2010	1684	SpA definition per clinical trial.	Risk of malignancy from global clinical trials of ADA in immune-mediated inflammatory diseases	GP	ADA (clinical trials)	Nearly 12 y of ADA exposure	All malignancies Lymphoma NMSC	SIR of malignancy in AS vs GP: 0.51(0.16–1.19) 1.93(0.03–10.7) 0.08(0.29–1.74)
Carmona et al,[20] 2011	Prospective cohort study- BIOBADASER 2.0 (ongoing cohort of patients with rheumatic diseases exposed to TNFi)	BIOBADASER (2001–2008)	761	Rheumatologist diagnosed rheumatic diseases starting treatment or were on a biologic response modifier	Cancer risk in RA, PsA, and AS patients exposed to TNFi	GP of Spain (source: GLOBOCON, WHO program 2002)	TNFi (IFX, ETN, ADA)	2288 PY	Colon and rectum Lung Prostate Bladder NHL Leukemia All sites but skin	SIR of cancer in AS pts exposed to TNFi: 2.38 (0.49–6.96) 1.66 (0.34–4.85) 1.10 (0.03–6.13) 0.96 (0.02–5.37) 2.72 (2.07–15.13) 3.97 (0.10–22.13) 0.92 (0.44–1.70)

(continued on next page)

Table 1
(continued)

Author, Year	Study Design	Study Period	No. of SpA Pts	SpA Definition	Relevant Study Questions	Comparison Group	Therapies	Follow-up Period, y	Types of Malignancies Reported	Estimate of Risk, Measure of Effect (95% CI)
Castro et al,[64] 2014	Cohort study from nationwide data registry (Sweden)	1964–2008	402462 (total autoimmune disease, AS NR separately)	ICD codes	Risk of hepatobiliary cancer after hospitalization with autoimmune diseases	Swedish population not hospitalized for autoimmune disease	NR	Until dx of cancer, death, emigration, or end of study (2008)	Hepatobiliary tract, Primary liver, Gallbladder, Extrahepatic bile duct, Ampulla of Vater	SIR of Hepatobiliary cancer in hospitalized patients with AS vs GP: SIR 1.50(0.87–2.41) SIR 1.70(0.81–3.14)
Chang et al,[28] 2017	Retrospective, cohort study from Taiwan National Health Insurance Research Database	2000–2008	5452	ICD-9-CM code 720.0	Association between AS and cancer	Non-AS pts in the database during the study period (age, sex-matched, n = 21,808)	NR	5.07 ± 2.07 y	All cancers, Digestive tract, Colon, Lung, Breast, Female genital system, Prostate cancer, Hematological, Upper respiratory tract	SIR of cancer in AS vs non-AS: 1.15(1.03–1.27) 1.01(0.79–1.27) 1.39(1.03–1.82) 1.07(0.79–1.43) 0.98(0.64–1.42) 0.78(0.49–1.18) 1.64(1.04–2.47) 2.10(1.32–3.19) 1.30(0.92–1.79)

Study	Study type	Period	N	Method	Objective	Comparator	TNFi	Follow-up	Cancer site	Results
Dreyer et al,[30] 2013	Cohort study (DANBIO arthritis cohort)	2000-2008.	861	Rheumatologist diagnosis	Incidence of overall and site-specific malignancies in TNFi-treated pts with AS	GP	TNFi	2.9 (mean).	All cancer sites	SIR: 0.82 (0.41-1.64) 8/861 pts at f/u
Fallah et al,[40] 2014 (HL)	Nationwide cohort study (Swedish Healthcare data registry)	1964-2010	17,641	ICD codes	Incidence of HL after autoimmune disease by age at dx and histologic subtype	GP (Sweden)	NR	~10 (190014 PY)	HL	SIR for HL in AS vs non-AS pts: Overall- 1.3 (0.4-3.0) Men- 1.3 (0.4-3.4) Women- 1.1 (0.0-6.1) SIR for HL stratified by age at dx and histologic subtype were not statistically significant
Fallah, 2014 (NHL)[39]	Nationwide cohort study (Swedish Healthcare data registry)	1964-2010	17,641	ICD codes	Incidence of NHL after autoimmune disease	GP (Sweden)	NR	10.4	NHL	SIR for NHL in AS vs non-AS pts: Overall- 1.0 (0.7-1.4) Men- 0.9 (0.6-1.4) Women- 1.2 (0.6-2.2)
Feltelius et al,[29] 2003	Population-based national cohort study (Swedish inpatient registry)	1965-1995	6621	ICD codes	Cancer incidence among AS pts in Sweden	GP	NR	67,885 PY	All cancers Rectal cancer Unspecified kidney cancer Cancer of digestive organ Respiratory cancer Cancer of female genital Prostate cancer Cancer of urinary organs Hematopoietic cancer	SIR of cancer in AS vs non-AS pts: 1.05; 95% CI 0.94-1.17). 0.41(0.15-0.89) 5.90 (1.61-15.1) 0.96(0.74-1.21) 1.05(0.73-1.47) 0.94(0.47-1.68) 1.02(0.77-1.33) 1.05(0.64-1.62) 1.34(0.93-1.89)

(continued on next page)

Table 1
(continued)

Author, Year	Study Design	Study Period	No. of SpA Pts	SpA Definition	Relevant Study Questions	Comparison Group	Therapies	Follow-up Period, y	Types of Malignancies Reported	Estimate of Risk, Measure of Effect (95% CI)
Hellgren et al,[22] 2014	Population-based, prospective cohort study from Swedish National Patient Register	2001-2010	8707	ICD codes for AS, PsA	Risk of malignant lymphoma in AS, PsA	Randomly selected from Swedish Population Register (matched for age-sex and county of residence)	TNFi MTX/ SSZ Oral GC	7790 PY	Malignant lymphoma	HR of lymphoma in PsA vs GP: Overall- 0.9 (0.5–1.6)
Hellgren et al,[15] 2017	Population-based, nationwide cohort study-ARTIS and DANBIO biologics registers, linked with the nationwide Swedish and Danish Cancer Registers	2001-2011	TNFi- 3078 TNFi naïve-7023	AS ICD-10 code (M45)	Cancer risk in SpA treated with TNFi	Swedish age-matched and sex-matched GP comparator cohort (n = 32,706)	TNFi treated TNFi naïve	Up to 10 y	Cancer overall Prostate Lung Colorectal Malignant lymphoma Breast Melanoma	TNFi naïve AS vs GP (RR): 1.1 (1.0–1.3) 1.3 (1.0–1.6) 1.0 (0.6–1.6) **0.4 (0.3–0.8)** 0.9 (0.5–1.6) 1.4 (1.0–2.0) 0.8 (0.5–1.5)

Study	Design	Years	N	Method	Aim	Comparator		PY	Cancer	SIR for cancer in AS vs GP:
Hemminki et al,[65] 2012 (Gynecological cancer)	Nationwide cohort study from Swedish Hospital Discharge Registry linked to Cancer Registry	1964–2008	1798	ICD codes	Effect of autoimmune diseases on risk and survival in female cancers	GP	NR	112824 PY	Breast cancer Cervical cancer Endometrial cancer Ovarian cancer Other female genital cancer	1.04 (0.79–1.35) 1.34(0.53–2.78) 1.34 (0.53–2.78) 0.94 (0.40–1.85) 2.18 (0.41–6.44)
Hemminki et al,[42] 2012 (Digestive tract)	Nationwide cohort study from Swedish Hospital Discharge Registry linked to Cancer Registry	1964–2008	5173	ICD codes	Risk of digestive tract cancer by histology in autoimmune disease	GP	NR	92,881 PY	Upper digestive tract Esophageal adeno cancer Esophageal squamous cell Stomach adeno cancer Colon adeno cancer Rectal adeno cancer Anal squamous cell cancer Carcinoid tumor-small intestine Carcinoid tumor-colorectal	1.05 (0.57–1.77) 2.99 (0.94–7.03) 0.73(0.07–2.70) 0.92 (0.49–1.57) **0.55 (0.32–0.88)** **0.35 (0.14–0.73)** 2.01 (0.19–7.41) 0.82 (0.00–4.72) 2.35 (0.22–8.63)
Hemminki et al,[34] 2012 (MM)	Nationwide cohort study from Swedish Hospital Discharge Registry linked to Cancer Registry	1964–2008.	6646	AS patients based on ICD codes.	Effect of autoimmune diseases on incidence and survival in subsequent MM	GP	NR	112824 PY 39,322 PY 73,502 PY	Multiple myeloma MM in AS between age 0-60 MM in AS at age 60+ MM in AS between 1964–1990 MM in AS between 1991–2008	2.02 (1.15–3.28) 3.31 (1.41–6.55) 1.45 0.62–2.87 1.73 (0.33–5.12) 2.09 (1.11–3.59)

(continued on next page)

Table 1
(continued)

Author, Year	Study Design	Study Period	No. of SpA Pts	SpA Definition	Relevant Study Questions	Comparison Group	Therapies	Follow-up Period, y	Types of Malignancies Reported	Estimate of Risk, Measure of Effect (95% CI)
Hemminki et al,[66] 2015 (unknown primary)	Nationwide cohort study from Swedish Hospital Discharge Registry, linkage with Swedish census data and National Swedish cancer registry	1964–2012	17,471	AS patients based on ICD codes.	Risk of cancer of unknown primary after hospitalization for autoimmune diseases	GP	Aspirin, NSAIDs or immunosuppressive medications (not specified)	189,971 PY of follow-up	Cancer of unknown primary after hospitalized for autoimmune diseases	SIR for cancer in AS vs GP: Overall- 0.68 (0.42–1.04) Female- 1.05 (0.52–1.89) Male- **0.49 (0.23–0.90)**
									Risk based on follow-up: <1 y 1–4 y 5+year	2.45 (0.64–6.33) 0.67 (0.17–1.74) **0.55 (0.29–0.95)**
									Risk based on age at dx: <60 y 60+ years	0.72 (0.41–1.17) 0.57 (0.18–1.35)
									Risk based on histology: Adenocarcinoma squamous cell cancer melanoma Undifferentiated	0.63 (0.30–1.16) 1.5 (0.28–4.44) 1.09 (0.9–3.99) 0.37 (0.03–1.36)
									Risk based on location: Respiratory system Liver Abdomen Unspecified	0.59 (0.15–1.53) 0.19 (0–1.06) 0.93 (0.24–2.39) 0.72 (0.29–1.5)

Study	Design	Years	N	Diagnosis/ICD	Objective	Controls/Population		Until	Malignancy	Results
Lee,[35] 2019 (abstract)	Nationwide population-based, cohort study from National Health Information Database in Korea	2010–2015	15,979	ICD-10-CM (M45.0)	Cancer risk in patients with AS	age- and sex-matched population without AS (1:3, n = 47,937)	NR	Until 2017	Lymphoma Leukemia MM	HR for AS vs non-AS patients: 3.05 (1.45–6.45) 2.32 (0.91–5.91) 2.83 (1.16–6.90). Risk of solid cancers was not statistically different between the 2 groups.
Lindqvist et al,[33] 2011	Population-based, case-control study from Sweden	1965–2004	19,112 (MM), 5403 (MGUS)	AS diagnosis based on ICD codes Hematological malignancy diagnosed by clinicians/pathologists and recorded in nationwide Swedish Cancer Register since 1958 (diagnostic accuracy 93%)	Risk of plasma cell disorder with personal and family history of immune-related conditions	96,617 matched control subjects, and 262931 first-degree relatives.	NR		MM MGUS	OR of MM and MGUS in AS patients: 1.2 (0.6–2.3) 2.7 (1.4–5.2) OR of MGUS with >5 y' latency in AS patient: 2.8 (1.3–5.9)

(continued on next page)

Table 1
(continued)

Author, Year	Study Design	Study Period	No. of SpA Pts	SpA Definition	Relevant Study Questions	Comparison Group	Therapies	Follow-up Period, y	Types of Malignancies Reported	Estimate of Risk, Measure of Effect (95% CI)
Liu et al,[67] 2013	Population-based, cohort study from national Swedish database	1964-2008	6646	AS patients based on ICD codes.	Risk of subsequent cancer in autoimmune diseases	Pts not hospitalized for autoimmune disease from Swedish discharge registry (expected number)	NR	112824 PY	Prostate Kidney Bladder	SIR and HR for subsequent urologic cancer in individuals hospitalized for autoimmune disease: SIR 1.09 (0.92–1.29) HR 0.96 (0.68–1.36) Before 1990: SIR 1.55 (0.97–2.35) 1991–2008: SIR 1.01 (0.66–1.47) SIR 1.51 (0.98–2.24) HR 0.30 (0.11–0.81) SIR 0.90 (0.61–1.28) HR 0.33 (0.08–1.31)
Melle-mkjaer et al,[41] 2008	A population-based case-control study from the Swedish Family-Cancer Database	1964-1998	Cases: 24,728 NHL pts in Denmark (1977-1997) and Sweden (1964-1998)	AS cases identified based on ICD codes (8 and 10) in discharge diagnosis	Risk of NHL associated with a personal or family history of autoimmune diseases	Randomly selected (1:2) from Family-Cancer Database (n = 55,632)	None	NA	NHL	OR of NHL with personal history of autoimmune disease >1 y before lymphoma diagnosis: 0.9 (0.6–1.5) OR of NHL with family history of autoimmune disease and related conditions: 0.8 (0.5–1.1)

Study	Design	Years	N	AS definition	Aim	Comparator		Follow-up	Outcomes	Results
Walsh et al,[27] 2018	Retrospective, observational cohort study from MarketScan and Medicare databases	2912–2014	6679	≥1 inpatient or ≥2 non-rule-out outpatient medical claims for AS (ICD-9-CM 720.0) >30 d apart but within ≤365 d of each other. Non-rule-out claims were defined as those not related to a diagnostic or rule-out procedure (eg, laboratory, pathology, or radiology)	Evaluation of comorbidity burden in AS pts in US	Pts without AS (matched on age, geographic region, index calendar year, and sex, n = 19,951)	NR	At least 12 mo after index date	Malignant neoplasms (malignant solid tumors) Hematologic malignancies, Neuroendocrine tumors	HR of overall malignancy in AS vs matched controls: 1.39 (1.19–1.62) Patients <45 y: 1.76 (1.06–2.91) Patients ≥45 to <65 y: 1.46 (1.18–1.79) Patients ≥65 y: 1.26 (0.98–1.63) HR of malignancy in male vs female pts with AS: 0.76 (0.62–0.94)

Abbreviations: ADA, adalimumab; ARTIS, Anti-Rheumatic Therapy in Sweden; AS, ankylosing spondylitis; ASAS-COMOSPA, Assessment of spondyloarthritis international society of comorbidities in SpA study; AxSpA, axial spondyloarthritis; AZT, azathioprine; BIOSPAR, Leuven spondyloarthritis biologics cohort; CASPAR, ClASsification criteria for Psoriatic ARthritis; CI, confidence interval; CM, Clinical Modification; CORRONA, Consortium of Rheumatology Researchers of North America registry; CPRD, Clinical Practice Research Datalink; DANBIO, Danish Biologics Registry; DMARDs, disease-modifying antirheumatic drugs; dx, diagnosis; ESR, erythrocyte sedimentation rate; ETN, etanercept; f/u, follow-up; GC, glucocorticoids; GP, general population; HL, Hodgkin lymphoma; HR, hazard ratio; ICD, International Classification of Diseases; IFX, infliximab; IQ, interquartile; IR, incidence rate; IRR, incidence rate ratio; MGUS, monoclonal gammopathy of undetermined significance; MM, multiple myeloma; mNY, modified New York; MTX, methotrexate; NA, not applicable; NHL, non-Hodgkin lymphoma; NMSC, nonmelanoma skin cancer; NR, not reported; NSAIDs, nonsteroidal anti-inflammatory drugs; OR, odds radio; PSA, prostate-specific antigen; PsA, psoriatic arthritis; PsO, psoriasis; pts, patients; PY, person years; RA, rheumatoid arthritis; RR, relative risk; SD, standard deviation; SIR, standardized incidence ratio; SMAHRT, Surveillance Epidemiology and End Results (SEER)-Medicare Assessment of Hematopoietic Malignancy Risk Traits Study; SpA, spondyloarthritis; SRR, Standardized risk ratios; SSZ, sulfasalazine; TNFi, tumor necrosis factor inhibitor; VA, Veterans Affairs; WHO, World Health Organization.

[a] Severe psoriasis defined as presence of referral to secondary care or use of systemic medications.

Data from Refs.[7,11–15,20,22,24,25,27–30,32–42,46,47,50,57,61–67]

conventional disease-modifying antirheumatic drugs (DMARDs) were found to have increased risk for cancer (RR 1.75; 95% CI 1.40–2.18), but not patients on biological DMARDs (RR 0.96; 95% CI 1.84–3.28). The studies, however, do not consistently specify the amount of drug exposure.

Skin Cancer in Psoriatic Arthritis

Skin cancer, particularly nonmelanoma skin cancer (NMSC) is among the most commonly reported cancers in patients with PsA. Subgroup analysis of cancer types in the meta-analysis by Luo and colleagues[5] showed an increased risk of NMSC (RR 2.46; 95% CI 1.84–3/28).[5] Similar results were also seen in the Consortium of Rheumatology Researchers of North America (CORRONA) PsA cohort in which the incidence of NMSC was elevated (0.21 per 100 patient years).[7] However, it remains unclear what portion of this risk is related to the skin psoriasis rather than the PsA itself. A recent meta-analysis found higher risk of NMSC (RR 1.72; 95% CI 1.46–2.02) in psoriasis compared with patients without psoriasis.[8] Several factors may impact the risk of NMSC in psoriasis. Phototherapy, including high-dose psoralen plus ultraviolet A (PUVA) and narrowband UVB, used in patients with psoriasis has a reported association with an increased risk of NMSC and melanoma. Studies in psoriasis report up to a sevenfold increase in the risk of skin cancer in patients treated with PUVA, methotrexate, and both combined,[9] with a dose-related effect of PUVA and methotrexate on the risk of squamous cell carcinoma (but not basal cell carcinoma).[10]

Although there are studies finding an increased risk of NMSC in PsA, this was not consistent across studies; several studies found no increased risk.[7,11–14] One long-term safety study of adalimumab found an increased risk of NMSC in psoriasis (SIR 1.76; 95% CI 1.26–2.39), but did not find a significant association in PsA (SIR 1.25; 95% CI 0.46–2.72).[13]

The risk of other skin cancers, such as melanoma, does not seem to be increased in PsA.[7,15,16] Edson-Heredia and colleagues[11] found significantly lower incidence of melanoma in PsA as compared with severe psoriasis (hazard ratio [HR] 0.12; 95% CI 0.02–0.90), but no statistically significant difference was seen between PsA and psoriasis as a whole for melanoma and NMSC. In a meta-analysis of malignancy risk in psoriasis, the risk of squamous cell carcinoma (SCC) was also significantly higher than those without psoriasis (RR 2.15; 95% CI 1.32–3.50), and the risk was much higher in the severe psoriasis subgroup (RR 11.74; 95% CI 1.52–90.66).[17] Similarly, the risk of basal cell carcinoma (BCC) was increased only in the severe psoriasis subgroup (RR 3.17; 95% CI 1.32–7.60) and not psoriasis as a whole (RR 1.29; 95% CI 0.73–2.26), suggesting this risk is tied to severity of skin disease. However, we did not find studies specifically addressing the risk of SCC or BCC in PsA (only reported as NMSC group); it is unclear if the risk is different in these 2 subgroups.

Hematologic Malignancies

Lymphoma is among the most worrisome cancers for rheumatologists, particularly given the perceived relationship with therapy and the known association with RA.[18,19] Unlike RA, most studies in PsA have not found an increased risk of lymphoma.[7,13,15,20–23] Only 2 studies found an increased risk of overall hematologic malignancies in patients with PsA. Data from Clinical Practice Research Datalink (CPRD), a general practice database in the United Kingdom, found an increased risk of hematologic malignancies in PsA compared with those without PsA (incidence rate ratio 1.52; 95% CI 1.10–2.10),[14] and a large, prospective cohort study from 4 Nordic countries (Sweden, Denmark, Iceland, and Finland) showed higher risk of lymphoma in patients with PsA on tumor necrosis factor inhibitors (TNFi) compared with the general population (SIR 1.84; 95% CI 1.20–2.82).[16] A higher prevalence of monoclonal gamm-opathy of unknown significance (MGUS) (9.7%, 35/361) was seen in a cross-sectional study from University of Toronto.[24] Only 1 of these patients was diagnosed as multiple myeloma. Another multicentric, longitudinal, prospective (CORRONA) study found no definite evidence of an increased risk of multiple myeloma in PsA (IRR 7.78; 95% CI 0.48–122.23).[7]

Solid Tumor Malignancies

Data on malignancies at other sites in PsA are inconsistent. A retrospective, population-based study in Olmsted County showed an increased risk of female breast cancer (HR 3.59; 95% CI 1.22–10.61) as well as overall malignancies, excluding NMSC, in patients with PsA (HR 1.64; 95% CI 1.03–2.61).[12] The risk of several other solid organ cancers (eye/orbit, female genital, urinary, NMSC, lung, prostate) was noted to be higher compared with subjects from the general population matched on age, sex, and calendar year in a retrospective cohort study (abstract) from British Columbia, Canada, that used health administrative data.[25] Lower risk of colon (IRR 0.84; 95% CI 0.72–0.99) and rectal carcinoma (IRR 0.79; 95% CI 0.64–0.98) was re-ported. Interestingly, unlike psoriasis, no increased risk of lymphoma and colorectal cancer was seen.[17] On the contrary, data from the CORRONA registry found similar risk of malignancy in PsA compared with RA (IRR 1.18; 95% CI 0.82–1.69).[7] Risk of malignancy by subtypes was not different, including that for NMSC and lymphoma. However, this study did not compare risk of malignancy to the general population.

RISK OF MALIGNANCY IN ANKYLOSING SPONDYLITIS

In AS, there seem to be more studies suggesting an increased risk for malignancy. A meta-analysis by Deng and colleagues[26] found an increased risk for overall malig-nancy (RR 1.14; 95% CI 1.03–1.25). Subgroup analysis in the study showed a higher risk in Asian populations, but not American or European populations. Also, the study design seems to influence the results, with cohort studies showing a higher risk than case-control studies and clinical trials. Another more recent study (not included in the meta-analysis) by Walsh and colleagues[27] also supports this conclusion, finding an overall risk for malignancy compared with population controls in MarketScan and Medicare (HR 1.39; 95% CI 1.19 to 1.62). However, several other studies did not show an overall increased risk of malignancy in AS.[13,15,20,28–30]

Hematologic Malignancies

In contrast to PsA, there may be a higher risk of hematological malignancies in AS although with some disagreement among individual studies within subtypes of hema-tologic malignancies (ie, lymphoma, multiple myeloma, and MGUS). Increased risk of malignancy was reported in axial SpA historically in patients undergoing radiation ther-apy where a threefold increase in risk of lymphoma was described with 28% higher mortality compared with the general population.[31] More recent studies have similarly found an increased risk of hematological malignancies, albeit with attenuated associ-ations. Chang and colleagues[28] noted a higher risk of overall hematological malig-nancies (SIR 2.10; 95% CI 1.32 to 3.19) in a study from the national Taiwan database. In addition, a meta-analysis found a higher risk of multiple myeloma (RR 1.92; 95% CI 1.37–2.69) and lymphoma (RR 1.32; 95% CI 1.11–1.57). An increased risk of MGUS and multiple myeloma in AS has been reported in several studies: Brown and colleagues[32] noted an increased risk of MGUS (RR 2.02; 95% CI 1.14–3.56) and multiple myeloma (RR 2.29; 95% CI 1.55–3.40) in patients with AS from US

Department of Veterans Affairs hospitals. In a case-control study from Sweden, Lindqvist and colleagues[33] noted an increased risk of MGUS (odds ratio [OR] 2.7; 95% CI 1.4–5.2), but not multiple myeloma (OR 1.2; 95% CI 0.6–2.3). Increased risk of multiple myeloma was also noted in several other studies.[34–36] Similarly, a higher risk of leukemia (SIR 1.44; 95% CI 1.24–1.65) and non-Hodgkin lymphoma (SIR 1.36; 95% CI 1.19–1.53) was reported among Medicare beneficiaries[36]; and Lee and colleagues[35] reported increased risk of lymphoma (HR 3.05; 95% CI 1.45–6.45), but not leukemia (HR 2.32; 95% CI 0.91–5.91) from the national database of Korea. However, several other studies included in our review did not report an increased risk of hematologic malignancies, such as lymphoma, in AS.[13,15,20,22,37–41]

Solid Tumor Malignancies

Although there is mixed reporting of the relationship between hematologic malignancies and AS, there remains an even more unclear association between solid organ malignancies and AS. Chang and colleagues[28] noted a higher risk of colon cancer (SIR 1.39; 95% CI 1.03–1.82) and prostate cancer (SIR 1.64; 95% CI 1.04–2.47) in patients with AS. In contrast, data from the Anti-Rheumatic Therapy in Sweden (ARTIS) and Danish Biologics (DANBIO) registries showed a lower risk of colorectal cancer (RR 0.40; 95% CI 0.3–0.8) in the TNFi-naïve patients with AS compared with the general population, and very few colorectal cancers were seen in those on TNFi (<5 events).[15] Lower risk of colorectal cancer was also reported in a study from the Medicare database (SIR 0.81; 95% CI 0.71–0.91)[36] and in a national Swedish study (colon adenocarcinoma: SIR 0.55; 95% CI 0.32–0.88; rectal adenocarcinoma: SIR 0.35; 95% CI 0.14–0.73).[42] Higher risk of renal carcinoma (SIR 5.90; 95% CI 1.61–15.1) was noted in a study from the Swedish inpatient registry.[29] A study on Medicare beneficiaries by Alehashemi and colleagues[36] reported very different results from the rest of the studies, finding higher SIR in AS compared with patients without AS for kidney, thyroid, prostate, esophagus, stomach, colorectal, and lung cancers, and melanoma.

Over the past 10 years, the nomenclature for AS has been changing. As we discuss these studies with regard to associations with malignancy, it is important to keep in mind that most studies to date have focused on AS (more recently referred to as radiographic AxSpA), and some use general codes for AS that mix the radiographic and nonradiographic AxSpA populations.[43,44] In our review of the literature, we did not find studies on the risk of malignancy in nonradiographic axial spondyloarthritis (nr-AxSpA). As we move forward, an important research objective should be to understand the potentially differential malignancy risk in each of these subgroups.

CANCER AND SPONDYLOARTHRITIS (COMBINED AXIAL SPONDYLOARTHRITIS AND PSORIATIC ARTHRITIS)

Although most studies have separately examined AS and PsA, several have examined malignancy risk across the SpA category. In the cross-sectional Assessment of SpondyloArthritis international Society of COMOrbidities in SpA (ASAS-COMOSPA) study, a cohort of patients fulfilling either axial or peripheral ASAS criteria,[45] the prevalence (at any point up to the study visit date) of overall malignancy was approximately 3% (95% CI 2.46–3.52). The most prevalent cancers identified were cervical cancer (1.2%), BCC (0.8%), and melanoma (0.7%).[46] A similar study in China did not find an increased prevalence of malignancies in SpA relative to the general poulation.[47] Disparate results could be related to the fact that patients in this study were relatively young, and very few patients with SpA had cervical smears or saw a dermatologist for skin check in China.[47] Also malignancy rates reported in Northern Europe and the

United States are generally higher than reported rates in Asian countries.[48] Similarly, Hellgren and colleagues[15] reported a slightly increased risk of prostate cancer in the biologic-naïve group in the ARTIS and DANBIO biologics registries compared with the general population (RR 1.2; 95% CI 1.1–1.4). These results suggest that the association with malignancy may not be a class effect of SpA, but rather results from a complex interaction of specific comorbidities (eg, severe psoriasis in PsA) and medication use. Therefore, it would be helpful to study the risk of malignancies separately in PsA and AxSpA, rather than lumping into a single SpA category.

ASSOCIATION OF PHARMACOTHERAPIES FOR SPONDYLOARTHRITIS WITH CANCER

Nonsteroidal anti-inflammatory drugs (NSAIDs) and TNFi are the most commonly used therapeutic agents in the treatment of AxSpA, with interleukin-17 inhibitors recently added (and thus with very few data on malignancy outside of clinical trials). In SpA, there are relatively few data on the risk of malignancy by therapy class, particularly when compared with the available literature in RA, which is also limited. Among the available studies, most have addressed the risk for malignancy among those using TNFi (**Table 2**).

Among patients with PsA on TNFi, no increased risk of overall malignancy was noted.[13,16,30,49] However, some studies noted increased risk of specific types of malignancies. A recent study from British Society for Rheumatology Biologics Register found an increased risk of NMSC among those using TNFi compared with general population (SIR 2.12; 95% CI 1.19–3.50) but this elevated risk was only among women (SIR 2.41; 95% CI 1.10–4.58) and not men (SIR 0.85; 95% CI 0.51–1.35).[49] An increased risk for NMSC was similarly found among patients with PsA using methotrexate compared with the general population in a study by Lange and colleagues[6] (SIR-5.91; 95% CI 3.56–9.22). Neither of these studies report prior phototherapy exposure. Besides skin cancer, a higher risk of breast cancer in patients with PsA treated with TNFi compared with TNFi-naïve patients (RR 1.8; 95% CI 1.1–2.9) but not compared with the general population (RR 0.9; 95% CI 0.8–1.1) was seen in the ARTIS and DANBIO registries.[15] Lange and colleagues[6] also reported a lower risk of prostate cancer in patients with PsA treated with TNFi compared with TNFi naïve (RR 0.4; 95% CI 0.2–0.8) and the general population (RR 0.4; 95% CI 0.2–0.8). A retrospective study from CPRD also noted an increased risk of solid organ malignancies, site not specified (IRR 1.84; 95% CI 1.46–2.32), and NMSC (IRR 2.54; 95% CI 1.84–3.51) in patients with PsA on methotrexate, sulfasalazine, or adalimumab compared with those with PsA not using these medications.[14] Finally, pooled data from long-term extension studies did not find a higher than expected risk of malignancies in patients with PsA on adalimumab.[13]

As noted previously, there is variability in the reported risk of hematological malignancies in PsA as a disease; and this is similarly true when examining therapies and the association with hematologic malignancies in PsA. No increased risk of hematologic malignancies was observed in patients with PsA on TNFi in most studies.[13,15,21–23,50] A retrospective cohort study using data from CPRD found increased risk of hematologic malignancies in PsA (IRR 3.59; 95% CI 1.96–6.60) on DMARDs/biologics (methotrexate, sulfasalazine, and adalimumab).[14] Similarly, a large prospective cohort study including patients from 4 Nordic countries (Sweden, Denmark, Iceland, and Finland) reported a higher risk of Hodgkin and non-Hodgkin lymphoma in patients with PsA ever treated with TNFi.[16]

Among patients with AS, none of the studies reported an increased risk of any cancer with immunosuppressive medications or TNFi.[15,21–23,51] We did not find any

Table 2
Summary of studies examining the risk of cancer with medications used to treat spondyloarthritis (SpA)

Author, Year	Study Design	Study Period	No. of SpA Pts	SpA Definition	Relevant Study Questions	Comparison Group	Therapies	Follow-up Period (y)	Types of Malignancies Reported	Estimate of Risk, Measure of Effect (95% CI)
SpA										
Atzeni et al,[54] 2018	Cohort study from GISEA registry, Italy	2003–2015	3321	Pts ≥18 y with physician diagnosis of RA, PsA, AS, enteropathic arthritis, undifferentiated SpA	Incidence of cancer in SpA treated with TNFi	GP (rates per Italian Association of Medical Oncology)	TNFi- ETN or ADA	12	56 malignancies including lung breast, colorectal, reproductive system malignancies.	Overall incidence of malignancies/1000 PY: SpA- 6.3 (4.7–8.2) PsA- 6.8 (4.5–9.7) AS-6.8 (4.2–10.4) Enteropathic arthritis- 6.7 (0.2–37.5) Undifferentiated SpA- 4.4 (1.4–10.3) GP- 5.1 (NR) HR of cancer in SpA with TNFi vs. SpA with no TNFi: TNFi- HR = **1.04 (1.01–1.06)** ADA- HR = 1.56 (0.8–3.2) ETN- HR = 1.05 (0.5–2.0) Previous neoplasia was a significant predictor of new malignancy, HR = 10.6 (4.2–27.0).

(continued on next page)

Table 2
(continued)

Author, Year	Study Design	Study Period	No. of SpA Pts	SpA Definition	Relevant Study Questions	Comparison Group	Therapies	Follow-up Period (y)	Types of Malignancies Reported	Estimate of Risk, Measure of Effect (95% CI)
Hellgren et al,[15] 2017	Population-based, nationwide cohort study-ARTIS and DANBIO biologics registers, linked with the nationwide Swedish and Danish Cancer Registers	2001–2011	TNFi-17406 TNFi naïve-28,164	AS ICD-10 code (M45) PsA ICD-10 code (L40.5)	Cancer risk in SpA treated with TNFi compared with biologic naïve and GP	Swedish age-matched and sex-matched GP comparator cohort (n = 131,687)	TNFi treated TNFi naïve	Up to 10 y	Cancer overall; Prostate; Lung; Colorectal; Malignant lymphoma; Breast; Melanoma; Cancer overall; Prostate; Lung; Colorectal; Malignant lymphoma; Breast; Melanoma	TNFi treated vs TNFi naïve SpA (RR): 0.8 (0.7–1.0); **0.5 (0.3–0.8)**; 0.6 (0.3–1.3); 1.0 (0.5–2.0); 0.8 (0.4–1.8); 1.3 (0.9–2.0); 1.4 (0.7–2.6); TNFi treated SpA vs GP (RR): 0.9 (0.7–1.0); **0.6 (0.4–0.9)**; 0.6 (0.3–1.2); 0.7 (0.4–1.2); 0.8 (0.4–1.9); 1.3 (0.9–1.9); 1.3 (0.7–2.3)
Westhovens et al,[53] 2014	Single-center, prospective, longitudinal cohort study (BIOSPAR)	Sep 2000-Mar 2010	231 (PsA-103)	Rheumatologist's diagnosis	Incidence of malignancy in SpA cohort treated with TNFi (BIOSPAR) compared with GP of Belgium	Belgian population of 2008 (45–50 y old), rates per Belgian Cancer Registry	TNFi (ETN, IFX, ADA, GOL)	1020.74 PY of treatment and 1199.83 PY F/U after the start of treatment.	All malignancies	SIR of malignancy in SpA on TNFi vs GP: Female- 1.54 (NR); Male- 1.31 (NR); 6/231 SpA patients (2.6%) developed malignancy

PsA

Study	Study design	Registry/ID	Diagnosis	Objective	Comparator	Treatment	PY/duration	Cancer sites	SIR results
Ballegaard,[16] 2019 (abstract)	Prospective, cohort study from ARTIS (Sweden), DANBIO (Denmark), ICEBIO (Iceland) or ROB-FIN (Finland) and linked to the national Cancer Registry in each country	NR	ARTIS-5218, DANBIO-2039, ICEBIO-270 and ROB-FIN-526	Rheumatologist's diagnosis	Risk of cancer in TNFi-treated PsA patients compared with standardized rates from the general population in Denmark, Finland, Iceland, and Sweden	GP	TNFi (ever treated)	44,041 PY across all 4 countries	All cancers; Colorectal; Hodgkin's and NHL; Lung; Malignant melanoma; Pancreas; Brain; Female breast; Corpus uteri; Prostate	SIR of malignancy in SpA with TNFi (ever treated) vs GP: 1.00 (0.89–1.13) 1.21 (0.85–1.71) **1.84 (1.20–2.82)** 0.79 (0.51–1.22) 1.07 (0.69–1.66) 1.21 (0.60–2.41) 0.95 (0.45–1.99) 1.20 (0.93–1.55) 0.67 (0.30–1.49) 0.70 (0.50–0.98)
Burmester et al,[13] 2013	Pooled data from clinical trials (Europe, North America, South America, Asia, Australia, New Zealand, and South Africa)	Through Nov 2010	837	SpA definition per clinical trial.	Risk of malignancy from global clinical trials of ADA in immune-mediated inflammatory diseases	GP	ADA (clinical trials)	Nearly 12 y of ADA exposure	All malignancies; Lymphoma; NMSC	SIR for cancer in PsA vs GP: 0.68 (0.22–1.59) 5.88 (0.66–21.2) 1.25 (0.46–2.72) Note: Melanoma <0.1/100 Pys SIR for cancer in psoriasis vs GP- 1.76 (1.26–2.39)
Carmona et al,[20] 2011	Prospective cohort study- BIOBADASER 2.0 (ongoing cohort of patients with rheumatic diseases exposed to TNFi)	BIOBADASER (2001–2008)	727	Rheumatologist diagnosed rheumatic diseases starting treatment or were on a biologic response modifier	Cancer risk in RA, PsA, and AS patients exposed to TNFi	GP of Spain (source: GLOBOCON, WHO program 2002)	TNFi (IFX, ETN, ADA)	2323 PY	Colon and rectum; Prostate; Bladder; NHL; All sites but skin	SIR for cancer in PsA pts exposed to TNFi: 1.28(0.15–4.62) 1.18(0.03–6.59) 2.06(0.25–7.42) 4.84(0.59–17.48) 0.73(0.33–1.39)

(continued on next page)

Table 2
(continued)

Author, Year	Study Design	Study Period	No. of SpA Pts	SpA Definition	Relevant Study Questions	Comparison Group	Therapies	Follow-up Period (y)	Types of Malignancies Reported	Estimate of Risk, Measure of Effect (95% CI)
Costa et al,[68] 2016	Prospective, single-center (University Federico II of Naples) cohort study	2001–2014	618	Pts fulfilling CASPAR criteria at the time of diagnosis (after 2006) or retrospectively (before 2006 and then obtaining first dx using Moll and Wright criteria)	Incidence of malignancies in PsA pts conventional DMARDs and TNFi	none	TNFi (ETN, ADA, IFX, GOL) Conventional DMARDs	9 (median)	Squamous cell Breast Meningioma Colorectal cancer Kidney cancer Ovarian cancer NHL Uterine cancer Seminoma Papillary thyroid cancer	Incidence of overall malignancy: TNFi-4.7% (2.8–7.8); IR- 0.52 cases/100 PY DMARD-9.3% (6.6–13.0); IR-1.03 cases/100 PY
Dreyer et al,[30] 2013	Cohort study (DANBIO arthritis cohort)	2000–2008.	656	Rheumatologist's diagnosis	Incidence of overall and site-specific malignancies in TNFi-treated pts with PsA	GP	TNFi	2.9 (mean).	All cancer sites	SIR of malignancy in PsA on TNFi vs GP: 1.16 (0.66–2.04) 12/656 pts during f/u HR of malignancy with PsA on TNFi vs no TNFi- NR.

Study	Design	Period	N	Diagnosis	Aim	Comparator	Treatment	Follow-up/PY	Cancer types	Results
Fagerli et al,[49] 2019	Cohort study from BSRBR	2002–2006	709 (males, n = 331, females, n = 378)	Rheumatologist's diagnosis	Malignancy and mortality rates in PsA pts requiring TNFi	GP	TNFi	8.4 (SD-1.5), followed until 2012	NMSC Malignant melanoma Genital cancer Lymphatic and hematological cancer Oropharyngeal cancer	SIR for PsA on TNFi vs GP: All malignancies - 0.94 (0.65–1.34) NMSC- **2.12 (1.19–3.50)** SIR for PsA on TNFi vs GP (males): All malignancies- 1.06 (0.61–1.72) NMSC- 0.85 (0.51–1.35) SIR for PsA on TNFi vs GP (females): All malignancies- 0.85(0.51–1.35) NMSC- **2.41(1.10–4.58)**
Hagberg et al,[14] 2016	Retrospective cohort study from CPRD, UK	1988–2012.	8943	PsA as diagnosed by general practitioner or specialist	Incidence rate of cancers in patients with PsA vs without PsA	Pts without PsA (n = 82,601)	Systemic therapies DMARDs/biologics (eg, MTX, SSZ, and ADA), immunosuppressants (eg, AZT and leflunomide),	Solid cancer- 3139 PY, Hematological cancer- 261 PY, NMSC- 1561 PY	Solid, hematologic, and NMSC	IRR of solid cancer in PsA on different drugs vs PsA with no drug: Any drug- 1.80 (1.44–2.27) DMARDs/ biologics- 1.84 (1.46–2.32)

(continued on next page)

Table 2
(continued)

Author, Year	Study Design	Study Period	No. of SpA Pts	SpA Definition	Relevant Study Questions	Comparison Group	Therapies	Follow-up Period (y)	Types of Malignancies Reported	Estimate of Risk, Measure of Effect (95% CI)
							and corticosteroids			Immuno-suppressant- 1.99 (1.02–3.87) 3.69 (1.37–9.91) IRR of hematologic cancer in PsA on different drugs vs PsA with no drug: Any drug- 3.50 (1.92–6.36) DMARDs/ biologics- 3.59 (1.96–6.60) Immuno-suppressant- 6.79 (2.04–22.62) IRR of NMSC in PsA on different drugs vs PsA with no drug: Any drug- 2.42 (1.76–3.34) DMARDs/ biologics- 2.54 (1.84–3.51) Immuno-suppressant- 2.63 (1.07–6.45)

										Corticosteroid- 4.19 (1.03–17.01) Drug exposure defined as first PsA drug prescription occurred at least 1 y before cancer dx date
Haynes et al,[21] 2013	Retrospective cohort study (SABER study)- Medicare, Medicaid, New Jersey's Pharmaceutical Assistance, Kaiser Permanente (US)[a]	1992–2007[a] (variable study periods in 4 different databases)	Total PsA- 2498 (PsA on TNFi, n = 1036)	ICD-9 diagnostic codes for PsA	Cancer risk with TNFi in chronic immune-mediated diseases	PsA with no TNFi (on MTX or sulfasalazine, n = 1462)	TNFi	618 PY	Any lymphoma, any hematologic cancer, any solid cancer other than nonmelanoma skin cancer, and nonmelanoma skin cancer, defined as squamous cell or basal cell cancer	HR of incident cancer for PsA on TNFi vs no TNFi: Any leukemia or lymphoma-<5 events Any solid cancer- 0.74 (0.20–2.76) NMSC-0.74 (0.06–8.72)

(continued on next page)

Table 2
(continued)

Author, Year	Study Design	Study Period	No. of SpA Pts	SpA Definition	Relevant Study Questions	Comparison Group	Therapies	Follow-up Period (y)	Types of Malignancies Reported	Estimate of Risk, Measure of Effect (95% CI)
Hellgren et al,[22] 2014	Population-based, prospective cohort study from Swedish National Patient Register	2001-2010	19,283	ICD codes for AS, PsA	Risk of malignant lymphoma in AS, PsA	Randomly selected from Swedish Population Register (matched for age-sex and county of residence)	TNFi MTX/SSZ Oral GC	10,912 PY	Malignant lymphoma	HR for lymphoma in PsA on drug vs no drug: MTX and/or SSZ- 1.7 (1.0–3.1). The numbers and incidence of lymphoma were not different in TNFi-exposed vs TNFi-naïve PsA patients, although the number of lymphoma was very small.

Author	Study	Period	N	Definition	Topic	Comparator	Treatment	Follow-up	Cancer	RR
Hellgren et al,[15] 2017	Population-based, nationwide cohort study- ARTIS and DANBIO biologics registers, linked with the nationwide Swedish and Danish Cancer Registers	2001–2011	TNFi-3833 TNFi naïve-15,908	ICD-10 code for PsA (L40.5)	Cancer risk in SpA treated with TNFi	Swedish age-matched and sex-matched GP comparator cohort (n = 74,010)	TNFi treated TNFi naïve	Up to 10 Y	**TNFi treated vs TNFi naïve PsA (RR):** Cancer overall / Prostate / Lung / Colorectal / Malignant lymphoma / Breast / Melanoma / **TNFi treated PsA vs GP (RR):** Cancer overall / Prostate / Lung / Colorectal / Malignant lymphoma / Breast / Melanoma / **TNFi naïve PsA vs GP (RR):** Cancer overall / Prostate / Lung / Colorectal / Malignant lymphoma / Breast / Melanoma	0.9 (0.7–1.1) / **0.4 (0.2–0.8)** / <5 events / 1.1 (0.5–2.4) / 1.0 (0.4–2.7) / 1.8 (1.1–2.9) / 1.7 (0.7–4.2) / 0.9 (0.7–1.1) / **0.4 (0.2–0.8)** / <5 events / 0.9 (0.4–1.8) / 1.1 (0.4–2.60) / 1.6 (1.0–2.5) / 1.5 (0.7–3.3) / 1.0 (0.9–1.1) / 1.1 (0.9–1.3) / 1.0 (0.7–1.3) / 0.8 (0.6–1.1) / 1.0 (0.6–1.4) / 0.9 (0.8–1.1) / 0.9 (0.6–1.3)
Lange, 2016[6]	Retrospective cohort study (2 private rheumatology practices in Hobart, Tasmania)	1978–2005	RA/PsA, n = 405; PsA, n = 60	Rheumatologist's diagnosis	NMSC risk with DMARDs in inflammatory arthritis (RA and PsA)	GP (expected rates)	MTX CSA + MTX Penicillamine D + MTX	First presentation to Dec 2005	NMSC	SIR of NMSC for PsA pts treated with MTX vs GP: 5.91 (3.56, 9.22)

(continued on next page)

Table 2
(continued)

Author, Year	Study Design	Study Period	No. of SpA Pts	SpA Definition	Relevant Study Questions	Comparison Group	Therapies	Follow-up Period (y)	Types of Malignancies Reported	Estimate of Risk, Measure of Effect (95% CI)
Rohekar et al,[50] 2008	Prospective cohort study from University of Toronto Psoriatic Arthritis Clinic	1978-2004	665	Rheumatologist's diagnosis	Prevalence of malignancy in PsA	GP (Ontario)	NSAID DMARD Immuno-suppressants	NR	All cancers	SIR for malignancy PsA vs GP: All cancers - 0.98 (0.77–1.24) Hematologic - 0.69 (0.26–1.83) Lung- 0.88 (0.46–1.69) Breast-1.55 (0.92–2.62) Prostate −0.65 (0.29–1.44) ESR, cm/h was the only significant predictor of malignancy in Cox regression, HR-1.13 (1.02–1.25). TNFi and DMARDs were not.

| Saad, 2011[69,70] | Prospective, multicenter, longitudinal, cohort study from BSRBR | 2002–2006 | 596 | Rheumatologist's diagnosis | Efficacy and safety of anti-TNF therapies in PsA | Seronegative RA control cohort in BSRBR receiving nonbiologic DMARDs, adjusting for age, sex, and baseline comorbidity | ETN (n = 333), IFX (n = 171) ADA (n = 92) | 1776.2 PY (median 3.07 per pt), | All cancers | IRR of cancer in PsA on TNFi vs seronegative RA on nonbiologic DMARDs: 0.9 (0.5–1.6)[b] In total, there were 81 malignancies reported at various sites (14 on anti-TNF and 67 on DMARD control). Of note, there were 5 cases of lymphoma in the control group and no cases in the anti-TNF group. 29 reports of skin cancer in total: 17 basal cell cancer (13 in controls, 4 in anti-TNF), 8 NMSC (6 in controls, 2 in anti-TNF) and 4 melanomas (2 in each group). |

(continued on next page)

Table 2
(continued)

Author, Year	Study Design	Study Period	No. of SpA Pts	SpA Definition	Relevant Study Questions	Comparison Group	Therapies	Follow-up Period (y)	Types of Malignancies Reported	Estimate of Risk, Measure of Effect (95% CI)
Saliba et al,[23] 2016	Disproportionality analysis (case/noncase study) from the French National Pharmaco Vigilance Database	2000–2010	128	Labeled indication of TNFi in database	Risk of cancer with TNFi + nonbiologic immuno suppressants (NBIS) vs NBIS only in autoimmune diseases (RA, AS, PsA, and IBD)	NBIS only	TNFi + NBIS NBIS only	Minimum 3 mo exposure to non-biologics	Overall Hematological cancer -Lymphoma Solid cancer	RR of malignancy with TNF + NBIS vs NBIS in psoriasis/PsA pts: 3.45 [1.09–10.92] 2.46 (0.52–11.62) 2.43 (0.36–16.68) 4.46 (0.84–23.82)
AxSpA										
Haynes et al,[21] 2013	Retrospective cohort study (SABER study)	1992–2007 [a](variable study periods in 4 different databases)	Total AS- 1486 (AS on TNFi, n = 783)	ICD-9 diagnostic codes for AS	Cancer risk with TNFi in chronic immune-mediated diseases	AS with no TNFi (on MTX or sulfasalazine, n = 703)	TNFi	433.1 PY	Any lymphoma, any hematologic cancer, any solid cancer other than nonmela- noma skin cancer, and nonme- lanoma skin cancer, defined as squamous cell or basal cell cancer	HR of incident cancer for AS on TNFi vs no TNFi: Any leukemia or lymphoma- <5 events Any solid cancer- 0.03 (0.002–0.45) NMSC <5 events

Study	Design	Period	Code	N	Aim	Comparator	Exposure	Follow-up	Outcome	Result
Hellgren et al,[22] 2014	Population-based, prospective cohort study from Swedish National Patient Register	2001-2010	ICD codes for AS, PsA	8707	Risk of malignant lymphoma in AS, PsA	Randomly selected from Swedish population register (matched for age-sex and county of residence)	TNFi MTX/SSZ Oral GC	7790 PY	Malignant lymphoma	HR for lymphoma in AS on DMARD vs no DMARD: MTX and/or SSZ- 1.2 (0.3-4.3) The numbers and incidence of lymphoma were not different in TNFi-exposed vs TNFi-naive AS patients, although the number of lymphoma was very small.
Hellgren et al,[15] 2017	Population-based, nationwide cohort study-ARTIS and DANBIO biologics registers, linked with the nationwide Swedish and Danish Cancer Registers	2001-2011	AS ICD-10 code (M45)	TNFi-3078 TNFi naive-7023	Cancer risk in SpA treated with TNFi	Swedish age-matched and sex-matched GP comparator cohort (n = 32,706)	TNFi treated TNFi naive	Up to 10 y	Cancer overall Prostate Lung Colorectal Malignant lymphoma Breast Melanoma Cancer overall Prostate Lung Colorectal Malignant lymphoma Breast Melanoma Cancer overall Prostate Lung Colorectal Malignant	TNFi treated vs TNFi naive AS (RR): 0.8 (0.6–1.1) 0.5 (0.2–1.1) <5 events <5 events <5 events 0.6 (0.2–1.6) 1.6 (0.5–4.6) TNFi treated AS vs GP: 1.0 (0.7–1.2) 0.6 (0.3–1.3) <5 events <5 events <5 events 0.9 (0.4–2.3)

(continued on next page)

**Table 2
(continued)**

Author, Year	Study Design	Study Period	No. of SpA Pts	SpA Definition	Relevant Study Questions	Comparison Group	Therapies	Follow-up Period (y)	Types of Malignancies Reported	Estimate of Risk, Measure of Effect (95% CI)
									lymphoma Breast Melanoma	1.4 (0.6–3.6) TNFi naive AS vs GP: 1.1 (1.0–1.3) 1.3 (1.0–1.6) 1.0 (0.6–1.6) **0.4 (0.3–0.8)** 0.9 (0.5–1.6) 1.4 (1.0–2.0) 0.8 (0.5–1.5)
Saliba et al,[23] 2016	Disproportionality analysis (case/noncase study) from the French National Pharmaco Vigilance Database	2000–2010	92	Labeled indication of TNFi in database	Risk of cancer with TNFi + nonbiologic immuno-suppressants vs nonbiologic immuno-suppressants only in autoimmune diseases (RA, AS, PsA, and IBD)	Nonbiologic immuno-suppressants only	TNFi + nonbiologic immuno-suppressants Nonbiologic immuno-suppressants only	Minimum 3 mo exposure to nonbiologics	Overall Hematological cancer -Lymphoma Solid cancer	RR of malignancy with TNF + NIBIS vs NBIS AS pts: 2.84 (0.32–24.87) – – 1.86 (0.16–22.05) RR adjusted for age, gender, year of reporting, history of cancer, exposure to TNFi and nonbiologic immuno-suppressants

van der Heijde et al,[51] 2014	A pooled analysis from 5 RCTs and 4 open label studies from Pfizer/Amgen	Dec 2001-Jan 2008	1323	Clinical trial definition of AS	Rates of malignancies in AS pts receiving ETN vs controls	GP (SEER database)	ETN SSZ	1131 PY of exposure to ETN	All malignancies NMSC -Basal cell cancer -Squamous cell cancer	SIR for malignancy in ETN treated pts vs GP: 1.47 (0.54–3.21) 0.12 (0.00–0.65) 0.56 (0.01–3.11)	Too few events to report RR for hematological cancer separately.

Abbreviations: ADA, adalimumab; ARTIS, Anti-Rheumatic Therapy in Sweden; AS, ankylosing spondylitis; AxSpA, axial spondyloarthritis; AZT, azathioprine; BIOSPAR, Leuven spondyloarthritis biologics cohort; BSRBR, British Society for Rheumatology Biologics Register; CASPAR, Clinical Classification of Psoriatic Arthritis; CI, confidence interval; CPRD, Clinical Practice Research Datalink; CSA, cyclosporine; DANBIO, Danish Biologics Registry; DMARDs, disease-modifying antirheumatic drugs; dx, diagnosis; ESR, erythrocyte sedimentation rate; ETN, etanercept; F/U, follow-up; GC, glucocorticoids; GISEA, Italian Group for the Study of Early Arthritis; GOL, golimumab; GP, general population; HR, hazard ratio; IBD, inflammatory bowel disease; ICD, International Classification of Diseases; ICEBIO, Icelandic nationwide database of biologic therapy; IFX, infliximab; IR, incidence rate; IRR, incidence rate ratio; MTX, methotrexate; NBIS, nonbiologic immunosuppressants; NHL, non-Hodgkin lymphoma; NMSC, nonmelanoma skin cancer; NR, not reported; NSAIDs, nonsteroidal anti-inflammatory drugs; PsA, psoriatic arthritis;; pts, patients; PY, person years; RA, rheumatoid arthritis; RCT, randomized controlled trial; ROB-FIN, Finnish Register of Biological Treatment; RR, relative risk; SABER, The Safety Assessment of Biological Therapeutics study using data from 4 sources: National Medicaid and Medicare databases, Tennessee Medicaid, pharmacy benefits plans for Medicare beneficiaries in New Jersey and Pennsylvania, and Kaiser Permanente Northern California; SD, standard deviation; SEER, surveillance, epidemiology, and end results; SIR, standardized incidence ratio; SpA, spondyloarthritis; SSZ, sulfasalazine; TNFi, tumor necrosis factor inhibitor; WHO, World Health Organization.

[a] (1) national Medicaid and Medicare databases (Medicaid Analytical eXtract, 2000–2005, excluding Tennessee; Medicare, 2000–2006; and Medicare Part D, 2006); (2) Tennessee Medicaid (TennCare, 1998–2005); (3) New Jersey's Pharmaceutical Assistance to the Aged and Disabled and Pennsylvania's Pharmaceutical Assistance Contract for the Elderly (1992–2006); and (4) Kaiser Permanente Northern California (1998–2007).

[b] Corrected data published as correction.

Data from Refs.[6,13–16,20–23,30,49–51,53,54,68–70]

studies examining the risk of cancer with NSAIDs in the SpA population (AS or PsA).The potential benefit of NSAIDs, in particular selective Cox-2 inhibitors, has been described in patients with recurrent colorectal cancer.[52] In a study by Hellgren and colleagues,[15] patients with AS who were TNFi naïve had a lower risk of colorectal cancer compared with the general population. It is possible that a high proportion of the TNFi-naïve population was using NSAID therapy, which may partially explain the results.

Few studies reported the risk of malignancy in relation to TNFi use in SpA population as a whole. Hellgren and colleagues[15] noted that the risk of malignancy was lower in patients with SpA on TNFi from ARTIS and DANBIO registries compared with the general population (RR 0.6; 95% CI 0.4–0.9) and compared with TNFi-naïve SpA (RR 0.6%, 95% 0.4–0.9). On the contrary, a study from the Leuven spondyloarthritis biologics cohort (BIOSPAR) reported an increased SIR of malignancy in SpA on TNFi compared with general population (SIR of 1.54 in women, and 1.31 in men, CI not reported).[53] A similar, although relatively lower, risk of malignancy in SpA treated with TNFi compared with the general population (HR 1.04; 95% CI 1.01–1.06) was also noted by the Italian Group for the Study of Early Arthritis (GISEA).[54]

In all studies examining the malignancy risk associated with pharmacotherapies, it is unclear if the effect seen is truly a medication effect or associated with features of disease that results in the patient receiving the medication (ie, confounding by indication).

RISK OF MALIGNANCY FOLLOWING THERAPEUTICS IN SPONDYLOARTHRITIS WITH PRIOR MALIGNANCY

Most of the studies included in the review are limited to study of the first occurrence of cancer and excluded patients with a history of malignancy (particularly for randomized controlled trials and their subsequent extension studies). Thus, little is known about treatment of patients with a prior malignancy. In a study from the Italian Group for the Study of Early Arthritis (GISEA) registry, history of neoplasia was a significant predictor of new malignancy in SpA patients on etanercept or adalimumab (HR 10.6; 95% CI 4.2–27.0); approximately 80% of which were solid organ malignancies and the rest NMSC.[54] In another study from the BIOBADASER study cohort, no significant risk of malignancy was reported in patients with previous cancers (IRR 5.22; 95% CI 0.79–34.34); however, only 1% of the patients in the cohort had a previous history of malignancy and more than 50% of patients had RA (results were not separately reported for SpA).[20] Finally, the risk for NMSC was greater among patients with a history of cancer (solid organ, hematologic, or NMSC); however, rates were similar in the PsA and non-PsA cohorts. More data are needed to better inform how to manage patients with SpA who have a prior history of malignancy.

OTHER RISK FACTORS FOR CANCER IN SPONDYLOARTHRITIS

There are relatively few studies specifically examining risk factors for malignancy in SpA, and those that exist have found risk factors that are also typical of those seen in the general population. Atzeni and colleagues[54] noted previous malignancy to be a significant predictor of new malignancy (HR 10.6; 95% CI 4.2–27, $P<.001$). Other risk factors noted in multivariate analysis were age at the time of diagnosis (HR 1.04; 95% CI 1.01–1.1) and Health Assessment Questionnaire-Disability Index score (HR 2.42; 95% CI 1.3–4.7).[54] Similarly, as would be expected, the rate of solid organ, hematologic cancers increased with age in a cohort study from CPRD, UK.[14] Female sex was associated with increased risk of overall malignancy in a population-based study from Olmsted County, MN (HR 2.17; 95% CI 1.05–4.48, $P = .037$).[12] Erythrocyte sedimentation rate (ESR) was the only significant predictor of malignancy in Cox regression (HR 1.13; 95% CI 1.02–1.25) in a prospective cohort study from University of Toronto Psoriatic Arthritis Clinic.[50] Longer disease duration (OR 1.04; 95% CI 1.01–1.07) and high ESR (OR 1.03; 95% CI 1.01–1.04) were associated with MGUS in PsA in a cross-sectional analysis.[24] Furthermore, the increased prevalence of known malignancy risk factors in SpA, such as obesity,[55,56] smoking,[46] and excess alcohol intake[57] may be a possible explanation for an association of SpA with malignancy in certain cohorts for particular cancers.

SPONDYLOARTHRITIS AND CANCER SCREENING

Regardless of whether there is a true increase in the risk for malignancy among patients with SpA, following general population guidelines for screening is important. Two studies found that cancer screening was suboptimal in at-risk patients with SpA (based on age and sex): 32% to 44% for breast cancer (>75% in most European countries, ~50% in China for the general population[58]), 40% for cervical cancer (~80% in Europe), 57% for prostate cancer, 33% for colon cancer (46.8% in Europe) and only 10.7% for skin cancer.[46,47] Patients with PsA should be referred for yearly skin checks with dermatology, especially those with severe psoriasis and on long-term phototherapy. The benefit of systematic screening for skin cancer in AxSpA has been reported in a prospective, 12-month randomized controlled trial.[59] The intervention consisted of nurse-led screening of 5 SpA comorbidities (ie, cardiovascular disease, osteoporosis, cancer, infection, and peptic ulcer), according to recommendations from the French Society of Rheumatology. Skin cancer screening rates increased in the intervention group (36.3% vs 17.2%; P = .04), and a decrease in comorbidity score (−3.20 vs −1.85) in the active nurse-led screening intervention group at 1 year was noted, although not statistically significant. This suggests possible short-term benefit of comorbidity screening even in this relatively young AxSpA population.

CONSIDERATIONS IN INTERPRETATION OF AVAILABLE DATA

Although most studies used a cohort design (ideal for studying the association of SpA with outcomes such as malignancy), a number of studies used case-control and cross-sectional designs. These may result in biased conclusions because of the inability to establish a temporal association. Data from TNFi trials were used for assessment as well, which typically have a shorter follow-up period and are thus not as helpful in studying the long-term risk of cancer. In observational studies, patients may have been exposed to multiple medications during or before the follow-up period, making it difficult to attribute the risk to a particular therapy or therapy class. Next, among studies of cancer in SpA, the definitions of SpA varied. Most often the diagnosis and outcomes were based on diagnostic codes, which may impact the validity of the results depending on the setting and validity of the individual codes used. Observation bias may also be problematic when comparing patients with SpA with the general population, and likewise when comparing patients on a particular therapy (ie, TNFi) given that they may be followed more closely than those without the disease. This bias may be exacerbated when reporting incidence of malignancy in one population versus an external general population (ie, not using internal matched controls). Most studies of SpA and malignancy reported an SIR in comparison with expected rates in the general population. Geographic, racial, and ethnic differences might exist; and screening practices across different countries might be highly variable. In addition, survival bias also has to be considered in the study of incident malignancies, as rapidly progressive malignancies might be underrepresented, as these patients might have died prematurely or patients may have died from other causes before diagnosis with malignancy. Finally, study of cancer subtypes is challenging, as some subtypes are quite rare and even large patient populations often lack power to detect differences in these rare outcomes.

Studies on the risk of malignancy with medications are especially difficult, as the results might be influenced by confounding by indication; that is, phototherapy, DMARDs, and TNFi are prescribed for those with severe or refractory disease, which in itself could be a risk factor. Similarly, in RA, older and less healthy patients seem to get conventional DMARDs as opposed to biological agents, leading to a channeling bias.[60]

CLINICS CARE POINTS

- In the literature, there are conflicting points about the association of malignancy with SpA/PsA. However, in caring for patients with PsA using biologic therapies or methotrexate, the increased risk for nonmelanoma skin cancers should be recognized.
- Age-appropriate cancer screening should be considered for all patients with SpA/PsA.

SUMMARY

In reviewing the literature, there is a mix of studies that support and refute an association between SpA and malignancies overall. However, there seems to be a higher incidence of NMSC in PsA, and increased incidence of both MGUS and multiple myeloma was noted in AS. Few studies showed a higher incidence of lymphoma in both PsA and AS, but the results were inconsistent. A higher risk of digestive tract cancers was noted in AS in some studies. No studies have addressed the risk of malignancy in nr-AxSpA. It is unclear if traditional immunosuppressive agents, TNFi or NSAIDs modulate the risk of cancer in SpA. However, overall, if there is an increased risk, it seems to be quite small.

Although no specific screening recommendations for malignancy in SpA are available at present, age-appropriate screening should be performed in all patients at minimum. In addition, annual dermatology checks for malignancy should be considered in PsA, especially in patients with moderate-to-severe psoriasis. Future studies of larger cohort studies with a better understanding of prior therapy history may help better understand the risk for malignancy in SpA.

DISCLOSURE

A. Ogdie has served as a consultant for AbbVie, Amgen, BMS, Celgene, Corrona, Janssen, Lilly, Novartis, and Pfizer and has received grants from Novartis and Pfizer to Penn and from Amgen to Forward.

REFERENCES

1. Mercer LK, Davies R, Galloway JB, et al. Risk of cancer in patients receiving non-biologic disease-modifying therapy for rheumatoid arthritis compared with the UK general population. Rheumatology (Oxford) 2013;52(1):91–8.
2. Balkwill F, Mantovani A. Inflammation and cancer: back to Virchow? Lancet 2001; 357(9255):539–45.
3. Chai EZP, Siveen KS, Shanmugam MK, et al. Analysis of the intricate relationship between chronic inflammation and cancer. Biochem J 2015;468(1):1–15.

4. Coates LC, FitzGerald O, Helliwell PS, et al. Psoriasis, psoriatic arthritis, and rheumatoid arthritis: Is all inflammation the same? Semin Arthritis Rheum 2016; 46(3):291–304.

5. Luo X, Deng C, Fei Y, et al. Malignancy development risk in psoriatic arthritis patients undergoing treatment: A systematic review and meta-analysis. Semin Arthritis Rheum 2019;48(4):626–31.

6. Lange E, Blizzard L, Venn A, et al. Disease-modifying anti-rheumatic drugs and non-melanoma skin cancer in inflammatory arthritis patients: a retrospective cohort study. Rheumatology (Oxford) 2016;55(9):1594–600.

7. Gross RL, Schwartzman-Morris JS, Krathen M, et al. A comparison of the malignancy incidence among patients with psoriatic arthritis and patients with rheumatoid arthritis in a large US cohort. Arthritis Rheumatol 2014;66(6):1472–81.

8. Wang X, Liu Q, Wu L, et al. Risk of non-melanoma skin cancer in patients with psoriasis: An updated evidence from systematic review with meta-analysis. J Cancer 2020;11(5):1047–55.

9. Mali-Gerrits MG, Gaasbeek D, Boezeman J, et al. Psoriasis therapy and the risk of skin cancers. Clin Exp Dermatol 1991;16(2):85–9.

10. Stern RS, Laird N. The carcinogenic risk of treatments for severe psoriasis. Photochemotherapy Follow-up Study. Cancer 1994;73(11):2759–64.

11. Edson-Heredia E, Zhu B, Lefevre C, et al. Prevalence and incidence rates of cardiovascular, autoimmune, and other diseases in patients with psoriatic or psoriatic arthritis: a retrospective study using Clinical Practice Research Datalink. J Eur Acad Dermatol Venereol 2015;29(5):955–63.

12. Wilton KM, Crowson CS, Matteson EL. Malignancy incidence in patients with psoriatic arthritis: a comparison cohort-based incidence study. Clin Rheumatol 2016; 35(10):2603–7.

13. Burmester GR, Panaccione R, Gordon KB, et al. Adalimumab: long-term safety in 23 458 patients from global clinical trials in rheumatoid arthritis, juvenile idiopathic arthritis, ankylosing spondylitis, psoriatic arthritis, psoriasis and Crohn's disease. Ann Rheum Dis 2013;72(4):517–24.

14. Hagberg KW, Li L, Peng M, et al. Rates of cancers and opportunistic infections in patients with psoriatic arthritis compared with patients without psoriatic arthritis. J Clin Rheumatol 2016;22(5):241–7.

15. Hellgren K, Dreyer L, Arkema EV, et al. Cancer risk in patients with spondyloarthritis treated with TNF inhibitors: a collaborative study from the ARTIS and DANBIO registers. Ann Rheum Dis 2017;76(1):105–11.

16. Ballegaard C, Hellgren K, Cordtz R, et al. OP0005 incidence of overall and sites-pecific cancers in tnf inhibitor treated patients with psoriatic arthritis: a population-based cohort study from 4 Nordic countries. Available at: https://ard.bmj.com/content/78/Suppl_2/67.3

17. Trafford AM, Parisi R, Kontopantelis E, et al. Association of psoriasis with the risk of developing or dying of cancer: a systematic review and meta-analysis. JAMA Dermatol 2019. https://doi.org/10.1001/jamadermatol.2019.3056.

18. Smitten AL, Simon TA, Hochberg MC, et al. A meta-analysis of the incidence of malignancy in adult patients with rheumatoid arthritis. Arthritis Res Ther 2008; 10(2):R45.

19. Simon TA, Thompson A, Gandhi KK, et al. Incidence of malignancy in adult patients with rheumatoid arthritis: a meta-analysis. Arthritis Res Ther 2015;17:212.

20. Carmona L, Abasolo L, Descalzo MA, et al. Cancer in patients with rheumatic diseases exposed to TNF antagonists. Semin Arthritis Rheum 2011;41(1):71–80.

21. Haynes K, Beukelman T, Curtis JR, et al. Tumor necrosis factor α inhibitor therapy and cancer risk in chronic immune-mediated diseases. Arthritis Rheum 2013; 65(1):48–58.

22. Hellgren K, Smedby KE, Backlin C, et al. Ankylosing spondylitis, psoriatic arthritis, and risk of malignant lymphoma: a cohort study based on nationwide prospectively recorded data from Sweden. Arthritis Rheumatol 2014;66(5): 1282–90.

23. Saliba L, Moulis G, Abou Taam M, et al. Tumor necrosis factor inhibitors added to nonbiological immunosuppressants vs. nonbiological immunosuppressants alone: a different signal of cancer risk according to the condition. A disproportionality analysis in a nationwide pharmacovigilance database. Fundam Clin Pharmacol 2016;30(2):162–71.

24. Eder L, Thavaneswaran A, Pereira D, et al. Prevalence of monoclonal gammopathy among patients with psoriatic arthritis. J Rheumatol 2012;39(3):564–7.

25. Risk of Cancer in Patients with Psoriasis/Psoriatic Arthritis: A Population-Based Study in the Province of British Columbia. ACR Meeting Abstracts. Available at: https://acrabstracts.org/abstract/risk-of-cancer-in-patients-with-psoriasis-psoriatic-arthritis-a-population-based-study-in-the-province-of-british-columbia/. Accessed January 15, 2020.

26. Deng C, Li W, Fei Y, et al. Risk of malignancy in ankylosing spondylitis: a systematic review and meta-analysis. Sci Rep 2016;6:32063.

27. Walsh JA, Song X, Kim G, et al. Evaluation of the comorbidity burden in patients with ankylosing spondylitis using a large US administrative claims data set. Clin Rheumatol 2018;37(7):1869–78.

28. Chang C-C, Chang C-W, Nguyen P-AA, et al. Ankylosing spondylitis and the risk of cancer. Oncol Lett 2017;14(2):1315–22.

29. Feltelius N, Ekbom A, Blomqvist P. Cancer incidence among patients with ankylosing spondylitis in Sweden 1965-95: a population based cohort study. Ann Rheum Dis 2003;62(12):1185–8.

30. Dreyer L, Mellemkjær L, Andersen AR, et al. Incidences of overall and site specific cancers in TNFα inhibitor treated patients with rheumatoid arthritis and other arthritides - a follow-up study from the DANBIO Registry. Ann Rheum Dis 2013; 72(1):79–82.

31. Darby SC, Doll R, Gill SK, et al. Long term mortality after a single treatment course with X-rays in patients treated for ankylosing spondylitis. Br J Cancer 1987;55(2): 179–90.

32. Brown LM, Gridley G, Check D, et al. Risk of multiple myeloma and monoclonal gammopathy of undetermined significance among white and black male United States veterans with prior autoimmune, infectious, inflammatory, and allergic disorders. Blood 2008;111(7):3388–94.

33. Lindqvist EK, Goldin LR, Landgren O, et al. Personal and family history of immune-related conditions increase the risk of plasma cell disorders: a population-based study. Blood 2011;118(24):6284–91.

34. Hemminki K, Liu X, Försti A, et al. Effect of autoimmune diseases on incidence and survival in subsequent multiple myeloma. J Hematol Oncol 2012;5:59.

35. Cancer Risk in Patients with Ankylosing Spondylitis: A Nationwide Population-based Dynamic Cohort Study from Korea. ACR Meeting Abstracts. Available at: https://acrabstracts.org/abstract/cancer-risk-in-patients-with-ankylosing-spondylitis-a-nationwide-population-based-dynamic-cohort-study-from-korea/. Accessed January 15, 2020.

36. Cancer Risk in Ankylosing Spondylitis in United States Medicare Beneficiaries: Detection of a Chronic Non Steroidal Anti-Inflammatory Drug Use Signature. ACR Meeting Abstracts. Available at: https://acrabstracts.org/abstract/cancer-risk-in-ankylosing-spondylitis-in-united-states-medicare-beneficiaries-detection-of-a-chronic-non-steroidal-anti-inflammatory-drug-use-signature/. Accessed January 15, 2020.

37. Anderson LA, Gadalla S, Morton LM, et al. Population-based study of autoimmune conditions and the risk of specific lymphoid malignancies. Int J Cancer 2009;125(2):398–405.

38. Becker N, Deeg E, Rüdiger T, et al. Medical history and risk for lymphoma: results of a population-based case-control study in Germany. Eur J Cancer 2005;41(1):133–42.

39. Fallah M, Liu X, Ji J, et al. Autoimmune diseases associated with non-Hodgkin lymphoma: a nationwide cohort study. Ann Oncol 2014;25(10):2025–30.

40. Fallah M, Liu X, Ji J, et al. Hodgkin lymphoma after autoimmune diseases by age at diagnosis and histological subtype. Ann Oncol 2014;25(7):1397–404.

41. Mellemkjaer L, Pfeiffer RM, Engels EA, et al. Autoimmune disease in individuals and close family members and susceptibility to non-Hodgkin's lymphoma. Arthritis Rheum 2008;58(3):657–66.

42. Hemminki K, Liu X, Ji J, et al. Autoimmune disease and subsequent digestive tract cancer by histology. Ann Oncol 2012;23(4):927–33.

43. Sieper J, Poddubnyy D. Axial spondyloarthritis. Lancet 2017;390(10089):73–84.

44. Boel A, Molto A, van der Heijde D, et al. Do patients with axial spondyloarthritis with radiographic sacroiliitis fulfil both the modified New York criteria and the ASAS axial spondyloarthritis criteria? Results from eight cohorts. Ann Rheum Dis 2019;78(11):1545–9.

45. Rudwaleit M, van der Heijde D, Landewé R, et al. The Assessment of SpondyloArthritis International Society classification criteria for peripheral spondyloarthritis and for spondyloarthritis in general. Ann Rheum Dis 2011;70(1):25–31.

46. Moltó A, Etcheto A, van der Heijde D, et al. Prevalence of comorbidities and evaluation of their screening in spondyloarthritis: results of the international cross-sectional ASAS-COMOSPA study. Ann Rheum Dis 2016;75(6):1016–23.

47. Jiang Y, Zhang P, Tu L, et al. Prevalence of comorbidities and evaluation of screening in Chinese patients with spondyloarthritis. Clin Rheumatol 2018;37(2):423–8.

48. Torre LA, Bray F, Siegel RL, et al. Global cancer statistics, 2012. CA Cancer J Clin 2015;65(2):87–108.

49. Fagerli KM, Kearsley-Fleet L, Mercer LK, et al. Malignancy and mortality rates in patients with severe psoriatic arthritis requiring tumour-necrosis factor alpha inhibition: results from the British Society for Rheumatology Biologics Register. Rheumatology (Oxford) 2019;58(1):80–5.

50. Rohekar S, Tom BDM, Hassa A, et al. Prevalence of malignancy in psoriatic arthritis. Arthritis Rheum 2008;58(1):82–7.

51. van der Heijde D, Zack D, Wajdula J, et al. Rates of serious infections, opportunistic infections, inflammatory bowel disease, and malignancies in subjects receiving etanercept vs. controls from clinical trials in ankylosing spondylitis: a pooled analysis. Scand J Rheumatol 2014;43(1):49–53.

52. Veettil SK, Lim KG, Ching SM, et al. Effects of aspirin and non-aspirin nonsteroidal anti-inflammatory drugs on the incidence of recurrent colorectal adenomas: a systematic review with meta-analysis and trial sequential analysis of randomized clinical trials. BMC Cancer 2017;17(1):763.

53. Westhovens I, Lories RJ, Westhovens R, et al. Anti-TNF therapy and malignancy in spondyloarthritis in the Leuven spondyloarthritis biologics cohort (BIOSPAR). Clin Exp Rheumatol 2014;32(1):71–6.

54. Atzeni F, Carletto A, Foti R, et al. Incidence of cancer in patients with spondyloarthritis treated with anti-TNF drugs. Joint Bone Spine 2018;85(4):455–9.

55. Maas F, Arends S, van der Veer E, et al. Obesity is common in axial spondyloarthritis and is associated with poor clinical outcome. J Rheumatol 2016;43(2): 383–7.

56. Queiro R, Lorenzo A, Tejón P, et al. Obesity in psoriatic arthritis. Medicine (Baltimore) 2019;98(28). https://doi.org/10.1097/MD.0000000000016400.

57. Kaine J, Song X, Kim G, et al. Higher incidence rates of comorbidities in patients with psoriatic arthritis compared with the general population using U.S. administrative claims data. J Manag Care Spec Pharm 2019;25(1):122–32.

58. Feng R-M, Zong Y-N, Cao S-M, et al. Current cancer situation in China: good or bad news from the 2018 Global Cancer Statistics? Cancer Commun 2019; 39(1):22.

59. Moltó A, Etcheto A, Poiraudeau S, et al. OP0303 Systematic screening of comorbidities improves vaccination rates, skin cancer screening and vitamin d supplementation in patients with axial spondyloarthritis: results of the comedspa prospective, controlled, one year randomised trial. Ann Rheum Dis 2018; 77(Suppl 2):198.

60. Frisell T, Baecklund E, Bengtsson K, et al. Patient characteristics influence the choice of biological drug in RA, and will make non-TNFi biologics appear more harmful than TNFi biologics. Ann Rheum Dis 2018;77(5):650–7.

61. Bautista-Molano W, Landewé R, Burgos-Vargas R, et al. Prevalence of comorbidities and risk factors for comorbidities in patients with spondyloarthritis in Latin America: a comparative study with the general population and data from the ASAS-COMOSPA Study. J Rheumatol 2018;45(2):206–12.

62. Fantò M, Peragallo MS, Pietrosanti M, et al. Risk of malignancy in patients with rheumatoid arthritis, psoriatic arthritis and ankylosing spondylitis under immunosuppressive therapy: a single-center experience. Intern Emerg Med 2016;11(1): 31–40.

63. Askling J, Klareskog L, Blomqvist P, et al. Risk for malignant lymphoma in ankylosing spondylitis: a nationwide Swedish case-control study. Ann Rheum Dis 2006;65(9):1184–7.

64. Castro FA, Liu X, Försti A, et al. Increased risk of hepatobiliary cancers after hospitalization for autoimmune disease. Clin Gastroenterol Hepatol 2014;12(6): 1038–45.e7.

65. Hemminki K, Liu X, Ji J, et al. Effect of autoimmune diseases on risk and survival in female cancers. Gynecol Oncol 2012;127(1):180–5.

66. Hemminki K, Sundquist K, Sundquist J, et al. Risk of cancer of unknown primary after hospitalization for autoimmune diseases. Int J Cancer 2015;137(12): 2885–95.

67. Liu X, Ji J, Forsti A, et al. Autoimmune disease and subsequent urological cancer. J Urol 2013;189(6):2262–8.

68. Costa L, Caso F, Del Puente A, et al. Incidence of malignancies in a cohort of psoriatic arthritis patients taking traditional disease modifying antirheumatic drug and tumor necrosis factor inhibitor therapy: an observational study. J Rheumatol 2016;43(12):2149–54.

69. Saad AA, Ashcroft DM, Watson KD, et al. Efficacy and safety of anti-TNF therapies in psoriatic arthritis: an observational study from the British Society for Rheumatology Biologics Register. Rheumatology (Oxford) 2010;49(4):697–705.

70. Saad AA, Ashcroft DM, Watson KD, et al. Efficacy and safety of anti-TNF therapies in psoriatic arthritis: an observational study from the British Society for Rheumatology Biologics Register. Rheumatology (Oxford) 2017;56(4):672–3.

Sjögren Syndrome and Cancer

Ann Igoe, MD[a,b], Sali Merjanah, MD[c], R. Hal Scofield, MD[b,d],*

KEYWORDS

- Sjögren syndrome • Malignancy • Lymphoma • Salivary glands • Amyloidosis
- Autoimmune disease • Lymphoproliferative disorders

KEY POINTS

- Patients with primary Sjögren syndrome (pSS) have a 10-fold to 44-fold greater risk of lymphoma than healthy individuals.
- Among lymphomas noted in pSS patients, 90% are due to mucosa-associated lymphoid tissue lymphoma, diffuse large B-cell lymphoma, or marginal zone lymphoma.
- Breast cancer can be overstaged due to misinterpretation of axillary metastasis.
- Head and neck cancers can present as rapidly developing neck lymphadenopathy.
- Lung cancer is found in excess among those with pulmonary disease.

Henrik Sjögren in 1933 presented clinical and histologic findings of 19 women who had symptomatic sicca.[1] The eponymous disease Sjögren syndrome (SS) ranges from only exocrine gland involvement with sicca to systemic, multiorgan autoimmune disease. SS is classified as either primary SS (pSS) or secondary SS, the latter accompanied by another connective tissue disease, such as systemic lupus erythematosus (SLE), with rheumatoid arthritis (RA) found most commonly.[2]

GENERAL CONSIDERATIONS

Among the systemic manifestations, benign or malignant lymphoproliferation may be a prominent part of this syndrome.[3] Several studies show a high incidence of

[a] Arthritis and Clinical Immunology Program, Oklahoma Medical Research Foundation, Department of Medicine, University of Oklahoma Health Sciences Center, MS 38, 825 Northeast 13th Street, Oklahoma City, OK 73104, USA; [b] Arthritis and Clinical Immunology Program, Oklahoma Medical Research Foundation, Departments of Medicine and Pathology, University of Oklahoma Health Sciences Center, MS 38, 825 Northeast 13th Street, Oklahoma City, OK 73104, USA; [c] The Metrohealth System, Case Western Reserve University, 2500 MetroHealth Drive, Cleveland, OH 44109, USA; [d] US Department of Veterans Affairs, Oklahoma City, OK, USA
* Corresponding author. Oklahoma Medical Research Foundation, 825 Northeast 13th Street, Oklahoma City, OK 73104.
E-mail address: hal-scofield@omrf.ouhsc.edu

Rheum Dis Clin N Am 46 (2020) 513–532
https://doi.org/10.1016/j.rdc.2020.05.004
0889-857X/20/© 2020 Elsevier Inc. All rights reserved.

rheumatic.theclinics.com

malignancy in SS, the most common being lymphoma.[4–6] When studied, no increased all-cause mortality was detected for patients with pSS compared with the general population (Supplemental Table 1). When pSS subgroups were compared, however, higher mortality due to lymphoproliferative malignancy was found in patients fulfilling the American-European Consensus Criteria for Sjögren's Syndrome, with the strongest predictor for an unfavorable outcome being low C3 and/or C4 levels at the time of diagnosis.[7] A study published in 2010 investigated tumors in pSS and noted that with a prevalence of 5%, lymphoma was the most common tumor.[8] This was confirmed further by Nishishinya and colleagues.[9] pSS patients have a 10-fold to 44-fold greater risk of lymphoma than healthy individuals. This risk is higher than that reported for SLE or RA.[10] Diagnosis of lymphoma prior to a diagnosis of an underlying or undiagnosed SS is not unusual; in a significant proportion of patients, particularly in men, pSS remains undiagnosed until after lymphoma diagnosis.[11] A summary of all studies of lymphoma in SS is given in **Table 1**.

MUCOSA-ASSOCIATED LYMPHOID TISSUE LYMPHOMA

Lymphoma is thought to occur due to the chronic stimulation of B cells by autoantigens in a cascade that is initiated by stimulation at the level of the target tissue by autoimmune damage of polyclonal B cells, especially B cells that secrete rheumatoid factor.[12] The risk of a malignant B-cell transformation is mediated by the likelihood that pro-oncogenic elements contribute to an aberrant increase in B-cell survival.[10,13] The World Health Organization (WHO) classification categorizes lymphomas into B-cell or T-cell/natural killer–cell neoplasms, which in turn are further designated into various subtypes.[14] T cells predominate in the infiltration of the salivary glands of patients with pSS.[15] Despite this, lymphomas that occur in pSS patients predominantly are of B-cell origin, with only a mere 2% of lymphomas attributable to T-cell lineage.[10]

Among lymphomas noted in pSS patients, 90% are due to mucosa-associated lymphoid tissue (MALT) lymphoma, diffuse large B-cell lymphoma, or marginal zone lymphoma.[16–21] Evidence shows that pSS patients have a 22-fold to 260-fold higher risk of developing parotid gland B-cell lymphoma and a 90-fold to 1000-fold higher risk of developing parotid gland MALT lymphoma in comparison with the general population.[10,22–24] Lymphoma, however, can target a range of tissues; the primary sites of lymphoma development in pSS patients in descending order include salivary; lungs; gastric; ocular; oral; spleen; liver; thymus/intestines; skin; and lastly bone.[10,25–32]

There are a variety of risk factors. Patients with young onset of the pSS develop lymphoma more frequently than those with a much later onset.[33,34] The glandular, cutaneous, and lymphadenopathy domains of EULAR Sjögren's syndrome disease activity index were noted to be the most prominent predictors.[10,35] A majority of pSS lymphomas arise in the parotid glands, and a history of parotid enlargement is a risk factor.[10] Enlarged lymph nodes along with a history of spleen enlargement have been reported as another risk marker for lymphoma.[10,16,17,36–39] In addition, low-grade fever, purpura, and skin ulcers have been associated with lymphoma.[10] There also is a notable association between monoclonal cryoglobulinemic vasculitis and lymphoma.[18,32,38–42]

CD4+ T cell lymphocytopenia has been reported as a significant predictor of lymphoproliferative disease, which is noted mainly in association with anti-Ro (or Sjogren's syndrome A) antibodies,[41] although having a positive antinuclear antibody test has not been implicated in lymphoma risk.[10,38,43,44] Controversy exists regarding the prognostic role of anti-Ro and anti-La (or Sjogren's syndrome B) antibodies. pSS negative for anti-Ro and anti-La antibodies is characterized by a lower risk of lymphoma, by a lower level of B-cell clonal expansion, and by a lower prevalence of

Table 1
Studies of lymphoma in Sjögren syndrome with calculated standardized incidence ratios and 95% CIs

Reference, Year	Location	Number Lymphoma/Cohort	Standardized Incidence Ratio (95% CI)	Follow-up Length/Patient-Years
Kassan et al,[124] 1978	USA	4/142	44.4 (16.7, 118.4)	8.1[a]/109
Kauppi et al,[125] 1997	Finland	22/676	8.7 (4.3, 15.5)	NG/5336
Valesini et al,[37] 1997	Italy	9/295	33.3 (17.3, 64.0)	5.9[a]/1756
Davidson et al,[29] 1999	UK	3/100	14.4 (4.7, 44.7)	8 (duration)
Pertovaara et al,[30] 2001	Finland	3/110	13 (2.7, 38)	15 (duration)/1015
Zintzaras et al,[20] 2005	Multiple	30/1300	18.8 (9.5–37.3)	22[b]
Lazarus et al,[5] 2006	UK	11/112	37.5 (20.7, 67.6)	10.8[a]/1210
Theander et al,[41] 2006	Sweden	11/286	15.57 (7.77, 27.85)	8[b]/2464
Brito-Zerón et al,[44] 2007	Spain	9/266	NG	8.66[a]
Zhang et al,[4] 2010	China	8/1320	48.1 (20.7, 94.76)	4.2[a]/5544
Baimpa et al,[16] 2009	Greece	40/536	NG	2.6[b]
Weng et al,[126] 2012	Taiwan	23/6911, 3/941	F: 7.08 (4.25, 10.3), M: 3.10 (0.64, 9.05)	3.5[a]/27,246
Solans-Laqué et al,[32] 2011	Spain	11/244	15.6 (8.7–28.2)	8.6[b]/NG
Johnsen et al,[27] 2013	Norway	7/443	9 (7.1, 26.3)	8[b]/3813
Liang et al,[6] 2014	Multiple	104/12,325	13.76 (8.53–18.99)	
Brito-Zerón et al,[20] 2017	Spain	12/1239	6.04 (3.43–10.64)	7.6[a]5.5[b]/9922

Follow-up is given as length (either mean or median) with total patient-years. For some studies, only the duration is given.
Abbreviations: NA, not applicable; NG, not given. F, female subjects; M, male subjects.
[a] Mean value.
[b] Median value.
Data from Refs.[4–6,16,20,27,29,30,32,37,41,44,124–126]

leukopenia.[45] Quartuccio and colleagues[45] performed univariate and multivariate analyses on 342 pSS patients. In the 2 groups that were compared, 342 patients were positive for both the histopathology (focal lymphocytic sialadenitis with a focus score of >1 per 4 mm^2) and for anti-Ro and/or anti-La, and 206 patients were positive for with a focus score less than 1 but negative for autoantibodies.

Cryoglobulin-related markers, such as serum cryoglobulins, C3 and C4 complement factors, and serum monoclonal immunoglobulins, are considered substantial predictors of lymphoma development in patients with pSS.[10] C4 hypocomplementemia, more so than C3 hypocomplementemia, is independently associated with the development of lymphoma,[39] poor survival, morbidity such as sialadenitis, and arthritis.[46,47] Low C4 also is associated with an elevated mortality risk (hazard ratio [HR] 2.82; 95% CI, 1.73–4.58; $P<.001$).[48] There also is an association between low complement levels and clinical features, such as fever, cutaneous vasculitis, and cryoglobulinemia.[46] Sicca did not correlate with the development of lymphoma.[27,38,49] In addition, hydroxychloroquine use was not associated with cancer risk in patients with pSS nor was hydroxychloroquine associated with any protective effect on the risk of lymphoma.[50]

The alliance between pSS and intracranial malignant lymphoma remains ambiguous. Nonetheless, despite being rare, MALT lymphoma should be considered a differential diagnosis of a central nervous system mass in the pSS population and in patients with a prior treated tumor because pseudoprogression and radionecrosis must be differentiated from the tumoral development.[51] Lesions due to inflammation, demyelination, infection, or vasculitis can manifest as intracranial masses that are pseudotumoral in nature. Pseudotumoral lesions are important to identify because treatment decision and ultimately disease course are impacted. There are a few case reports of pseudotumor secondary to pSS.[52–55]

MALT lymphoma of the central nervous system is uncommon and can occur in part associated with autoimmune diseases or inflammatory sequela.[56–58] By nature, this lymphoma is indolent and treated with excision and radiotherapy. Pathologically, central nervous system MALT lymphoma is characterized by an extranodal lymphoma composed of a proliferation of centrocyte-like cells and plasmacytoid cells with lymph follicle formation resembling chronic inflammation.[57] There have been reports of intracranial primary MALT lymphoma in SS.[59,60] One such report documents the development of such lesions in the cerebellopontine angle in a female pSS patient. The tumor demonstrated inflammatory features of reactive lymphocytic infiltration with follicle formation, with slightly atypical lymphocytes and plasmacytes with diffuse dense sheets of B cells evidenced by CD20 immunostaining. These cells invaded reactive follicles, showing follicular colonization, and demonstrated aberrant expression of CD43. This all supported the diagnosis of lymphoma.[57]

MALT lymphomas involving the breast are uncommon (<0.5% of all breast malignancies). This is due to the lack of MALT in the breast. Belfeki and colleagues[61] described an unusual mammary MALT lymphoma with amyloid light chain (AL) amyloidosis in the setting of SS. Breast MALT lymphoma is reported in 1.7% to 2.2% of extranodal breast lymphoma.[62]

Cutaneous vasculitis is more frequent in pSS with non-Hodgkin lymphoma (NHL) than in the general pSS population.[63] MALT lymphomas are known to be associated with localized peritumoral amyloidosis in internal organs. It is postulated that AL-type localized nodular cutaneous amyloidosis is a manifestation of MALT lymphoma of the skin.[64] The clinical phenotype and course reflect those of primary cutaneous marginal zone lymphoma. The lymphoplasmacytic variant is now included among the larger group of extranodal B-cell lymphomas of MALT.[64]

OTHER LYMPHOMAS AND LEUKEMIAS

In addition to elevated risk of NHL in pSS (standardized incidence ratio [SIR] 11.5; 95% CI, 8.4–15.4),[49] several studies have suggested that pSS is associated with a higher risk for developing Hodgkin lymphoma.[20,65] Brito-Zerón and colleagues[20] formed the Autoimmune Diseases Study Group (GEAS) that collected a large series of Spanish patients with pSS. Among 1300 consecutive patients who fulfilled the 2002 classification criteria for pSS, 4 pSS patients had Hodgkin lymphoma (SIR 19.41; 95% CI, 7.29–51.72). The control group consisted of sex-specific and age-specific incidence rates of cancer for Spain and were estimated from national mortality data from 2012 by modeling, using a set of age-specific, sex-specific, and site-specific incidence. Mortality ratios were obtained by the aggregation of recorded data from 12 Spanish cancer registries. For Hodgkin lymphoma, mortality ratios for pSS compared with the Spanish controls were 2.6 for men and 2.2 women (age-standardized rates, per 100,000).[20] Although rare, T-cell cutaneous involvement is not completely unheard of in pSS.[66,67] Nonetheless, a majority of T-cell lymphomas associated with SS are angioimmunoblastic T-cell lymphomas.[68] Difficult to diagnose pleomorphic T-cell lymphoma also has been reported in pSS.[67]

T-cell (CD3þ) large granular lymphocyte (LGL) leukemia has been described as associated with pSS.[69] In this study, all patients at a single medical center with LGL leukemia were evaluated for pSS. Among 48 of these patients, 21 had sicca and 13 (27%) had pSS. No patient was diagnosed with pSS prior to the evaluation performed in this study. Thus, sicca as well as pSS are common among patients with LGL leukemia but the prevalence of this leukemia among a cohort of pSS patients and the relative risk for LGL leukemia in pSS are unknown.

The inclination for pSS-related lymphoma to target the parotid glands is supported by several studies.[70–72] In a conducted pooled analysis of 12 case-control studies, including 29,423 participants, SS was found associated with a 1000-fold increase in the risk of parotid gland marginal zone lymphoma and a 6.5-fold increase in the risk of NHL overall.[23]

MULTIPLE MYELOMA

Multiple myeloma is found in excess among cohorts of pSS (**Table 2**). In particular, monoclonal gammopathy in patients with pSS is reported to carry an elevated risk of developing multiple myeloma compared with pSS patients without this finding,[73] but this risk compared with the general population with monoclonal gammopathy is unknown. A recent study from Scandinavia followed 1009 pSS patients for an average of 10 years.[74] Four were diagnosed with multiple myeloma. Each pSS subject had 10 age-specific, sex-specific and residency-matched controls, among whom there were 14 diagnoses of multiple myeloma. All pSS patients with multiple myeloma had anti-Ro and 3 of the 4 had anti-La (HR 6.2 compared with controls). Both Brom and colleagues[75] and Brito- Zerón and colleagues[20] found increased multiple myeloma when comparing pSS to the general population, with SIRs of 35 to 45. Yang and colleagues[76] found monoclonal gammopathy most frequent among pSS patients compared with other inflammatory rheumatic diseases. These workers suggested screening for monoclonal gammopathy and for multiple myeloma as indicated by the presence of monoclonal gammopathy.[76] The authors conclude, given the high risk, that screening likely is warranted.

LUNG CANCER

The pulmonary manifestations of pSS include an array of airway abnormalities.[77] Pulmonary involvement of SS is now regarded both clinically and histopathologically as a

Table 2
Studies of multiple myeloma in Sjögren syndrome with calculated standardized incidence ratios and the 95% CIs

Reference, Year	Location	Number Tumor/ Cohort		Standardized Incidence Ratio (95% CI)	Follow-up Length/ Patient-Years
Kauppi et al,[125] 1997	Finland	2	676	3.4 (0.4–12.4)	22 (duration)/ 5336
Pertovaara et al,[30] 2001	Finland	1	110	8.3 (0.2–48)	15 (duration)/ 1015
Theander et al,[41] 2006	Sweden	1	286	3.27 (0.08–18.23)	8[b]/2464
Zhang et al,[4] 2010	China	2	1320	37.9 (4.58, 136.7)	4.2[a]/5544
Weng et al,[126] 2012	Taiwan	5	6911	F: 6.09 (1.98, 14.2)	3.5[a]/27,246
Brito-Zerón et al,[20,c] 2017	Spain	31	1239	36.17 (25.44, 51.43)	7.6[a], 5.5[b]/9922

Follow-up is given as length (either mean or median) with total patient-years. F, female subjects only in this study.
[a] Mean value.
[b] Median value.
[c] This study included both multiple myeloma and other immunoproliferative diseases.
Data from Refs.[4,20,30,41,125,126]

wide spectrum of lung lymphoproliferative disorders ranging from benign to malignant. The incidence rate of lung cancer in pSS has been reported to be 0.477%, with similar studies confirming this and supporting the concept that pSS has an increased risk of lung cancer (**Table 3**), with SIR 4.51 compared with the general population's incidence.[4,41,75,78]

In patients with pSS and in the SS group as a whole, there are independent and significant associations between lung cysts and anti-La seropositivity or clonally derived lymphoproliferative disorder. Lung cysts noted on chest CT could serve as a prognostic predictor of clonally derived lymphoproliferative disorder in patients with SS.[79] Another study suggested that lung cancer might be derived from cystic lesions associated with SS.[80] Lung adenocarcinoma has been associated with another entity distinct from cysts, lymphocytic interstitial pneumonitis (LIP) caused by pSS.[81] A small study examining pSS patients with lung cancer noted women were seen more frequently with adenocarcinoma as the most common pathologic type of lung cancer. pSS patients with lung cancer were noted to be significantly older than those who did not develop lung cancer, and immunosuppressant treatment might be associated with lung cancer.[78]

Unusual combinations of lung cancer have occurred in conjunction with SS. Such examples include lung adenocarcinoma in LIP associated with pSS[81] as well as a rare association of pulmonary carcinoid, lymphoma, and SS.[82] Regarding lung adenocarcinoma in LIP, histopathologic diagnosis of nodular lesion revealed papillary adenocarcinoma in LIP with marked mononuclear infiltration adjacent to papillary adenocarcinoma. This infiltrate was composed of mature plasma cells resembling plasma cell interstitial pneumonitis. Although plasma cell interstitial pneumonitis frequently is classified separately from LIP, most investigators believe that it represents a variant of LIP.[81,83] The mechanisms of plasma cell predominance, however, with respect to papillary adenocarcinoma remains to be elucidated. Nonetheless, primary lung tumors should be considered in the differential diagnosis of nodular lesions in patients with LIP associated with pSS.[81]

Table 3
Studies of lung cancer in Sjögren syndrome with calculated standardized incidence ratios and 95% CI

Reference, Year	Location	Number Tumor	/Cohort	Standardized Incidence Ratio (95% CI)	Follow-up Length/ Patient-Years
Theander et al,[41] 2006	Finland	4	286	2.71 (0.74–6.94)	8[b]/2464
Weng et al,[126] 2012	Taiwan	20	6911	F: 1.40 (0.85–2.16)	3.5[a]/27,246
		9	941	M: 1.23 (0.56, 2.33)	
Brito-Zerón et al,[20] 2017	Spain	6	1239	1.29 (0.58, 2.87)	7.6[a], 5.5[b]/9922

Follow-up is given as length (either mean or median) with total patient-years. F, female subects; M, male subjects.
[a] Mean value.
[b] Median value.
Data from Refs.[20,41,126]

Other deposition diseases that can infiltrate lung tissue are seen in conjunction with SS. According to the 2008 WHO Classification of Tumors of Hematopoietic and Lymphoid Tissues, light chain deposition disease (LCDD) belongs to the group of monoclonal immunoglobulin deposition diseases.[84,85] This disease is indolent in nature and can be the first manifestation of a previously undetected plasma cell disorder or low-grade lymphoma with plasma cell differentiation.[86] Localized LCDD is rare and often associated with a B-lymphoproliferative or plasma cell neoplasm.[85,87–92] Nodular pulmonary LCDD (NPLCDD) is uncommon and typically limited to the lung. NPLCDD frequently is seen in association with SS and/or low-grade B cell lymphoproliferative disorder.[85]

THYMUS MASSES

True thymic hyperplasia demonstrates an enlarged but histologically normal tissue, which is cured with excision,[93] whereas thymic lymphoid hyperplasia usually does not show thymic enlargement but an increased number of lymphoid follicles with hyperplastic germinal centers.[93,94] With an abnormal thymus in pSS, the differential diagnosis may include MALT lymphoma, Castleman disease, and lymphocyte predominant thymoma (type B1).[95] Multilocular thymic cysts are thought to be the consequence of cystic transformation of medullary epithelium induced by an acquired inflammatory process.[96] Thymic lesions in pSS primarily consist of extranodal MALT lymphoma and rarely consist of thymoma, thymic carcinoma, or lymphoid hyperplasia.[97] A handful of cases reporting thymic lymphoid hyperplasia associated with pSS have been documented and all were accompanied by multilocular thymic cysts.[97–100] One case report noted a diagnosis of thymic lymphoid hyperplasia with multilocular thymic cysts that subsequently led to a new diagnosis of SS based on sicca symptoms, positive serology, and pathology.[95] Multilocular thymic cysts are rare acquired multicystic lesions generally associated with autoimmune disorders (myasthenia gravis and SLE), tumors (thymoma and lymphoma), and human immunodeficiency virus infection.[101] Uncommonly multilocular thymic cysts have been noted in pSS,[100] although there are no reports of sicca symptoms improving upon thymectomy.[95]

SKIN CANCER

Skin complications of pSS are well established and include xerosis, epidermal IgG deposits, cutaneous vasculitis, and cutaneous B-cell lymphoma. To a lesser degree, alopecia, vitiligo, and papular lesions also have been attributed to pSS.[63] Regarding malignancy, a recent study has noted that patients with SLE or pSS have a significantly increased risk of nonmelanoma skin cancer. The patients most at risk were those receiving higher cumulative doses of corticosteroids and hydroxychloroquine.[102] An expedited progression of skin malignancy was not reported; however, 1 case report discussed a male pSS patient without mention of immunosuppressive treatment who rapidly developed a succession of cutaneous squamous cell carcinoma skin lesions despite undergoing surgical resection to remove the cutaneous squamous cell carcinoma on 3 separate occasions.[103]

OTHER CANCERS, INCLUDING BREAST

A summary of studies of nonlymphoma cancers among SS is given in Supplemental Table 2. Other nonlymphoid cancers, including breast cancer, also can occur in SS patients; however, an increase in the incidence of these cancers has not been demonstrated in every study.[5,75] SS has been associated with a statistically significantly reduced risk of breast cancer in a Swedish study[104]; however, another study found no difference in risk for pSS subjects compared with the general population.[105] Hemminki and colleagues[104] studied breast, uterine, and ovarian cancers among 200,000 subjects with 1 of 33 autoimmune diseases. The SIR for breast cancer among pSS patients was only 0.49; meanwhile, the HR for endometrial cancer was increased approximately 4-fold. In another large study of 209,929 US patients with breast cancer at greater than 66 years of age, however, there was no association with pSS compared with age-matched and sex-matched controls from the same database. A recent study of an Argentinian pSS cohort (n = 157) showed increased SIRs for tongue, breast, uterus, and lung cancers. Historical population controls were used as a comparison group.[75] Although an association between pSS and thyroid cancer might exist, further investigations are needed.[106] A study from China of 1320 pSS patients used historical population controls and found an increased SIR for thyroid cancer. There was 1 thyroid cancer, however, among the pSS patients. Furthermore, pSS patients likely undergo a radiological and physical examination of the neck at a much greater rate than the general population. Thus, the data are mixed and confounded concerning an association of pSS to carcinoma. The differences in these studies may be due to methodology. For instance, the use of historical population controls instead of a contemporaneous control group. In addition, ethnic differences could be important.

Diagnosis of breast cancer can be a challenge in pSS. Localized amyloidosis should be suspected in patients with consistently high serologic activity and suggestive lesions[107] because amyloid tumor of the breast has been reported in pSS, which may be suggestive of breast cancer. If nonstructural substances are noted with hematoxylin-eosin staining, Congo red staining should be added.[108] Physicians should keep in mind the possibility of overstaged breast cancer due to misinterpretation of axillary metastasis in patients with SS presenting with a breast mass. It is wise to obtain axillary node status first to correctly establish tumor stage situation of SS patient with breast cancer.[109]

In patients with pSS and a history of rapidly developing neck lymphadenopathy, potential malignancies other than lymphoma should be entertained. This includes involvement of the nasopharynx.[110] In such an instance, a biopsy of the nasopharynx is necessary to make a definitive diagnosis. The coexistence of SS with nasopharyngeal carcinoma (NPC), however, rarely has been reported.[111] Nonetheless, with pSS and NPC, significantly elevated antibody titers for Epstein-Barr virus viral capsid antigen and early antigen can be found.[111] Both pSS and NPC are related to previous Epstein-Barr virus infection.[112,113] Reduced radiation dose may need to be considered to lessen the risk of developing cranial nerve palsy in patients with pSS and head/neck carcinoma.[111]

Other areas in the head and neck region possibly are involved in an association of pSS with cancer, but diagnoses other than cancer may be found for a mass in this region. A patient with an eyelid mass subsequently was diagnosed with both pSS and localized amyloidosis of the lacrimal gland.[114] There is a report of 64-year-old woman diagnosed with pseudolymphoma of the lacrimal gland and pSS.[115] An Argentinian study of cancer in pSS found an SIR for tongue cancer approximately 50 times that found in a matched general population, but there was only 1 pSS with tongue cancer.[75] Nonetheless, tongue cancer might be increased but still uncommon among pSS patients.

Vaginal dryness can be attributed to SS. Despite a higher prevalence of dyspareunia and vaginal dryness in SS patients, no significant differences were observed between SS and the control group who were evaluated by using cervical cytology, colposcopy examination, and human papillomavirus DNA tests.[116] These data suggest that cervical cancer is not increased among pSS patients.

SARCOMA

Parotid liposarcomas have been reported rarely in adults. There has only been 1 known association with SS and parotid liposarcoma.[117] Thus, with only a single report, the authors conclude that there is no association between parotid sarcoma and pSS.

Angioimmunoblastic lymphadenopathy is a rare lymphoproliferative disorder marked by the clinical features of lymphadenopathy, hepatosplenomegaly, rash, and hypergammaglobulinemia.[118] A case report describing a patient with immunoblastic lymphadenopathy and features of SS and SLE has been reported. Clinical features included sicca syndrome, enlarged parotids, generalized lymphadenopathy, rash, alopecia, and synovitis, with positive serology (positive antinuclear antibody test, double-stranded DNA, and positive lupus band test) and hemolytic anemia. At autopsy, immunoblastic sarcoma was found that had invaded the myocardium, which stained for both κ and λ light chains by immunoperoxidase techniques.[119]

CANCER THERAPY AND SJÖGREN SYNDROME

Immunotherapy for cancer produces autoimmune disease, and the development of autoimmunity is associated with the responsiveness of the cancer. Generally organ-specific autoimmune disease, however, has been reported.[120–122] One case concerned a long-term survivor with metastatic colon carcinoma with node and lung metastases, who developed clinical, pathologic, and immunologic SS during maintenance treatment with low-dose subcutaneous metronomic interleukin (IL)-2 and granulocyte-macrophage colony-stimulating factor, which is part of GOLFIG treatment. Her symptoms of keratoconjunctivitis and sicca remained stable until the end of the maintenance treatment with IL-2 and disappeared completely a few weeks later. This case shows a possible correlation between the efficacy of treatment, long-term survival, and the occurrence of autoimmunity in a patient who received chemoimmunotherapy regimen.[123]

SUMMARY

Clinicians should closely pay attention to the possibilities of the various cancers in pSS patients. Currently recommended screening testing based on age and sex should be pursued. Cancer screening for patients with pSS should focus on NHL and multiple myeloma.[4] Skin cancer should be considered increased among pSS patients, such that thorough cancer-associated examinations with skin biopsy when appropriate should be routine. Respiratory symptoms should prompt a thorough history and physical examination. Furthermore, chest CT scanning is important for the diagnosis and assessment of lung cancer in pSS patients. Clinical stages and individualized treatments for pSS patients with possible cancer should be determined carefully.

CLINICS CARE POINTS

- There is a high risk of lymphoma, especially MALT-associated disease.
- Lymphoma most commonly affects parotid gland.
- Multiple myeloma occurs more commonly in SS. Patients should be screened for monoclonal gammopathy.
- Diagnosis and staging of breast cancer may be difficult in SS.
- Lung cancer is 5 times more frequent in SS.
- Lung cancer is associated with lung cysts.

DISCLOSURE

The authors have no commercial or financial conflicts of interest. This work was supported in part by NIH grants AR053483, AI0822714, and GM104938.

REFERENCES

1. Sjogren, H. A New Conception of Keratoconjunctivitis Sicca (Keratitis Fili- formis in Hypofunction of the Lacrymal Glands). (Translated by J. Bruce Hamilton.) Australasian Medical Publishing Company, Ltd. Glebe, N.S.W., Australia, I943.
2. Haga H, Naderi Y, Moreno AM, et al. A study of the prevalence of sicca symptoms and secondary Sjögren's syndrome in patients with rheumatoid arthritis , and its association to disease activity and treatment profile. Int J Rheum Dis 2012;15:284–8.
3. Yoshimura, Koizumi K, Satani K, et al. Gallium-67 scintigraphic findings in a patient with breast lymphoma complicated with Sjögren syndrome. Ann Nucl Med 2000;14:227–9.
4. Zhang W, Feng S, Yan S, et al. Incidence of malignancy in primary Sjögren's syndrome in a Chinese cohort. Rheumatology (Oxford) 2010;49:571–7.
5. Lazarus MN, Robinson D, Mak V, et al. Incidence of cancer in a cohort of patients with primary Sjögren's syndrome. Rheumatology (Oxford) 2006;45:1012–5.
6. Liang Y, Yang Z, Qin B, et al. Primary Sjögren's syndrome and malignancy risk: A systematic review and meta-analysis. Ann Rheum Dis 2014;73:1151–6.
7. Theander E, Manthorpe R, Jacobsson LTH. Mortality and Causes of Death in Primary Sjögren's Syndrome: A Prospective Cohort Study. Arthritis Rheum 2004;50:1262–9.
8. Kovács L, Szodoray P, Kiss E. Secondary tumours in Sjögren's syndrome. Autoimmun Rev 2010;9:203–6.
9. Nishishinya MB, Pereda CA, Muñoz-Fernández S, et al. Identification of lymphoma predictors in patients with primary Sjögren's syndrome: A systematic literature review and meta-analysis. Rheumatol Int 2015;35:17–26.
10. Retamozo S, Brito-Zerón P, Ramos-Casals M. Prognostic markers of lymphoma development in primary Sjögren syndrome. Lupus 2019;28:923–36.
11. Vasaitis L, Nordmark G, Theander E, et al. Comparison of patients with and without pre-existing lymphoma at diagnosis of primary Sjögren's syndrome. Scand J Rheumatol 2019;48:207–12.
12. Nocturne G, Virone A, Ng W-F, et al. Rheumatoid Factor and Disease Activity Are Independent Predictors of Lymphoma in Primary Sjögren's Syndrome. Arthritis Rheumatol 2016;68:977–85.

13. Schenone LN, Pellet AC, Mamani M, et al. Development of lymphoma in patients with primary Sjögren syndromes. Int J Clin Rheumtol 2019;14:69–74.

14. Jaffe ES, Harris NL, Stein H, et al. Classification of lymphoid neoplasms: The microscope as a tool for disease discovery. Blood 2008;112:4384–99.

15. Brito-Zerón P, Baldini C, Bootsma H, et al. Sjögren syndrome. Nat Rev Dis Primers 2016;2:16047.

16. Baimpa E, Dahabreh IJ, Voulgarelis M, et al. Hematologic manifestations and predictors of lymphoma development in primary sjögren syndrome: Clinical and pathophysiologic aspects. Medicine (Baltimore) 2009;88:284–93.

17. Voulgarelis M, Ziakas PD, Papageorgiou A, et al. Prognosis and outcome of non-hodgkin lymphoma in primary sjögren syndrome. Medicine (Baltimore) 2012;91:1–9.

18. Risselada AP, Kruize AA, Bijlsma JWJ. Clinical features distinguishing lymphoma development in primary Sjögren's syndrome-A retrospective cohort study. Semin Arthritis Rheum 2013;43:171–7.

19. Navarro-Mendoza EP, Aguirre-Valencia D, Posso-Osorio I, et al. Cytokine markers of B lymphocytes in minor salivary gland infiltrates in Sjögren's syndrome. Autoimmun Rev 2018;17:709–14.

20. Brito-Zerón P, Kostov B, Fraile G, et al. Characterization and risk estimate of cancer in patients with primary Sjögren syndrome. J Hematol Oncol 2017;10:90.

21. De Vita S, Gandolfo S, Zandonella Callegher S, et al. The evaluation of disease activity in Sjögren's syndrome based on the degree of MALT involvement: Glandular swelling and cryoglobulinaemia compared to ESSDAI in a cohort study. Clin Exp Rheumatol 2018;36:S150–6.

22. Anderson LA, Gadalla S, Morton LM, et al. Population-based study of autoimmune conditions and the risk of specific lymphoid malignancies. Int J Cancer 2009;125:398–405.

23. Ekström Smedby K, Vajdic CM, Falster M, et al. Autoimmune disorders and risk of non-Hodgkin lymphoma subtypes: A pooled analysis within the InterLymph Consortium. Blood 2008;111:4029–38.

24. Engels EA, Parsons R, Besson C, et al. Comprehensive evaluation of medical conditions associated with risk of non-Hodgkin lymphoma using medicare claims ('MedWAS'). Cancer Epidemiol Biomarkers Prev 2016;25:1105–13.

25. Zucca E, Conconi A, Pedrinis E, et al. Nongastric marginal zone B-cell lymphoma of mucosa-associated lymphoid tissue. Blood 2003;101:2489–95.

26. Voulgarelis M, Dafni UG, Isenberg DA, et al. Malignant lymphoma in primary Sjögren's syndrome: A multicenter, retrospective, clinical study by the European concerted action on Sjögren's syndrome. Arthritis Rheum 1999;42:1765–72.

27. Johnsen SJ, Brun JG, Gøransson LG, et al. Risk of non-Hodgkin's lymphoma in primary Sjögren's syndrome: A population-based study. Arthritis Care Res 2013;65:816–21.

28. Tzioufas AG, Boumba DS, Skopouli FN, et al. Mixed monoclonal cryoglobulinemia and monoclonal rheumatoid factor cross-reactive idiotypes as predictive factors for the development of lymphoma in Primary Sjögren's Syndrome. Arthritis Rheum 1996;39:767–72.

29. Davidson BKS, Kelly CA, Griffiths ID. Primary Sjogren's syndrome in the North East of England: A long-term follow-up study. Rheumatology (Oxford) 1999;38:245–53.

30. Pertovaara M, Pukkala E, Laippala P, et al. A longitudinal cohort study of Finnish patients with primary Sjögren's syndrome: Clinical, immunological, and epidemiological aspects. Ann Rheum Dis 2001;60:467–72.

31. Lazarus MN, Isenberg DA. Development of additional autoimmune diseases in a population of patients with primary Sjögren's syndrome. Ann Rheum Dis 2005; 64:1062–4.

32. Solans-Laqué R, López-Hernandez A, Bosch-Gil JA, et al. Risk, Predictors, and Clinical Characteristics of Lymphoma Development in Primary Sjögren's Syndrome. Semin Arthritis Rheum 2011;41:415–23.

33. Brito-Zerón P, Acar-Denizli N, Ng W-F, et al. How immunological profile drives clinical phenotype of primary Sjögren's syndrome at diagnosis: Analysis of 10,500 patients (Sjögren Big Data Project). Clin Exp Rheumatol 2018;36:S102–11.

34. Ramos-Casals M, Cervera R, Font J, et al. Young onset of primary Sjogren's syndrome: Clinical and immunological characteristics. Lupus 1998;7:202–6.

35. Seror R, Ravaud P, Bowman SJ, et al. EULAR Sjögren's syndrome disease activity index: Development of a consensus systemic disease activity index for primary Sjögren's syndrome. Ann Rheum Dis 2010;69:1103–9.

36. Golovach IY, Yehudina YD. Prognostic markers of lymphoma in primary Sjogren's syndrome. Pract Oncol 2019;2:9–23.

37. Valesini G, Priori R, Bavoillot D, et al. Differential risk of non-Hodgkin's lymphoma in Italian patients with primary Sjögren's syndrome. J Rheumatol 1997;24:2376–80.

38. Ioannidis JPA, Vassiliou VA, Moutsopoulos HM. Long-term risk of mortality and lymphoproliferative disease and predictive classification of primary Sjögren's syndrome. Arthritis Rheum 2002;46:741–7.

39. Fragkioudaki S, Mavragani CP, Moutsopoulos HM. Predicting the risk for lymphoma development in Sjogren syndrome. Medicine (Baltimore) 2016;95:1–8.

40. Skopouli FN, Dafni U, Ioannidis JPA, et al. Clinical evolution, and morbidity and mortality of primary Sjögren's syndrome. Semin Arthritis Rheum 2000;29:296–304.

41. Theander E, Henriksson G, Ljungberg O, et al. Lymphoma and other malignancies in primary Sjögren's syndrome: A cohort study on cancer incidence and lymphoma predictors. Ann Rheum Dis 2006;65:796–803.

42. Abrol E, González-Pulido C, Praena-Fernández JM, et al. A retrospective study of long-term outcomes in 152 patients with primary Sjögren's syndrome: 25-Year experience. Clin Med (Lond) 2014;14:157–64.

43. Quartuccio L, Isola M, Baldini C, et al. Biomarkers of lymphoma in Sjögren's syndrome and evaluation of the lymphoma risk in prelymphomatous conditions: Results of a multicenter study. J Autoimmun 2014;51:75–80.

44. Brito-Zerón P, Ramos-Casals M, Bove A, et al. Predicting adverse outcomes in primary Sjögren's syndrome: Identification of prognostic factors. Rheumatology (Oxford) 2007;46:1359–62.

45. Quartuccio L, Baldini C, Bartoloni E, et al. Anti-SSA/SSB-negative Sjögren's syndrome shows a lower prevalence of lymphoproliferative manifestations, and a lower risk of lymphoma evolution. Autoimmun Rev 2015;14:1019–22.

46. Brito-Zerón P, Retamozo S, Ramos-Casals M. Phenotyping Sjögren's syndrome: Towards a personalised management of the disease. Clin Exp Rheumatol 2018;36: S198–209.

47. Maślińska M, Wojciechowska B, Mańczak M, et al. Serum immunoglobulin G4 in Sjögren's syndrome: a pilot study. Rheumatol Int 2020;40:555–61.

48. Brito-Zerón P, Kostov B, Solans R, et al. Systemic activity and mortality in primary Sjögren syndrome: Predicting survival using the EULAR-SS Disease Activity Index (ESSDAI) in 1045 patients. Ann Rheum Dis 2016;75:348–55.

49. Fallah M, Liu X, Ji J, Försti A, et al. Autoimmune diseases associated with non-Hodgkin lymphoma: a nationwide cohort study. Ann Oncol 2014;25:2025–30.

50. Fang Y-F, Chen Y-F, Chung T-T, et al. Hydroxychloroquine and risk of cancer in patients with primary Sjögren syndrome: Propensity score matched landmark analysis. Oncotarget 2017;8:80461–71.
51. Leclercq D, Trunet S, Bertrand A, et al. Cerebral tumor or pseudotumor? Diagn Interv Imaging 2014;95:906–16.
52. Sassi SB, Nabli F, Boubaker A, et al. Pseudotumoral brain lesion as the presenting feature of primary Sjögren's syndrome. J Neurol Sci 2014;339:214–6.
53. Telenti-Rodríguez G, Medrano-Martínez V, Terán-Villagrá N, et al. Cerebelous Pseudotumor due to a Localized Vasculitis as First Presentation of Sjögren Syndrome. J Neurol Neurosci 2018;9:253.
54. Sanahuja J, Ordoñez-Palau S, Begué R, et al. Primary Sjögren syndrome with tumefactive central nervous system involvement. Am J Neuroradiol 2008;29:1878–9.
55. Michel L, Toulgoat F, Desal H, et al. Atypical Neurologic Complications in Patients with Primary Sjögren's Syndrome: Report of 4 Cases. Semin Arthritis Rheum 2011;40:338–42.
56. Dong R, Ji J, Liu H, et al. Primary spinal mucosa-associated lymphoid tissue lymphoma: A case report. Medicine (Baltimore) 2018;97:e9329.
57. Itoh T, Shimizu M, Kitami K, et al. Primary extranodal marginal zone B-cell lymphoma of the mucosa-associated lymphoid tissue type in the CNS. Neuropathology 2001;21:174–80.
58. Garcia-Serra A, Mendenhall NP, Hinerman RW, et al. Management of neurotropic low-grade B-cell lymphoma: Report of two cases. Head Neck 2003;25:972–6.
59. Kumar S, Kumar D, Kaldjian EP, et al. Primary low-grade B-cell lymphoma of the dura: A mucosa associated lymphoid tissue-type lymphoma. Am J Surg Pathol 1997;21:81–7.
60. Kambham N, Chang Y, Matsushima A. Primary low-grade B-cell lymphoma of mucosa-associated lymphoid tissue (MALT) arising in dura. Clin Neuropathol 1998;17:311–7.
61. Belfeki N, Bellefquih S, Bourgarit A. Breast MALT lymphoma and AL amyloidosis complicating Sjögren's syndrome. BMJ Case Rep 2019;12 [pii:e227581].
62. Hissourou M III, Zia SY, Alqatari M, et al. Primary MALT Lymphoma of the Breast Treated with Definitive Radiation. Case Rep Hematol 2016;2016:1–6.
63. Roguedas AM, Misery L, Sassolas B, et al. Cutaneous manifestation of primary Sjögren's syndrome are underestimated. Clin Exp Rheumatol 2004;22:632–6.
64. Walsh N, Lano IM, Hanly JG, et al. 164 Sjogren's syndrome and localisedlocalized nodular cutaneous amyloidosis: new insights into the link between the two. BMJ 2017. https://doi.org/10.1136/lupus-2017-000215.164.
65. Martín-Santos JM, Carretero L, Armentia A, et al. Hodgkin's disease occurring in primary Sjogren's syndrome. Ann Rheum Dis 1990;49:646–7.
66. Rustin MH, Isenberg DA, Griffiths MH, et al. Sjögren's syndrome and pleomorphic T-cell lymphoma presenting with skin involvement. J R Soc Med 1988;81:47–9.
67. Van Der Valk PGM, Hollema H, Van Voorst Vander PC, et al. Sjögren's syndrome with specific cutaneous manifestations and multifocal clonal T-cell populations progressing to a cutaneous pleomorphic T-cell lymphoma. Am J Clin Pathol 1989;92:357–61.
68. Saito M, Fukuda T, Shiohara T, et al. Angioimmunoblastic T-cell lymphoma: A relatively common type of T-cell lymphoma in Sjögren's syndrome. Clin Exp Rheumatol 2005;23(6):888–90.
69. Friedman J, Schattner A, Shvidel L, et al. Characterization of T-Cell Large Granular Lymphocyte Leukemia Associated with Sjogren's Syndrome-An Important but Underrecognized Association. Semin Arthritis Rheum 2006;35:306–11.

70. Singh A, Umarani M, Muttagi S. Refractory Sjögren's Syndrome: Is parotidectomy justified? Natl J Maxillofac Surg 2019;10:257.
71. Dispenza F, Cicero G, Mortellaro G, et al. Primary Non-Hodgkins lymphoma of the parotid gland. Braz J Otorhinolaryngol 2011;77:639–44.
72. Zenone T. Parotid gland non-Hodgkin lymphoma in primary Sjögren syndrome. Rheumatol Int 2012;32:1387–90.
73. Tomi AL, Belkhir R, Nocturne G, et al. Brief Report: Monoclonal Gammopathy and Risk of Lymphoma and Multiple Myeloma in Patients with Primary Sjögren's Syndrome. Arthritis Rheumatol 2016;68:1245–50.
74. Mofors J, Björk A, Smedby KE, et al. Increased risk of multiple myeloma in primary Sjögren's syndrome is limited to individuals with Ro/SSA and La/SSB autoantibodies. Ann Rheum Dis 2020;79:307–8.
75. Brom M, Moyano S, Gandino IJ, et al. Incidence of cancer in a cohort of patients with primary Sjögren syndrome in Argentina. Rheumatol Int 2019;39:1697–702.
76. Yang Y, et al. Monoclonal gammopathy in rheumatic diseases. Clin Rheumatol 2018;37:1751–62.
77. Flament T, Bigot A, Chaigne B, et al. Pulmonary manifestations of Sjögren's syndrome. Eur Respir Rev 2016;25:110–23.
78. Xu Y, Fei Y, Zhong W, et al. The Prevalence and clinical characteristics of primary Sjogren's syndrome patients with lung cancer: An analysis of ten cases in China and literature review. Thorac Cancer 2015;6:475–9.
79. Watanabe M, Naniwa T, Hara M, et al. Pulmonary manifestations in Sjögren's syndrome: Correlation analysis between chest computed tomographic findings and clinical subsets with poor prognosis in 80 patients. J Rheumatol 2010;37:365–73.
80. Uji M, Matsushita H, Watanabe T, et al. A case of primary Sjögren's syndrome complicated with lung adenocarcinoma. Nihon Kokyuki Gakkai Zasshi 2007; 45:409–12.
81. Takabatake N. Lung adenocarcinoma in lymphocytic interstitial pneumonitis associated with primary Sjögren's syndrome. Respirology 1999;4:181–4.
82. Taylor WSJ, Vaughan P, Trotter S, et al. A rare association of pulmonary carcinoid, lymphoma, and Sjögren syndrome. Ann Thorac Surg 2013;95:1086–7.
83. Vath RR, Alexander CB, Fulmer JD. The lymphocytic infiltrative lung diseases. Clin Chest Med 1982;3:619–34.
84. Campo E, Swerdlow SH, Harris NL, et al. The 2008 WHO classification of lymphoid neoplasms and beyond: Evolving concepts and practical applications. Blood 2011;117:5019–32.
85. Arrossi AV, Merzianu M, Farver C, et al. Nodular pulmonary light chain deposition disease: An entity associated with Sjögren syndrome or marginal zone lymphoma. J Clin Pathol 2016;69:490–6.
86. Vidal R, Goñi F, Stevens F, et al. Somatic mutations of the L12a gene in V-κ1 light chain deposition disease: Potential effects on aberrant protein conformation and deposition. Am J Pathol 1999;155:2009–17.
87. Bhargava P, Rushin JM, Rusnock EJ, et al. Pulmonary light chain deposition disease: Report of five cases and review of the literature. Am J Surg Pathol 2007;31:267–76.
88. Colombat M, Stern M, Groussard O, et al. Pulmonary Cystic Disorder Related to Light Chain Deposition Disease. Am J Respir Crit Care Med 2006;173:777–80.
89. Colombat M, Holifanjaniaina S, Guillonneau F, et al. Mass Spectrometry–based Proteomic Analysis: A Good Diagnostic Tool for Cystic Lung Light Chain Deposition Disease. Am J Respir Crit Care Med 2013;188:404–5.

90. Makis W, Derbekyan V, Novales-Diaz JA. Pulmonary light and heavy chain deposition disease: A pitfall for lung cancer evaluation with F-18 FDG PET/CT. Clin Nucl Med 2010;35:640–3.

91. Rho L, Qui L, Strauchen JA, et al. Pulmonary manifestations of light chain deposition disease. Respirology 2009;14:767–70.

92. Hirschi S, Colombat M, Kessler R, et al. Lung Transplantation for Advanced Cystic Lung Disease Due to Nonamyloid Kappa Light Chain Deposits. Ann Am Thorac Soc 2014;11:1025–31.

93. Thymic Hyperplasia - Surgical Pathology Criteria - Stanford University School of Medicine. Available at: http://surgpathcriteria.stanford.edu/thymus/thymic-hyperplasia/. Accessedth January 12, 2020.

94. Shimosato Y, Mukai K, Matsuno Y. AFIP atlas of tumor pathology: tumors of the mediastinum. Arlington, Virginia, USA: American Registry of Pathology Press; 2010.

95. Minato H, Kinoshita E, Nakada S, et al. Thymic lymphoid hyperplasia with multilocular thymic cysts diagnosed before the Sjögren syndrome diagnosis. Diagn Pathol 2015;10:4–9.

96. Suster S, Rosai J. Multilocular thymic cyst: an acquired reactive process. Study of 18 cases. Am J Surg Pathol 1991;15:388–98.

97. Izumi H, Nobukawa B, Takahashi K, et al. Multilocular thymic cyst associated with follicular hyperplasia: Clinicopathologic study of 4 resected cases. Hum Pathol 2005;36:841–4.

98. Kobayashi H, Ozeki Y, Aida S. Pulmonary and thymic lymphoid hyperplasia in primary Sjögren's syndrome. Jpn J Radiol 2009;27:107–10.

99. Kondo K, Miyoshi T, Sakiyama S, et al. Multilocular thymic cyst associated with Sjögren's syndrome. Ann Thorac Surg 2001;72:1367–9.

100. Gorospe L, García-Villanueva MJ, García-Cosío-Piqueras M, et al. Multilocular thymic cyst in a patient with Sjögren syndrome. Rheumatology (Oxford) 2019;58:369.

101. Goldman RL. Multilocular thymic cyst. Am J Surg Pathol 1992;16:89.

102. Tseng H-W, Huang W-C, Lu L-Y. The influence of immunosuppressants on the non-melanoma skin cancer among patients with systemic lupus erythematosus and primary Sjögren's syndrome: a nationwide retrospective case-control study in Taiwan. Clin Exp Rheumatol 2019;37(6):946–52.

103. Teh LS, Lai JC, Lian JC. Rapidly developed multiple face and neck skin cancers in a patient with Sjögren's syndrome: A case report. Am J Case Rep 2017;18:347–50.

104. Hemminki K, Liu X, Ji J, et al. Effect of autoimmune diseases on risk and survival in female cancers. Gynecol Oncol 2012;127:180–5.

105. Schairer C, Pfeiffer RM, Gadalla SM. Autoimmune diseases and breast cancer risk by tumor hormone-receptor status among elderly women. Int J Cancer 2018;142:1202–8.

106. Pego-Reigosa JM, Restrepo Vélez J, Baldini C, et al. Comorbidities (excluding lymphoma) in Sjögren's syndrome. Rheumatology (Oxford) 2019. https://doi.org/10.1093/rheumatology/key329.

107. Hernandez-Molina G, Faz-Munoz D, Astudillo-Angel M, et al. Coexistence of Amyloidosis and Primary Sjögren's Syndrome: An Overview. Curr Rheumatol Rev 2018;14:231–8.

108. Mori M, Kotani H, Sawaki M, et al. Amyloid tumor of the breast. Surg Case Reports 2019;5:31.

109. Cipe G, Genc V, Genc A, et al. Clinically positive axillary lymphadenopathy may lead to false diagnosis of overstaged breast cancer in patients with sjögren's syndrome: A case report. J Breast Cancer 2011;14:337–9.

110. Lal P, Gupta SD, Thakar A. Sjogren's syndrome masquerading as nasopharyngeal carcinoma. Am J Otolaryngol 2009;30:209–11.
111. Lai WS, Liu FC, Wang CH, et al. Unusual cancer in primary Sjögren syndrome. Can Fam Physician 2014;60:912–5.
112. Raab-Traub N. Epstein-Barr virus in the pathogenesis of NPC. Semin Cancer Biol 2002;12:431–41. Academic Press.
113. Igoe A, Scofield RH. Autoimmunity and infection in Sjögren's syndrome. Curr Opin Rheumatol 2013;25:480–7.
114. Kweon S-M, Koh JH, Lee H-N, et al. Primary Sjogren syndrome diagnosed simultaneously with localized amyloidosis of the lacrimal gland. Medicine (Baltimore) 2018;97:e11014.
115. Takeshita S, Sugai S, Ogawa Y, et al. A case of Sjögren's syndrome with an eyelid tumor, a so-termed pseudolymphoma of the lacrimal gland. Ryumachi 1996;36:43–9.
116. Cirpan T, Guliyeva A, Onder G, et al. Comparison of human papillomavirus testing and cervical cytology with colposcopic examination and biopsy in cervical cancer screening in a cohort of patients with Sjogren's syndrome. Eur J Gynaecol Oncol 2007;28:302–6.
117. Madiha M, Khaled K. Association rare: Syndrome de Sjögren et liposarcome de la parotide. Pan Afr Med J 2015;20:8688.
118. Vaseer S, Chakravarty EF. Musculosketal syndromes in Malignancy. In: Firestein GS, Gabriel SE, McInnes IB, et al, editors. Kelley and Firestein's Textbook of Rheumatology (tenth edition). New York: Elsiver; 2017. p. 2062–3.
119. Pierce DA, Stern R, Jaffe R, et al. Immunoblastic sarcoma with features of sjögren's syndrome and systemic lupus erythematosus in a patient with immunoblastic lymphadenopathy. Arthritis Rheum 1979;22:911–6.
120. Boutros C, Tarhini A, Routier E, et al. Safety profiles of anti-CTLA-4 and anti-PD-1 antibodies alone and in combination. Nat Rev Clin Oncol 2016;13:473–86.
121. Horvat TZ, Adel NG, Dang T-O, et al. Immune-related adverse events, need for systemic immunosuppression, and effects on survival and time to treatment failure in patients with melanoma treated with ipilimumab at memorial sloan kettering cancer center. J Clin Oncol 2015;33:3193–8.
122. Weber JS, Hodi FS, Wolchok JD, et al. Safety profile of nivolumab monotherapy: A pooled analysis of patients with advanced melanoma. J Clin Oncol 2017;35:785–92.
123. Tenti S, Correale P, Conca R, et al. Occurrence of Sjögren syndrome in a long-term survivor patient with metastatic colon carcinoma treated with GOLFIG regimen. J Chemother 2012;24:245–6.
124. Kassan SS, Thomas TL, Moutsopoulos HM, et al. Increased risk of lymphoma in sicca syndrome. Ann Intern Med 1978;89:888–92.
125. Kauppi M, Pukkala E, Isomäki H. Elevated incidence of hematologic malignancies in patients with Sjogren's syndrome compared with patients with rheumatoid arthritis (Finland). Cancer Causes Control 1997;8:201–4.
126. Weng MY, Huang YT, Liu MF, et al. Incidence of cancer in a nationwide population cohort of 7852 patients with primary Sjögren's syndrome in Taiwan. Ann Rheum Dis 2012;71:524–7.
127. Thomas E, Brewster DH, Black RJ, et al. Risk of malignancy among patients with rheumatic conditions. Int J Cancer 2000;502:497–502.
128. Landgren AM, Landgren O, Gridley G, et al. Autoimmune disease and subsequent risk of developing alimentary tract cancers among 4.5 million US male veterans. Cancer 2011;117:1163–71.

SUPPLEMENTAL TABLE 1: COMPARISON OF STANDARDIZED INCIDENCE RATIOS FOR OVERALL MALIGNANCY INCIDENCE IN PATIENTS WITH SJÖGREN SYNDROME

Author, Year	Country	Standardized Incidence Ratio (95% CI)	Malignancy (no.)	Total Number of Patients	Follow-up Time (Person- Year)
Kassan et al,[124] 1978 Only women	USA	2.2	15	142	8.1 (mean) 22 (duration) (1099)
Thomas et al,[127] 2000	Scotland	M: 0.66 (0.21, 1.54) F: 1.36 (0.98, 1.83)	M: 5 43	M: 106 F: 576	5.3 (mean) (652,133)
Pertovaara et al,[30] 2001	Finland	1.1 (0.5–2.2)	8	110	15 (duration) (1015)
Zhang et al,[4] 2010	China	3.25 (2.12, 4.52)	29	1320	4.2 (mean) (5544)
Lazarus et al,[5] 2006	Britain	2.63 (1.73, 3.99)	25	112	10.8 (mean) (1210)
Theander et al,[41] 2006	Sweden	1.42 (0.98–2.00)	33	286	8 (median) (2464)
Weng et al,[126] 2012	Taiwan	1.04 (0.91–1.18)	277	7852	3.5 (mean) (27,246)
Liang et al,[6] 2014 (up to 12/2013	Multiple	1.53 (1.17–1.88		11,889 (from 8 studies)	
Brito-Zerón et al,[20] 2017	Spain	1.91 (1.59–2.27	121	1239	7.6 (mean) 5.5 (median) (9922)

Data from Refs.[4–6,20,30,41,124,126,127]

SUPPLEMENTAL TABLE 2: STUDIES OF NONLYMPHOMA MALIGNANCY IN SJÖGREN SYNDROME

Cancer Type	Study, Year	Country	Standardized Incidence Ratio (95% CI)	Cancer Patients (no.)	Total Patients (no.)	Follow-up Time, (Person- Year)
Non-Hodgkin lymphoma	Lazarus et al,[5] 2006	Britain	1.53 (0.89–2.63)	13	112	8 (median) (2464)
Hodgkin lymphoma	Brito-Zerón et al,[20] 2017	Spain	19.41 (7.29–51.72)	4	1239	7.6 (mean) 5.5 (median) (9922)

(continued on next page)

(continued)

Cancer Type	Study, Year	Country	Standardized Incidence Ratio (95% CI)	Cancer Patients (no.)	Total Patients (no.)	Follow-up Time, (Person-Year)
Multiple myeloma	Kauppi et al,[125] 1997	Finland	3.4 (0.4–12.4)	2	676	22 (duration) (5336)
	Pertovaara et al,[30] 2001	Finland	8.3 (0.2–48)	1	110	15 (duration) (1015)
	Theander et al,[41] 2006	Sweden	3.27 (0.08–18.23	1	286	8 (median) (2464)
	Zhang et al,[4] 2010	China	37.9 (4.58, 136.7)	2	1320	4.2 (mean) (5544)
	Weng et al,[126] 2012	Taiwan	F: 6.09 (1.98–14.2)	5	6911	3.5 (mean) (27,246)
	Brito-Zerón et al,[20] 2017 (multiple myeloma and immunop-roliferative disease)	Spain	36.17 (25.44–51.43)	31	1239	7.6 (mean) 5.5 (median) (9922)
Solid tumors	Kauppi et al,[125] 1997	Finland	1.1 (0.8–1.5)	41	676	22 (duration) (5336)
	Zhang et al,[4] 2010	China	2.12 (1.27, 3.31)	19	1320	4.2 (mean) (5544)
	Brito-Zerón et al,[20] 2017	Spain	1.13 (0.88–1.46)	60	1239	7.6 (mean) 5.5 (median) (9922)
Leukemia	Kauppi et al,[125] 1997	Finland	3.6(0.8–10.6)	3	676	22 (duration) (5336)
	Brito-Zerón et al,[20] 2017	Spain	2.02 (0.65, 6.26)	3	1239	7.6 (mean) 5.5 (median) (9922)
Gastroin-testinal	Theander et al,[41] 2006	Finland	1.75 (0.76–3.46)	8	286	8 (median) (2464)
	Weng et al,[126] 2012	Taiwan	F: 1.56 (0.75, 2.86)	10	6911	3.5 (mean) (27,246)
	Brito-Zerón et al,[20] 2017 (stomach)	Spain	F: 2.53 (1.05, 6.07)	5	1145	7.6 (mean) 5.5 (median) (9922)

(continued on next page)

(continued)

Cancer Type	Study, Year	Country	Standardized Incidence Ratio (95% CI)	Cancer Patients (no.)	Total Patients (no.)	Follow-up Time, (Person-Year)
Colon	Weng et al,[126] 2012	Taiwan	F: 0.22 (0.05–0.65)	3	6911	3.5 (mean) (27,246)
	Landgren et al,[128] 2012	USA (VA)	0.99 (0.55, 1.79)	12	7349	7.47 (mean)
	Brito-Zerón et al,[20] 2017	Spain	0.89 (0.46, 1.72)	9	1239	7.6 (Mean) 5.5 (median) (9922)
Breast	Theander et al,[41] 2006	Finland	0.51 (0.10–1.48)	3	286	8 (median) (2464)
	Hemminki et al,[104] 2012	Sweden	0.46 (0.26, 0.75)	16	1516	(16,700)
	Weng et al,[126] 2012	Taiwan	0.99 (0.70, 1.36)	37	6911	3.5 (mean) (27,246)
	Brito-Zerón et al,[20] 2017	Spain	0.89 (0.53, 1.51)	14	1239	7.6 (mean) 5.5 (median) (9922)
Cervical cancer	Hemminki et al,[104] 2012	Sweden	0.83 (0.08–3.06)	2	1516	(16,700)
	Weng et al,[126] 2012	Taiwan	0.65 (0.26–1.34)	7	6911	3.5 (mean) (27,246)
	Brito-Zerón et al,[20] 2017	Spain	0.72 (0.1, 5.1)	1	1239	7.6 (mean) 5.5 (median) (9922)
Mouth and throat	Theander et al,[41] 2006	Finland	3.03 (0.08–16.88)	1	286	8 (median) (2464)
	Weng et al,[126] 2012	Taiwan	F: 1.42 (0.29, 4.16)	3	6911	3.5 (mean) (27,246)
	Landgren et al,[128] 2012	USA	1.41 (0.90, 2.22)	20	7349	7.47 (mean)
	Brito-Zerón et al,[20] 2017	Spain	F: 4.81 (1.81–12.83)	4	1145	7.6 (mean) 5.5 (median) (9922)
Thyroid	Theander et al,[41] 2006	Finland	6.86 (0.17–38.21)	1	286	8 (median) (2464)
	Weng et al,[126] 2012	Taiwan	F: 2.56 (1.40, 4.30)	14	6911	3.5 (mean) (27,246)
	Brito-Zerón et al,[20] 2017	Spain	F: 5.17 (1.94–13.79)	4	1145	7.6 (Mean) 5.5 (median) (9922)

(continued on next page)

(continued)

Cancer Type	Study, Year	Country	Standardized Incidence Ratio (95% CI)	Cancer Patients (no.)	Total Patients (no.)	Follow-up Time, (Person-Year)
Lung	Theander et al,[41] 2006	Finland	2.71 (0.74–6.94)	4	286	8 (median) (2464)
	Weng et al,[126] 2012	Taiwan	F: 1.40 (0.85–2.16) M: 1.23 (0.56, 2.33)	20 9	6911 941	3.5 (mean) (27,246)
	Brito-Zerón et al,[20] 2017	Spain	1.29 (0.58, 2.87)	6	1239	7.6 (mean) 5.5 (median) (9922)
Nonmelanoma skin cancer	Theander et al,[41] 2006	Finland	1.93 (0.23–6.98)	2	286	8 (median) (2464)
	Weng et al,[126] 2012	Taiwan	F: 1.56 (0.42–3.99)	4	6911	3.5 (mean) (27,246)
Melanoma of the skin	Brito-Zerón et al,[20] 2017	Spain	1.16 (0.29, 4.62)	2	1239	7.6 (mean) 5.5 (median) (9922)
Kidney and urinary tract	Theander et al,[41] 2006	Finland	0.77 (0.02–4.29)	1	286	8 (median) (2464)
	Weng et al,[126] 2012	Taiwan	F: 1.18 (0.38–2.76)	5	6911	3.5 (mean) (27,246)
	Brito-Zerón et al,[20] 2017	Spain	1.8 (0.58, 5.57)	3	1239	7.6 (mean) 5.5 (median) (9922)
Bladder	Weng et al,[126] 2012	Taiwan	1.77 (0.65–3.84)	6	6911	3.5 (mean) (27,246)
	Brito-Zerón et al,[20] 2017	Spain	0.95 (0.24, 3.8)	2	1239	7.6 (mean) 5.5 (median) (9922)

Data from Refs.[4–6,20,30,41,104,125,126,128]

Cancer and Systemic Lupus Erythematosus

Alexandra Ladouceur, MD, PhD[a], Basile Tessier-Cloutier, MD[b],
Ann E. Clarke, MD, MSc[c], Rosalind Ramsey-Goldman, MD, DrPh[d],
Caroline Gordon, MD[e], James E. Hansen, MD, MS[f], Sasha Bernatsky, MD, PhD[a,g],*

KEYWORDS

- Systemic lupus erythematosus • Cancer • Malignancy • Epidemiology

KEY POINTS

- Systemic lupus erythematosus (SLE) is associated with a small overall increased cancer risk compared with the general population. This risk includes a 4-fold increased risk of non-Hodgkin lymphoma, but a decreased risk of other cancers (such as breast cancer).
- The pathophysiology underlying the increased risk of hematologic cancer is not fully understood, but many potential mechanisms have been proposed, including dysfunction of the tumor necrosis factor and other pathways. Recent evidence suggests that higher disease activity itself may be associated with lymphoma risk in SLE, but not with nonhematologic malignancies.
- A decreased risk of breast, ovarian, and endometrial cancer might be driven by hormonal factors or lupus-related antibodies, but these links have not been proved.
- Cyclophosphamide may be a risk factor for hematological cancers in SLE, but this does not entirely explain the altered cancer risk profile in SLE. Exposure to hydroxychloroquine may be inversely related to breast and possibly other cancers.
- Cancer preventive methods, such as smoking cessation and regular cancer screening, remain important in the SLE population.

[a] Department of Medicine, McGill University, 1001 Decarie Boulevard, Suite D05-2212, Montreal, Quebec H4A 3J1, Canada; [b] Department of Pathology and Laboratory Medicine, University of British Columbia, Room G227 – 2211 Wesbrook Mall, Vancouver, British Columbia V6T 2B5, Canada; [c] Division of Rheumatology, University of Calgary, 3330 Hospital Drive Northwest, Calgary, Alberta T2N 4N1, Canada; [d] Division of Rheumatology, Northwestern University Feinberg School of Medicine, McGaw Pavilion, 240 East Huron Street, Suite M-300, Chicago, IL 60611, USA; [e] Rheumatology Research Group, Institute of Inflammation and Ageing, College of Medical and Dental Sciences, University of Birmingham, Birmingham, B15 2TT, UK; [f] Department of Therapeutic Radiology, Yale School of Medicine, 333 Cedar Street, New Haven, CT 06520, USA; [g] Division of Clinical Epidemiology, Research Institute of McGill University Health Centre, 5252 de Maisonneuve West, 3rd Floor, Montreal, Quebec H4A 3S5, Canada
* Corresponding author. Division of Clinical Epidemiology, Research Institute of the McGill University Health Centre, 5252 de Maisonneuve West, Office 3F.51, Montreal, Quebec H4A 3S5, Canada.
E-mail address: sasha.bernatsky@mcgill.ca

Rheum Dis Clin N Am 46 (2020) 533–550
https://doi.org/10.1016/j.rdc.2020.05.005
0889-857X/20/© 2020 Elsevier Inc. All rights reserved.

rheumatic.theclinics.com

INTRODUCTION

Over the last 2 decades, there has been an increasing interest in links between autoimmune disorders such as systemic lupus erythematosus (SLE) and cancer risk. The most recent evidence comparing SLE with the general population shows a slight increase in cancer risk overall (standardized incidence ratio [SIR], 1.14; 95% confidence interval [CI], 1.05–1.23).[1] Many recent large cohort studies and meta-analyses have also shown an increased risk of malignancy.[2–6] The underlying pathophysiologic mechanisms are still not fully understood, but possible factors include lupus-related medications, inherent immune system abnormalities,[7] overlap with Sjögren syndrome,[8] viral infections, and/or traditional cancer risk factors.[9] Although the risk in SLE for hematologic cancers, especially non-Hodgkin lymphoma (NHL), is increased about 4-fold,[1,2,10,11] breast, endometrial, and possibly ovarian cancers seem to be associated with a decreased risk in the SLE population.[1,2,12–15] This article first focuses on hematologic, lung, and other cancers with an increased risk in SLE, and then reviews the data regarding cancers for which patients with SLE may have a decreased risk.

HEMATOLOGIC CANCERS
Epidemiology

A link between hematologic cancer and SLE was initially suggested more than 3 decades ago[16] and has been supported by many studies, which suggest an increased risk of about 3-fold[1,2,10,11,17] (**Table 1**). Based on incidence and mortality data generated from the large, multicenter, international SLE cohort contributed by the Systemic Lupus International Collaborating Clinics (SLICC) and other investigators, it was observed that NHL incidence (SIR, 4.39; 95% CI, 3.48–5.49) and mortality caused by NHL (standardized mortality ratio [SMR] 2.8; 95% CI, 1.2–5.6) were particularly increased in patients with SLE, compared with the general population.[1,18] A recent systematic literature review confirmed that both lymphoma incidence and mortality are increased in SLE.[19]

Diffuse large B-cell lymphoma (DLBCL) is the most common subtype of NHL[6] and patients with SLE may present at more advanced stages at diagnosis and have a worse prognosis.[20] As in the general population, lymphoma risk in SLE increases with age.[21] Patients with SLE are also at increased risk of Hodgkin lymphoma (HL)[5,22,23] and leukemia.[1,2,10] Although many individual cohort studies were not able to show an increased risk of multiple myeloma (MM) in SLE,[1,2,6] the frequency of monoclonal gammopathy was higher than expected in 1 study[24] and a recent meta-analysis reported a moderate increased risk of MM in SLE (pooled SIR, 1.48; 95% CI, 1.02–2.14).[5] In a review of SLE MM cases, 80% of the patients were of black race/ethnicity.[22] It was not clear whether this may be caused by race/ethnicity itself versus disease activity, medication exposures, or other factors.

Pathophysiology

Increased disease activity
Disease activity has been invoked as a potential factor to explain the increased lymphoma risk in SLE (**Table 2**). One analysis has suggested that higher disease activity in SLE may be associated with greater risk of hematologic cancers, but a possible decreased risk for other cancer types.[25] Although increased disease activity has been associated with higher lymphoma risk in certain other autoimmune disorders (eg, rheumatoid arthritis [RA][26]), the association in SLE is less clear,[21,27] but there is a growing body of circumstantial evidence, which is reviewed later.

Table 1
Cancer risk profiles in systemic lupus erythematosus

Cancer Type	Risk Compared with the General Population	References
Hematologic (lymphoma, leukemia, multiple myeloma)	At least 3-fold increased risk	[1,2,10,11,17]
NHL	About 4-fold higher risk	[1,18,21]
Lung	Several studies report an increased risk	[3]
Cervical	Increased risk of squamous intraepithelial lesions (preceding cancer)	[64]
Vulva/vagina	At least 1 study found an increased risk	[1]
Head and neck	At least 1 study found an increased risk	[84]
Thyroid	Several studies report an increased risk	[5]
Bladder and kidney	A meta-analysis reported an increased risk	[5]
Liver	Several studies report an increased risk	[3]
Nonmelanoma skin	Several studies report an increased risk	[4]
Breast Ovarian Endometrial	Several studies report a decreased risk	[1,13]

Data from Refs.[1–5,10,11,13,17,18,21,64,84]

High expression of a proliferation-inducing ligand

DLBCL is the most common lymphoma subtype in SLE.[13] Because DLBCL lesions arise from activated lymphocyte (the cell line responsible for most of the inflammation in autoimmune disorders such as SLE), it may be that the chronic inflammatory state seen in patients with SLE contributes to the cancer risk. Furthermore, DLBCL lesions that develop in patients with SLE were shown to highly express APRIL (a proliferation-inducing ligand), a cytokine from the tumor necrosis factor (TNF) ligand superfamily that is essential for B-cell survival and development.[7] The investigators proposed that APRIL might mediate the development of lymphoma in SLE and other rheumatic diseases, possibly by allowing NHL B cells to escape apoptosis (see **Table 2**).[28] DLBCL is classified by gene expression into 2 major groups according to the cell of origin: germinal center B cell (GCB) or non-GCB.[29] In the general population, the GCB subtype is the most common.[30] However, most (60%) DLBCLs in SLE are non-GCB.[31] Non-GCB DLBCLs are defined by activation of the nuclear factor (NF)-κB and Janus kinase/signal transducers and activators of transcription (JAK-STAT) pathways, which are both involved in SLE through dysfunctions of A20, TNF superfamily 4 (TNFSF4), and other molecular pathways.[32]

Polymorphism of tumor necrosis factor alpha–induced protein 3 and other genetic factors

Given findings that the link between SLE and NHL may be bidirectional, potentially shared genetic risk factors are of great interest.[33] One particularly interesting potential

Table 2
Factors that have been suggested as mediating cancer risk in systemic lupus erythematosus

Cancer Type	Mechanisms Potentially Involved	References
Hematologic (including all lymphomas, leukemias, and MM)	Potential effect of disease activity (for lymphoma), but still unclear	21
	High expression of APRIL could possibly allow NHL B cells to escape apoptosis	28
	For DLBCL, single nucleotide polymorphisms including TNFSF4 and SLE IRF5. Importance of polygenic risk scores remains unclear although 1 gene (TERT) was identified as associated with both SLE and chronic lymphocytic leukemia	35,36
	SLE has increased levels of IL-6 and IL-10 and these cytokines are associated with increased NHL in the general population	44
	EBV: no clear evidence	19
	Secondary Sjögren syndrome may explain some of the increased risk	21
	Possibly increased risk with cyclophosphamide	53
Lung	Smoking is associated with increased risk	57
	No clear association with the exposure to immunosuppressive therapy	57,58
	Lung fibrosis may be associated with increased risk	57
	Genetic factors, possibly polygenic	36,58,62
Cervical and vulva/vagina	HPV infection and immunosuppressants	11,72
Head and neck	Smoking is a major risk factor in the general population, but more studies are needed to establish its role in SLE	—
	Possible decreased clearance of oncogenic viruses such as HPV and EBV	85,86
Thyroid	Thyroid antibodies are more frequent in SLE with thyroid cancer vs cancer-free patients, but their significance is unclear	89
Bladder and kidney	The role of cyclophosphamide as a causative agent in SLE remains unclear	68
Liver	Possible decreased clearance of HBV and HCV	—
Skin	Antimalarials may decrease risk, cyclophosphamide may increase risk	99
Breast	Later menarche and earlier menopause in SLE vs the general population	13
	In the general population, black and Asian people have greater risk of SLE and these race/ethnic groups have lower breast cancer risk than white people. This finding may invoke genetic factors, but to date none have been specifically identified	109
	Antimalarials might decrease the risk of breast cancer	99
	Possible subset of anti-DNA antibodies may decrease risk	110
	Highly expressed regulatory T cells may favor efficient antitumor response	115

(continued on next page)

Table 2 (continued)		
Cancer Type	**Mechanisms Potentially Involved**	**References**
Ovarian	Later menarche and earlier menopause in SLE vs the general population	13
Endometrial	Later menarche and earlier menopause in SLE vs the general population	13

Abbreviations: APRIL, a proliferation-inducing ligand; EBV, Epstein-Barr virus; HPV, human papilloma virus; IL, interleukin; IRF5, interferon regulatory factor 5; TNF, tumor necrosis factor; TNFSF4, tumor necrosis factor superfamily 4.
Data from Refs.[11,13,19,21,28,35,36,44,53,57,58,62,68,72,85,86,89,99,109,110,115]

mechanism linking lymphoma risk to autoimmune rheumatic disease is via polymorphisms of TNF-alpha–induced protein 3 (TNFAIP3), related to the A20 protein, which is important in NF-κB activation. Polymorphisms of that protein have been found in mucosa-associated lymphoid tissue lymphoma in primary Sjögren as well as in HL in RA.[34] However, in our analyses of genome-wide association studies (GWAS), data could not confirm a strong relationship with the lupus-related TNFAIP3 single nucleotide polymorphism (SNP) rs7749323 specifically for DLBCL; this could be explained by a lack of power caused by the sample size.[35] In those GWAS analyses, the rs2205960 SNP, related to TNFSF4, was associated with an odds ratio (OR) per risk allele of 1.07 (95% CI, 1.00–1.16). SLE interferon regulatory factor (IRF) risk allele rs12537284 (chromosome 7q32, IRF5 gene) was associated with an OR of 1.08 (95% CI, 0.99–1.18). The signal transducer and activator of transcription 4 (STAT4) lupus risk SNP rs7582694 was not clearly associated with DLBCL, although this could also be a sample size issue. A recent evaluation of polygenic risk scores using multiple GWAS datasets suggested that complex genetic risk factors may be shared between autoimmune diseases (including SLE) and NHL, but ultimately the autoimmune disease–related polygenic risk scores were not highly predictive of NHL risk, although in SLE a link between 1 gene (TERT) and chronic lymphocytic leukemia was noted.[36]

Polymorphism of the Fas gene and close relationships between Fas and Sle1 genes have been reported in SLE,[37–42] and defective Fas-mediated apoptosis of lymphocytes contributes to the pathophysiology of autoimmune lymphoproliferative syndrome (ALPS), a rare autosomal dominant disorder with increased risk of both autoimmunity (including many SLE manifestations: rash, nephritis, arthritis, and autoantibodies) and lymphoma. Although ALPS is an example of how a genetic defect can increase an individual's risk for both autoimmune disease and lymphoma, this specific genetic disorder does not explain most of the lymphoma cases that arise in SLE. As mentioned earlier, recent analyses of autoimmune disease GWAS data (including SLE) found more genetic commonalities with NHL than with solid cancers.[35]

Our conclusion is that TNF superfamily and perhaps interferon pathways warrant more study to determine their potential role in mediating the risk of DLBCL (particularly non-GCB type) in SLE.

The role of cytokines

Cytokines also potentially play a role in the increased risk of NHL in SLE. Patients with SLE have increased levels of interleukin (IL)-6[43] and IL-10, and these cytokines are also associated with NHL risk in the general population,[44] particularly non-GCB DLBCL,[45] the most frequent DLBCL subtype in SLE (see **Table 2**).[31,46]

Epstein-Barr virus

The Epstein-Barr virus (EBV) is suggested to have a role in the pathophysiology of SLE,[47–49] and because it is also associated with some cancers in the general population, EBV has been proposed as a potential risk factor driving cancers in SLE. EBV seropositivity is only slightly increased in patients with SLE compared with the general population, but some data indicate altered ability to clear this viral infection in SLE.[50] Increased viral load, EBV messenger RNA expression, EBV-directed antibodies, and decreased EBV-directed cell immunity have all been shown in patients with SLE compared with healthy controls.[49,50] This finding is relevant to studies of the association of SLE and cancer because EBV has been associated with several cancers known to be increased in SLE, including HL, DLBCL, and some head and neck cancers.[51] The mechanisms by which EBV promotes malignancy may involve B-cell immortalization; manipulation of host chromatin-remodeling machinery; and promoting cell migration and resistance to apoptosis through p53, BCL-2, A20, and Fas modulation.[51,52] Although links between EBV and SLE-related malignancies are interesting, there is no clear evidence of a strong role of EBV as a driver in cancer risk in SLE (see **Table 2**).[19]

Secondary Sjögren syndrome

It has been suggested that lupus-induced secondary Sjögren syndrome could account for some of the heightened risk of hematologic malignancies. Our case-cohort analyses based on the large multicenter international SLE cohort showed a trend supporting an increased risk for lymphoma development in patients with Sjögren syndrome (hazard ratio [HR], 1.79; 95% CI, 0.88–3.62).[21] Here, Sjögren syndrome was based on clinical judgment, as opposed to requiring patients to fulfill specific criteria, and thus may have been subject to nondifferential misclassification of the exposure, which could have biased this result toward the null value. Thus, it remains possible that secondary Sjögren syndrome may explain some (but not all) of the increased lymphoma risk in SLE (see **Table 2**).

Immunosuppressive therapy

Another potential cause of increased hematological malignancy is the effect of immunosuppressive therapy. Our multicenter case-cohort study reported an increased risk of hematological cancer with immunosuppressant exposure (HR, 2.29, 95% CI, 1.02–5.15).[53] When the effect was decomposed to specifically assess each drug separately, the risk after cyclophosphamide exposure was 3.55 (95% CI, 0.94–13.37); after azathioprine, 1.02 (95% CI, 0.34–3.03); and, after methotrexate, 2.57 (95% CI, 0.80–8.27). In a case-cohort study published later, most of the patients who developed lymphoma (56%) were never exposed to cyclophosphamide, azathioprine, methotrexate, or mycophenolate[21] (see **Table 2**). Moreover, the cases and the controls did not differ in their exposure to immunosuppressive treatment except for a slightly more frequent exposure to cyclophosphamide in patients diagnosed with lymphoma compared with controls (20% vs 16.8%). One of the difficulties in interpreting these results is that patients with SLE receiving potent immunosuppressive therapies, especially cyclophosphamide, are sicker and probably have higher disease activity. There is a strong association between disease activity and the increased risk of lymphoma in RA,[26] and, although the contribution of disease activity to lymphoma risk in SLE remains unclear,[21,53] it is a confounding variable that needs to be controlled for.

LUNG CANCERS
Epidemiology

Studies have systematically reported an increased risk of lung cancer with autoimmune rheumatologic conditions, including SLE,[1,3,54] RA,[55] and scleroderma.[56] It is the second most frequent cancer in SLE.[57] Patients with SLE are at increased risk not only of developing lung cancer (see **Table 1**)[3] but also of dying of it.[18] Although a potential trend toward overrepresentation of rarer types (including bronchoalveolar and carcinoid) was identified in 1 study, the overall histologic distribution was comparable with that of the general population.[58]

Pathophysiology

Smoking

Smoking may represent a shared environmental risk factor between both lung cancer and SLE. Data support an association between lupus and smoking,[59] because most lung cancer in SLE occurs in smokers.[58] In analyses of data from 49 incident lung cancer cases from a multicenter SLE cohort, 84.2% of patients were smokers compared with 40.8% of patients with SLE without lung cancer, and the association persisted in multivariate analyses (see **Table 2**).[57]

Fibrosis and inflammation

The proven link between lung cancer, inflammation, and fibrosis in the general population[60,61] invokes the possibility that alveolitis and/or pulmonary fibrosis in SLE may drive lung cancer risk. In case-cohort analyses of the multicenter international SLE dataset, there was a trend toward an increased lung malignancy risk in the patients who developed pulmonary fibrosis (unadjusted HR, 3.29; 95% CI, 0.86–12.6; and adjusted HR, 2.41; 95% CI, 0.63–9.22) (see **Table 2**).[57]

Genetic factors

Genetic associations are an interesting possible explanation for the association between SLE and lung cancer, including shared susceptibility loci on chromosome 4 (p15.1–15.3) and 6 (p21).[58] More precisely, rs13194781 and rs1270942 on the gene region 6p21-22 are of great interest, because they play a role in pathophysiologic pathways of both SLE and lung cancer (see **Table 2**).[62] Although it remains unclear how much of the increased risk of lung cancer in SLE these genetic factors may play, 1 study did suggest polygenic links between SLE and lung adenocarcinoma.[36]

Immunosuppressive therapy

There is no clear association between the risk of lung cancer and medication use in SLE. In our multicohort study assessing lung cancer risk in SLE, none of the patients who developed a lung cancer were exposed to cyclophosphamide.[57] In addition, only 20% of patients affected by lung cancer from the large international SLE cohort had previously been exposed to immunosuppressive therapy[58]; this may suggest that drugs are not the primary cause of lung cancer in patients with SLE (see **Table 2**).

CERVICAL AND VULVAR CANCERS
Epidemiology

It has constantly been shown that patients with SLE are at increased risk of developing the squamous intraepithelial lesions that precede cervical cancer development.[63–66] A recent meta-analysis reported a higher risk of high-grade squamous intraepithelial lesions in patients with SLE (OR, 8.66; 95% CI, 3.75–20.00) (see **Table 1**).[64] The magnitude of risk may vary from one country to another, because studies from countries where cervical cancer screening is effectively implemented report a considerably lower risk than the countries where the screening program is less accessible,[67] because screening identifies early-stage lesions that can be treated before progression to more advanced stages. The low incidence of cervical cancer in countries with effective screening programs (about 6.6 per 100,000 North American women) makes it a challenge to assess its relation to SLE with sufficient power. There may also be ascertainment issues, because cancer registries often do not record noninvasive malignancies, which may explain why a systematic review found a higher risk of squamous intraepithelial lesions in SLE but was not able to conclude that patients with SLE have a higher risk of cervical cancer than the general population.[63] Patients with SLE have increased risk of other malignancies that are also strongly associated with human papilloma virus (HPV),[1,11,17,54] including vulvar (SIR, 3.78; 95% CI, 1.52–7.78) and anal carcinoma (SIR, 26.9; 95% CI, 8.7–83.4).[1,68]

Pathophysiology

Human papilloma virus

It has been hypothesized that patients with SLE are more vulnerable to developing cervical dysplasia because patients with SLE are more vulnerable to infection with HPV,[11,68] particularly the high-risk aggressive variants that are linked to cervical dysplasia and cancer.[69,70] Furthermore, immunosuppressants may cause reduced clearance of HPV in SLE[71] and predispose to cervical dysplasia[71–74] (see **Table 2**). A vaccine against HPV is available and, despite the fact that the immune response engendered might be lower in patients with SLE versus the general populations, studies suggest it is safe and efficient in patients with autoimmune diseases, including SLE.[75,76] Moreover, studies of the vaccine against HPV suggested that immunogenicity at 5 years is maintained in most patients with SLE.[77] Accordingly, the US Centers for Disease Control and Prevention recommends the vaccine for any immunocompromised patients up to age 26 years.[78] The 2019 update of European League Against Rheumatism (EULAR) recommends that all patients with SLE should be vaccinated against HPV according to the recommendations for the general population.[79] In the latest recommendations for the assessment and monitoring of SLE, the Canadian Rheumatology Association does not comment on HPV vaccination.[80] As with cervical dysplasia, poor HPV clearance, caused by baseline defects and/or immunosuppression, could drive the risk of vulvar and anal cancer in SLE.[74,81]

Routine screening for cervical dysplasia is important for patients with SLE, and these examinations could also bring to clinical attention the more rare vulvar and vaginal malignancies. However, 1 study observed that female patients with SLE with the most severe disease burden (based on SLICC/American College of Rheumatology damage index scores) were the least likely to have undergone cervical screening.[82] Recent Canadian SLE guidelines recommend Pap tests annually in patients from the time they begin sexual activity until the age of 69 years.[80] EULAR guidelines recommend annual Pap tests in heavily immunosuppressed patients with SLE (eg, exposure to cyclophosphamide) but to follow local guidelines for low-risk patients.[83]

OTHER CANCERS WITH INCREASED RISK

Patients with SLE are at increased risk of other types of malignancy, including head and neck, thyroid, and liver (see **Table 1**). A recent study[84] reported an SIR for head and neck cancers of 2.16 (95% CI, 1.13–4.13) in SLE, consistent with previous data.[17] However, both of these studies were in Asian populations (which have a higher general population risk for head and neck malignancy), therefore the relevance of these data to North American and European SLE populations is uncertain. Nevertheless, a recent systematic review also found an increased risk of oropharynx and larynx cancer in SLE, indicating that these data may be generalizable to other populations.[5] Again, because head and neck malignancies may be associated with HPV[85] and potentially, in some immunosuppressed individuals, EBV,[86–88] altered viral clearance in SLE may be a risk factor for this malignancy type. Smoking cigarettes remains a major risk factor for the development of oral cancers in general, and further studies are required to determine the potential contribution of smoking specifically in SLE.

In a recent review, thyroid cancer was consistently increased in patients with SLE.[5] One study found that thyroid antibodies (antithyroglobulin and anti–thyroid peroxidase) were more frequent in patients with SLE with concomitant thyroid cancer (80%) than in cancer-free patients with SLE (31%) (see **Table 2**).[89] A similar association between thyroid autoantibodies and thyroid cancer has also been described in scleroderma.[90] The prevalence of hypothyroidism, which is often itself a manifestation of autoimmune disease, is increased in SLE, but hypothyroidism per se is not associated with an increase in the risk of developing thyroid malignancy in either lupus, scleroderma, or the general population.[91]

The conclusions of a recent meta-analysis also suggest a higher risk of both kidney (SIR, 2.10; 95% CI, 1.11–3.96) and bladder cancers (SIR, 1.86; 95% CI, 1.16–2.99).[5] Cyclophosphamide is known to increase the risk of bladder cancer in the general population,[92] although its role in SLE-related bladder cancer remains unclear.[68] Cyclophosphamide, particularly oral and high cumulative dose, has also been associated with bladder cancer in granulomatosis with polyangiitis, RA, and NHL.[93] A single study reported that the risk of bladder cancer in SLE is highest with daily oral cyclophosphamide, especially when the cumulative dose was greater than 6 g.[94] However, in SLE, intravenous cyclophosphamide is generally used, and there has long been a trend toward use of lower cumulative doses. These factors may explain why cyclophosphamide has not been found to be strongly associated with renal or bladder cancer in SLE. However, it is recommended that patients with SLE who have received cyclophosphamide should be monitored lifelong with annual urine cytology with prompt investigation of any abnormal cytology.[95]

An increased risk of liver cancer in SLE is also consistently reported in the literature; a recent meta-analysis found an SIR of 2.37 (95% CI, 1.37–3.38).[5] Although it has been proposed that decreased clearance of both hepatitis B virus (HBV) and hepatitis C virus (HCV) could contribute to this, their role in SLE remains unclear.

Many cohort studies have reported an increased risk of nonmelanoma skin cancer.[10,17,68] In a recent systematic review and meta-analysis, Song and colleagues[5] also found an increased risk of nonmelanoma skin cancer but a decreased risk of melanoma, with a pooled SIR of 0.72 (95% CI, 0.56–0.93). This finding is consistent with a previous meta-analysis that also found a lower risk of melanoma.[4] In immunosuppressed organ transplanted patients, the risks of both melanoma and nonmelanoma skin cancers are increased.[96] The increased risk in nonmelanoma skin cancer has been related to immunosuppressive therapies in inflammatory bowel disease,[97,98] and 1 study suggested an association with cyclophosphamide in SLE.[99]

DECREASED CANCER RISK IN SYSTEMIC LUPUS ERYTHEMATOSUS
Epidemiology

Patients with SLE may have a decreased incidence rate of certain cancers compared with the general population.[15] One meta-analysis of studies primarily involving patients with clinically confirmed SLE found a decreased risk of breast cancer,[13] although another meta-analysis (which included several administrative-database studies that did not clinically confirm SLE) found a pooled SIR for breast cancer of 0.89, with a CI that just included the null value (95% CI, 0.77–1.04).[5] However, in the general population, black and Asian women have lower breast cancer risk than white women; because black and Asian women may be more susceptible to SLE, some of the lower breast cancer risk in SLE could be driven by race/ethnicity (via genetic or other factors).

Several studies including a meta-analysis have suggested that ovarian and endometrial cancers may be decreased in SLE (see **Table 1**)[1,13] although 1 meta-analysis (which included large administrative-database studies that did not clinically confirm SLE) found a pooled SIR of 0.70 (95% CI, 0.46–1.07) for ovarian cancers where the 95% CI barely included the null value.[5]

Pathophysiology

Hormonal factors

Multiparity is a protective factor against ovarian cancer,[100] and long-term use of a combined oral contraceptive (COC) is associated with a decreased risk of ovarian as well as endometrial cancer in the general population.[100] However, patients with SLE tend to have fewer children than the general population, and COC use is low in SLE.[101] Because breast, endometrial, and possibly ovarian cancers are often driven by hormonal factors, it has been suggested that altered estrogen metabolism in SLE could at least in part explain the negative association between SLE and these cancers. Patients with SLE are known to have their menarche at an older age and their menopause at a younger age compared with the general population.[13,102] The result may equal a total endogenous estrogen exposure in patients with SLE, possibly explaining why they seem less inclined to develop some cancers, particularly hormone receptor–positive breast cancer.

As in the general population, the most frequent breast cancer type in SLE is ductal carcinoma, but breast cancers in SLE are more often estrogen receptor and progesterone receptor negative.[95] Although it is possible that the cancer type is influenced by the young age of patients with SLE, 1 study reported a tendency toward an increased prevalence of triple-negative breast cancers (ie, breast cancers that do not express estrogen, progesterone, and HER2 receptors) in patients with lupus.[103] These observations suggest a complex interplay of influential mechanisms, possibly linking the immune and endocrine systems to cancer risk in SLE.

Medications

There is also speculation regarding a possible protective role of certain medications used in treating patients with SLE, such as antimalarials (ie, hydroxychloroquine), in long-term cancer risk.[104] The proposed mechanism involves its role in promoting the autophagy (a form of self-induced cell death) of malignant cells.[105,106] Emerging evidence suggests that antimalarials may decrease risk of breast cancer in SLE (see **Table 2**).[99] In addition, aspirin and nonsteroidal antiinflammatory drugs (NSAIDs) have been linked with a decreased risk of some cancers in the general population.[107,108] However, there is at present no robust evidence of a clear effect of aspirin and NSAIDs on cancer risk in SLE.

Genetic factors

As noted earlier, it is possible that the cancer risk profile in SLE may be, at least in part, genetically mediated. However, analyses of GWAS data did not show any differences in the frequency of 10 SLE-related SNPs in patients with breast cancer (in the general population) compared with cancer-free controls. If decreased breast cancer risk in SLE is influenced by genetic profiles, this may be caused by complex interactions and/or epigenetic factors.[109]

Autoantibodies

Another potential explanation for the decreased risk of breast cancer in women with SLE is that lupus autoantibodies may be suppressing the emergence of certain types of malignant cells. A cell-penetrating, lupus-related, anti-DNA antibody was shown to inhibit DNA repair and to be toxic to cancer cells with intrinsic defects in DNA repair.[110] Triple-negative breast cancers are known to harbor defects in DNA repair and thus are likely to be particularly susceptible to the effects of such lupus autoantibodies. It is thus possible that suppression of triple-negative and BRCA-deficient breast cancers by anti-DNA antibodies may partly account for the lower-than-expected rates of breast cancer in women with SLE. This line of reasoning is supported by a trend for decreased ductal carcinomas in SLE, which are predominantly triple-negative breast cancers.[14,111] A cell-penetrating monoclonal antibody from a lupus mouse model that targets single-stranded DNA has received particular attention in this regard.[112] In abnormal, cancer-promoting cells carrying double-strand DNA breaks, this cell-penetrating antibody promotes cell death.[113] However, only a subset of anti-DNA antibodies are cell penetrating, and, so far, there has been no clear role for anti-DNA antibodies mediating cancer risk in SLE (see **Table 2**).[114]

Regulatory T cells

Regulatory T cells (T_{regs}) may also play a role in suppressing the development of breast cancer in SLE. T_{regs} are responsible for attenuating immune responses and in some cases may protect malignant cells from the immune system's role in deleting abnormal cancer cells, such as breast cancers. T_{regs} that are highly expressed in some breast tumors in patients who do not have lupus are associated with a poor prognosis.[115] However, because T_{reg} functions are altered in SLE, it is possible that this favors a more effective antitumor response (in SLE) from unopposed helper T cells (see **Table 2**). This specific hypothesis is still unproved.

SUMMARY

This article summarizes data published in the last decade regarding SLE and malignancy. The data regarding the relationship between medications used to treat SLE and cancer risk suggest that cyclophosphamide may be a risk factor for hematological and nonmelanoma skin cancers in SLE, but even this drug exposure only explains a small proportion of the altered cancer risk profile in SLE. Antimalarial drugs may be associated with lower risk of breast and skin cancers in SLE. Many molecular mechanisms, such as increased expression of APRIL, higher levels of IL-6 and IL-10, and polymorphism of TNFAIP3, are possibly involved in the increased risk of hematological cancers in SLE. The possible mechanism of SLE-related cell-penetrating anti-DNA antibodies in suppression of breast cancer in SLE provides a useful direction for future research. At present, promotion of preventive measures such as smoking cessation and encouraging HPV vaccination and regular cancer screening programs (particularly for cervical dysplasia) are common-sense interventions for patients with SLE.

CLINICS CARE POINTS

- At present, promotion of preventive measures such as smoking cessation and regular cancer screening programs (particularly for cervical dysplasia) are common-sense interventions for patients with SLE.

- Smoking is associated with increased lung cancer risk; Lung fibrosis may be associated with increased risk. No specific screening tests are recommended at this time.
- It has constantly been shown that patients with SLE are at increased risk of developing the squamous intraepithelial lesions that precede cervical cancer development. Patients with SLE have increased risk of other malignancies that are also strongly associated with human papilloma virus, including vulvar and anal carcinoma.
- Screening for cervical dysplasia is important for patients with SLE, and these examinations could also bring to clinical attention the more rare vulvar and vaginal malignancies. Recent Canadian SLE guidelines recommend Pap tests annually in patients from the time they begin sexual activity until the age of 69 years. EULAR guidelines recommend annual Pap tests in heavily immunosuppressed patients with SLE (eg, exposure to cyclophosphamide) but to follow local guidelines for low-risk patients
- Regarding bladder cancer, it is recommended that patients with SLE who have received cyclophosphamide should be monitored lifelong with annual urine cytology with prompt investigation of any abnormal cytology
- Skin cancer- antimalarials may decrease risk, cyclophosphamide may increase risk. No specific screening is recommended at this time.

DISCLOSURE

None.

REFERENCES

1. Bernatsky S, Ramsey-Goldman R, Labrecque J, et al. Cancer risk in systemic lupus: an updated international multi-centre cohort study. J Autoimmun 2013; 42:130–5.
2. Parikh-Patel A, White RH, Allen M, et al. Cancer risk in a cohort of patients with systemic lupus erythematosus (SLE) in California. Cancer Causes Control 2008; 19(8):887–94.
3. Ni J, Qiu LJ, Hu LF, et al. Lung, liver, prostate, bladder malignancies risk in systemic lupus erythematosus: evidence from a meta-analysis. Lupus 2014;23(3): 284–92.
4. Cao L, Tong H, Xu G, et al. Systemic lupus erythematous and malignancy risk: a meta-analysis. PLoS One 2015;10(4):e0122964.
5. Song L, Wang Y, Zhang J, et al. The risks of cancer development in systemic lupus erythematosus (SLE) patients: a systematic review and meta-analysis. Arthritis Res Ther 2018;20(1):270.
6. Tallbacka KR, Pettersson T, Pukkala E. Increased incidence of cancer in systemic lupus erythematosus: a Finnish cohort study with more than 25 years of follow-up. Scand J Rheumatol 2018;1–4. https://doi.org/10.1080/03009742. 2017.1384054.
7. Lofstrom B, Backlin C, Pettersson T, et al. Expression of APRIL in diffuse large B cell lymphomas from patients with systemic lupus erythematosus and rheumatoid arthritis. J Rheumatol 2011;38(9):1891–7.
8. Kassan SS, Thomas TL, Moutsopoulos HM, et al. Increased risk of lymphoma in sicca syndrome. Ann Intern Med 1978;89(6):888–92.

9. Bernatsky S, Boivin JF, Joseph L, et al. Prevalence of factors influencing cancer risk in women with lupus: social habits, reproductive issues, and obesity. J Rheumatol 2002;29(12):2551–4.
10. Bjornadal L, Lofstrom B, Yin L, et al. Increased cancer incidence in a Swedish cohort of patients with systemic lupus erythematosus. Scand J Rheumatol 2002; 31(2):66–71.
11. Mellemkjaer L, Andersen V, Linet MS, et al. Non-Hodgkin's lymphoma and other cancers among a cohort of patients with systemic lupus erythematosus. Arthritis Rheum 1997;40(4):761–8.
12. Dey D, Kenu E, Isenberg DA. Cancer complicating systemic lupus erythematosus–a dichotomy emerging from a nested case-control study. Lupus 2013;22(9): 919–27.
13. Bernatsky S, Ramsey-Goldman R, Foulkes WD, et al. Breast, ovarian, and endometrial malignancies in systemic lupus erythematosus: a meta-analysis. Br J Cancer 2011;104(9):1478–81.
14. Tessier Cloutier B, Clarke AE, Ramsey-Goldman R, et al. Breast cancer in systemic lupus erythematosus. Oncology 2013;85(2):117–21.
15. Gadalla SM, Amr S, Langenberg P, et al. Breast cancer risk in elderly women with systemic autoimmune rheumatic diseases: a population-based case-control study. Br J Cancer 2009;100(5):817–21.
16. Green JA, Dawson AA, Walker W. Systemic lupus erythematosus and lymphoma. Lancet 1978;2(8093):753–6.
17. Chen YJ, Chang YT, Wang CB, et al. Malignancy in systemic lupus erythematosus: a nationwide cohort study in Taiwan. Am J Med 2010;123(12):1150.e1-6.
18. Bernatsky S, Boivin JF, Joseph L, et al. Mortality in systemic lupus erythematosus. Arthritis Rheum 2006;54(8):2550–7.
19. Klein A, Polliack A, Gafter-Gvili A. Systemic lupus erythematosus and lymphoma: Incidence, pathogenesis and biology. Leuk Res 2018;75:45–9.
20. Knight JS, Blayney DW, Somers EC. Patients with systemic lupus erythematosus and haematological malignancy at a tertiary care centre: timing, histopathology and therapy. Lupus Sci Med 2014;1(1):e000051.
21. Bernatsky S, Ramsey-Goldman R, Joseph L, et al. Lymphoma risk in systemic lupus: effects of disease activity versus treatment. Ann Rheum Dis 2014; 73(1):138–42.
22. Lu M, Bernatsky S, Ramsey-Goldman R, et al. Non-lymphoma hematological malignancies in systemic lupus erythematosus. Oncology 2013;85(4):235–40.
23. Bernatsky S, Ramsey-Goldman R, Rajan R, et al. Non-Hodgkin's lymphoma in systemic lupus erythematosus. Ann Rheum Dis 2005;64(10):1507–9.
24. Ali YM, Urowitz MB, Ibanez D, et al. Monoclonal gammopathy in systemic lupus erythematosus. Lupus 2007;16(6):426–9.
25. Ladouceur A, Clarke AE, Ramsey-Goldman R, et al. Hematologic and non-hematologic cancer risk in a large inception SLE cohort. Canadian Rheumatology Association (CRA). Victoria, British Columbia, Canada, February 26–29, 2020.
26. Baecklund E, Iliadou A, Askling J, et al. Association of chronic inflammation, not its treatment, with increased lymphoma risk in rheumatoid arthritis. Arthritis Rheum 2006;54(3):692–701.
27. Koyama T, Tsukamoto H, Miyagi Y, et al. Raised serum APRIL levels in patients with systemic lupus erythematosus. Ann Rheum Dis 2005;64(7):1065–7.
28. He B, Chadburn A, Jou E, et al. Lymphoma B cells evade apoptosis through the TNF family members BAFF/BLyS and APRIL. J Immunol 2004;172(5):3268–79.

29. Rosenwald A, Wright G, Chan WC, et al. The use of molecular profiling to predict survival after chemotherapy for diffuse large-B-cell lymphoma. N Engl J Med 2002;346(25):1937–47.

30. Ennishi D, Mottok A, Ben-Neriah S, et al. Genetic profiling of MYC and BCL2 in diffuse large B-cell lymphoma determines cell-of-origin-specific clinical impact. Blood 2017;129(20):2760–70.

31. Tessier-Cloutier B, Twa DD, Baecklund E, et al. Cell of origin in diffuse large B-cell lymphoma in systemic lupus erythematosus: molecular and clinical factors associated with survival. Lupus Sci Med 2019;6(1):e000324.

32. Compagno M, Lim WK, Grunn A, et al. Mutations of multiple genes cause deregulation of NF-kappaB in diffuse large B-cell lymphoma. Nature 2009;459(7247): 717–21.

33. Wang LH, Wang WM, Lin SH, et al. Bidirectional relationship between systemic lupus erythematosus and non-Hodgkin's lymphoma: a nationwide population-based study. Rheumatology (Oxford) 2019. https://doi.org/10.1093/rheumatology/kez011.

34. Nocturne G, Boudaoud S, Miceli-Richard C, et al. Germline and somatic genetic variations of TNFAIP3 in lymphoma complicating primary Sjogren's syndrome. Blood 2013;122(25):4068–76.

35. Bernatsky S, Velasquez Garcia HA, Spinelli JJ, et al. Lupus-related single nucleotide polymorphisms and risk of diffuse large B-cell lymphoma. Lupus Sci Med 2017;4(1):e000187.

36. Din L, Sheikh M, Kosaraju N, et al. Genetic overlap between autoimmune diseases and non-Hodgkin lymphoma subtypes. Genet Epidemiol 2019;43(7): 844–63.

37. Lu MM, Ye QL, Feng CC, et al. Association of FAS gene polymorphisms with systemic lupus erythematosus: A case-control study and meta-analysis. Exp Ther Med 2012;4(3):497–502.

38. Shi X, Xie C, Kreska D, et al. Genetic dissection of SLE: SLE1 and FAS impact alternate pathways leading to lymphoproliferative autoimmunity. J Exp Med 2002;196(3):281–92.

39. Pettersson T, Pukkala E, Teppo L, et al. Increased risk of cancer in patients with systemic lupus erythematosus. Ann Rheum Dis 1992;51(4):437–9.

40. Moss KE, Ioannou Y, Sultan SM, et al. Outcome of a cohort of 300 patients with systemic lupus erythematosus attending a dedicated clinic for over two decades. Ann Rheum Dis 2002;61(5):409–13.

41. Cibere J, Sibley J, Haga M. Systemic lupus erythematosus and the risk of malignancy. Lupus 2001;10(6):394–400.

42. Lofstrom B, Backlin C, Sundstrom C, et al. A closer look at non-Hodgkin's lymphoma cases in a national Swedish systemic lupus erythematosus cohort: a nested case-control study. Ann Rheum Dis 2007;66(12):1627–32.

43. Arenas-Padilla M, Mata-Haro V. Regulation of TLR signaling pathways by microRNAs: implications in inflammatory diseases. Cent Eur J Immunol 2018;43(4): 482–9.

44. Makgoeng SB, Bolanos RS, Jeon CY, et al. Markers of Immune Activation and Inflammation, and Non-Hodgkin Lymphoma: A Meta-Analysis of Prospective Studies. JNCI Cancer Spectr 2018;2(4):pky082.

45. Qiu H, Gong S, Xu L, et al. MYD88 L265P mutation promoted malignant B cell resistance against T cell-mediated cytotoxicity via upregulating the IL-10/ STAT3 cascade. Int Immunopharmacol 2018;64:394–400.

46. Tamma R, Ingravallo G, Albano F, et al. STAT-3 RNAscope Determination in Human Diffuse Large B-Cell Lymphoma. Transl Oncol 2019;12(3):545–9.

47. James JA, Neas BR, Moser KL, et al. Systemic lupus erythematosus in adults is associated with previous Epstein-Barr virus exposure. Arthritis Rheum 2001; 44(5):1122–6.

48. James JA, Kaufman KM, Farris AD, et al. An increased prevalence of Epstein-Barr virus infection in young patients suggests a possible etiology for systemic lupus erythematosus. J Clin Invest 1997;100(12):3019–26.

49. Moon UY, Park SJ, Oh ST, et al. Patients with systemic lupus erythematosus have abnormally elevated Epstein-Barr virus load in blood. Arthritis Res Ther 2004;6(4):R295–302.

50. Draborg AH, Duus K, Houen G. Epstein-Barr virus in systemic autoimmune diseases. Clin Dev Immunol 2013;2013:535738.

51. Pattle SB, Farrell PJ. The role of Epstein-Barr virus in cancer. Expert Opin Biol Ther 2006;6(11):1193–205.

52. Saha A, Robertson ES. Epstein-Barr virus-associated B-cell lymphomas: pathogenesis and clinical outcomes. Clin Cancer Res 2011;17(10):3056–63.

53. Bernatsky S, Joseph L, Boivin JF, et al. The relationship between cancer and medication exposures in systemic lupus erythaematosus: a case-cohort study. Ann Rheum Dis 2008;67(1):74–9.

54. Hemminki K, Liu X, Ji J, et al. Effect of autoimmune diseases on risk and survival in histology-specific lung cancer. Eur Respir J 2012;40(6):1489–95.

55. De Cock D, Hyrich K. Malignancy and rheumatoid arthritis: Epidemiology, risk factors and management. Best Pract Res Clin Rheumatol 2018;32(6):869–86.

56. Maria ATJ, Partouche L, Goulabchand R, et al. Intriguing Relationships Between Cancer and Systemic Sclerosis: Role of the Immune System and Other Contributors. Front Immunol 2018;9:3112.

57. Bernatsky S, Ramsey-Goldman R, Petri M, et al. Smoking Is the Most Significant Modifiable Lung Cancer Risk Factor in Systemic Lupus Erythematosus. J Rheumatol 2018;45(3):393–6.

58. Bin J, Bernatsky S, Gordon C, et al. Lung cancer in systemic lupus erythematosus. Lung Cancer 2007;56(3):303–6.

59. Ekblom-Kullberg S, Kautiainen H, Alha P, et al. Smoking and the risk of systemic lupus erythematosus. Clin Rheumatol 2013;32(8):1219–22.

60. Franks AL, Slansky JE. Multiple associations between a broad spectrum of autoimmune diseases, chronic inflammatory diseases and cancer. Anticancer Res 2012;32(4):1119–36.

61. Hubbard R, Venn A, Lewis S, et al. Lung cancer and cryptogenic fibrosing alveolitis. A population-based cohort study. Am J Respir Crit Care Med 2000; 161(1):5–8.

62. Rosenberger A, Sohns M, Friedrichs S, et al. Gene-set meta-analysis of lung cancer identifies pathway related to systemic lupus erythematosus. PLoS One 2017;12(3):e0173339.

63. Santana IU, Gomes Ado N, Lyrio LD, et al. Systemic lupus erythematosus, human papillomavirus infection, cervical pre-malignant and malignant lesions: a systematic review. Clin Rheumatol 2011;30(5):665–72.

64. Zard E, Arnaud L, Mathian A, et al. Increased risk of high grade cervical squamous intraepithelial lesions in systemic lupus erythematosus: A meta-analysis of the literature. Autoimmun Rev 2014;13(7):730–5.

65. Kim SC, Glynn RJ, Giovannucci E, et al. Risk of high-grade cervical dysplasia and cervical cancer in women with systemic inflammatory diseases: a population-based cohort study. Ann Rheum Dis 2015;74(7):1360–7.

66. Wadstrom H, Arkema EV, Sjowall C, et al. Cervical neoplasia in systemic lupus erythematosus: a nationwide study. Rheumatology (Oxford) 2017;56(4):613–9.

67. Dugue PA, Lynge E, Rebolj M. Increased risk of high-grade squamous intraepithelial lesions in systemic lupus erythematosus: additional data from Denmark. Autoimmun Rev 2014;13(12):1241–2.

68. Dreyer L, Faurschou M, Mogensen M, et al. High incidence of potentially virus-induced malignancies in systemic lupus erythematosus: a long-term followup study in a Danish cohort. Arthritis Rheum 2011;63(10):3032–7.

69. Nath R, Mant C, Luxton J, et al. High risk of human papillomavirus type 16 infections and of development of cervical squamous intraepithelial lesions in systemic lupus erythematosus patients. Arthritis Rheum 2007;57(4):619–25.

70. Lee YH, Choe JY, Park SH, et al. Prevalence of human papilloma virus infections and cervical cytological abnormalities among Korean women with systemic lupus erythematosus. J Korean Med Sci 2010;25(10):1431–7.

71. Tam LS, Chan PK, Ho SC, et al. Risk factors for squamous intraepithelial lesions in systemic lupus erythematosus: a prospective cohort study. Arthritis Care Res (Hoboken) 2011;63(2):269–76.

72. Bernatsky S, Ramsey-Goldman R, Gordon C, et al. Factors associated with abnormal Pap results in systemic lupus erythematosus. Rheumatology (Oxford) 2004;43(11):1386–9.

73. Klumb EM, Araujo ML Jr, Jesus GR, et al. Is higher prevalence of cervical intraepithelial neoplasia in women with lupus due to immunosuppression? J Clin Rheumatol 2010;16(4):153–7.

74. Tam LS, Chan AY, Chan PK, et al. Increased prevalence of squamous intraepithelial lesions in systemic lupus erythematosus: association with human papillomavirus infection. Arthritis Rheum 2004;50(11):3619–25.

75. Grein IH, Groot N, Lacerda MI, et al. HPV infection and vaccination in Systemic Lupus Erythematosus patients: what we really should know. Pediatr Rheumatol Online J 2016;14(1):12.

76. Mok CC, Ho LY, Fong LS, et al. Immunogenicity and safety of a quadrivalent human papillomavirus vaccine in patients with systemic lupus erythematosus: a case-control study. Ann Rheum Dis 2013;72(5):659–64.

77. Mok CC, Ho LY, To CH. Long-term immunogenicity of a quadrivalent human papillomavirus vaccine in systemic lupus erythematosus. Vaccine 2018; 36(23):3301–7.

78. Markowitz LE, Dunne EF, Saraiya M, et al. Human papillomavirus vaccination: recommendations of the Advisory Committee on Immunization Practices (ACIP). MMWR Recomm Rep 2014;63(Rr-05):1–30.

79. Furer V, Rondaan C, Heijstek MW, et al. 2019 update of EULAR recommendations for vaccination in adult patients with autoimmune inflammatory rheumatic diseases. Ann Rheum Dis 2020;79(1):39–52.

80. Keeling SO, Alabdurubalnabi Z, Avina-Zubieta A, et al. Canadian Rheumatology Association Recommendations for the Assessment and Monitoring of Systemic Lupus Erythematosus. J Rheumatol 2018;45(10):1426–39.

81. Tam LS, Chan PK, Ho SC, et al. Natural history of cervical papilloma virus infection in systemic lupus erythematosus - a prospective cohort study. J Rheumatol 2010;37(2):330–40.

82. Bernatsky SR, Cooper GS, Mill C, et al. Cancer screening in patients with systemic lupus erythematosus. J Rheumatol 2006;33(1):45–9.

83. Andreoli L, Bertsias GK, Agmon-Levin N, et al. EULAR recommendations for women's health and the management of family planning, assisted reproduction, pregnancy and menopause in patients with systemic lupus erythematosus and/or antiphospholipid syndrome. Ann Rheum Dis 2017;76(3):476–85.

84. Chang SL, Hsu HT, Weng SF, et al. Impact of head and neck malignancies on risk factors and survival in systemic lupus erythematosus. Acta Otolaryngol 2013;133(10):1088–95.

85. Koslabova E, Hamsikova E, Salakova M, et al. Markers of HPV infection and survival in patients with head and neck tumors. Int J Cancer 2013;133(8):1832–9.

86. Sisk EA, Bradford CR, Carey TE, et al. Epstein-Barr virus detected in a head and neck squamous cell carcinoma cell line derived from an immunocompromised patient. Arch Otolaryngol Head Neck Surg 2003;129(10):1115–24.

87. Asten P, Barrett J, Symmons D. Risk of developing certain malignancies is related to duration of immunosuppressive drug exposure in patients with rheumatic diseases. J Rheumatol 1999;26(8):1705–14.

88. Knight A, Askling J, Granath F, et al. Urinary bladder cancer in Wegener's granulomatosis: risks and relation to cyclophosphamide. Ann Rheum Dis 2004; 63(10):1307–11.

89. Antonelli A, Mosca M, Fallahi P, et al. Thyroid cancer in systemic lupus erythematosus: a case-control study. J Clin Endocrinol Metab 2010;95(1):314–8.

90. Antonelli A, Ferri C, Ferrari SM, et al. Increased risk of papillary thyroid cancer in systemic sclerosis associated with autoimmune thyroiditis. Rheumatology (Oxford) 2016;55(3):480–4.

91. Lim H, Devesa SS, Sosa JA, et al. Trends in Thyroid Cancer Incidence and Mortality in the United States, 1974-2013. JAMA 2017;317(13):1338–48.

92. International Agency of Research on Cancer. IARC monographs on the evaluation of carcinogenic risks to humans. In: Muir CS, Wagner G, editors. Some antineoplastic and immunosuppressive agents, Vol 26. Lyon (France): International Agency for Research on Cancer; 1981. p. 411.

93. Monach PA, Arnold LM, Merkel PA. Incidence and prevention of bladder toxicity from cyclophosphamide in the treatment of rheumatic diseases: a data-driven review. Arthritis Rheum 2010;62(1):9–21.

94. Kang KY, Kim HO, Yoon HS, et al. Incidence of cancer among female patients with systemic lupus erythematosus in Korea. Clin Rheumatol 2010;29(4):381–8.

95. Tessier-Cloutier B, Clarke AE, Pineau CA, et al. What investigations are needed to optimally monitor for malignancies in SLE? Lupus 2015;24(8):781–7.

96. Collins L, Quinn A, Stasko T. Skin cancer and immunosuppression. Dermatol Clin 2019;37(1):83–94.

97. Hagen JW, Pugliano-Mauro MA. Nonmelanoma Skin Cancer Risk in Patients With Inflammatory Bowel Disease Undergoing Thiopurine Therapy: A Systematic Review of the Literature. Dermatol Surg 2018;44(4):469–80.

98. Moran GW, Lim AW, Bailey JL, et al. Review article: dermatological complications of immunosuppressive and anti-TNF therapy in inflammatory bowel disease. Aliment Pharmacol Ther 2013;38(9):1002–24.

99. Bernatsky S, Ramsey-Goldman R, Urowitz M, et al. Cancer risk in a large inception SLE cohort: effects of age, smoking and medications. ACR/ARP Annual meeting. Atlanta, GA, November 8–13, 2019.

100. Bermas BL, Sammaritano LR. Fertility and pregnancy in rheumatoid arthritis and systemic lupus erythematosus. Fertil Res Pract 2015;1:13.

101. Petri M, Kim MY, Kalunian KC, et al. Combined oral contraceptives in women with systemic lupus erythematosus. N Engl J Med 2005;353(24):2550–8.

102. Cooper GS, Dooley MA, Treadwell EL, et al. Hormonal and reproductive risk factors for development of systemic lupus erythematosus: results of a population-based, case-control study. Arthritis Rheum 2002;46(7):1830–9.

103. Chan K, Clarke AE, Ramsey-Goldman R, et al. Breast cancer in systemic lupus erythematosus (SLE): receptor status and treatment. Lupus 2018;27(1):120–3.

104. Ruiz-Irastorza G, Ugarte A, Egurbide MV, et al. Antimalarials may influence the risk of malignancy in systemic lupus erythematosus. Ann Rheum Dis 2007;66(6):815–7.

105. Amaravadi RK. Autophagy-induced tumor dormancy in ovarian cancer. J Clin Invest 2008;118(12):3837–40.

106. Rahim R, Strobl JS. Hydroxychloroquine, chloroquine, and all-trans retinoic acid regulate growth, survival, and histone acetylation in breast cancer cells. Anti-cancer Drugs 2009;20(8):736–45.

107. Akhmedkhanov A, Toniolo P, Zeleniuch-Jacquotte A, et al. Aspirin and lung cancer in women. Br J Cancer 2002;87(1):49–53.

108. Moran EM. Epidemiological and clinical aspects of nonsteroidal anti-inflammatory drugs and cancer risks. J Environ Pathol Toxicol Oncol 2002;21(2):193–201.

109. Bernatsky S, Easton DF, Dunning A, et al. Decreased breast cancer risk in systemic lupus erythematosus: the search for a genetic basis continues. Lupus 2012;21(8):896–9.

110. Hansen JE, Chan G, Liu Y, et al. Targeting cancer with a lupus autoantibody. Sci Transl Med 2012;4(157):157ra142.

111. Pathology of familial breast cancer: differences between breast cancers in carriers of BRCA1 or BRCA2 mutations and sporadic cases. Breast Cancer Linkage Consortium. Lancet 1997;349(9064):1505–10.

112. Rattray Z, Dubljevic V, Rattray NJW, et al. Re-engineering and evaluation of anti-DNA autoantibody 3E10 for therapeutic applications. Biochem Biophys Res Commun 2018;496(3):858–64.

113. Noble PW, Bernatsky S, Clarke AE, et al. DNA-damaging autoantibodies and cancer: the lupus butterfly theory. Nat Rev Rheumatol 2016;12(7):429–34.

114. Bernatsky S, Ramsey-Goldman R, Petri M, et al. Breast cancer in systemic lupus. Lupus 2017;26(3):311–5.

115. Bates GJ, Fox SB, Han C, et al. Quantification of regulatory T cells enables the identification of high-risk breast cancer patients and those at risk of late relapse. J Clin Oncol 2006;24(34):5373–80.

Cancer and Scleroderma

Emma Weeding, MD, Livia Casciola-Rosen, PhD,
Ami A. Shah, MD, MHS*

KEYWORDS

- Scleroderma • Malignancy • Autoantibodies • Epidemiology • Cancer screening

KEY POINTS

- Scleroderma may be a paraneoplastic phenomenon in unique patient subgroups, including those with anti-RNA polymerase III antibodies or those who are negative for centromere, topoisomerase 1, or RNA polymerase III antibodies.
- All patients with new-onset scleroderma should undergo comprehensive physical examination and age-based, sex-based, and risk factor–based cancer screening tests.
- Recent data suggest that autoantibody and cutaneous subtype may define cancer risk, type, and timing in scleroderma. If validated, these findings may inform the development of targeted cancer screening guidelines.

EPIDEMIOLOGY OF CANCER IN PATIENTS WITH SCLERODERMA

Most epidemiologic studies have shown that individuals with scleroderma have an increased age-adjusted and sex-adjusted risk of developing cancer, with this risk generally ranging from 1.5 to 4 times higher than that of the general population.[1–14] Although it is beyond the scope of this article to discuss all of these studies, particular attention is drawn to 3 meta-analyses that have both quantified the magnitude of cancer risk and examined the particular tumor types that are enriched in scleroderma.

Onishi and colleagues[9] examined 6 population-based cohort studies comprising a total of 6641 people with scleroderma from Australia, northern Europe, Taiwan, and the United States. They found a pooled standardized incidence ratio (SIR) of 1.41 for cancer overall, with a trend toward a greater risk in men than women (SIR, 1.85 vs 1.33 respectively). With regard to particular tumors types that were enriched in these cohorts, they found an increased risk of lung, liver, and hematologic cancers overall, as well as an increased risk of bladder cancer in women and nonmelanomatous skin cancer in men. In contrast, there was no increased risk of breast cancer,

Funding: This work was supported by grants from the NIH/NIAMS (R01 AR073208) and the Donald B. and Dorothy L. Stabler Foundation.
Division of Rheumatology, Johns Hopkins University School of Medicine, 5200 Eastern Avenue, Mason F. Lord Building, Center Tower, Suite 4100, Baltimore, MD 21224, USA
* Corresponding author.
E-mail address: Ami.Shah@jhmi.edu

although the investigators excluded cases of cancer that were diagnosed before the onset of scleroderma. The temporal clustering of breast cancer and scleroderma, with either diagnosis arising shortly before the other, has been well described in the literature and is discussed in more detail later.[15–18] They likewise did not find an increased risk of other sex-specific cancers such as prostate, cervical, or uterine cancer. A contemporaneous meta-analysis by Zhang and colleagues[14] found similar results, with increased SIRs for lung cancer, hematopoietic cancer, and non-Hodgkin lymphoma, but not breast cancer.

Bonifazi and colleagues[2] conducted the largest meta-analysis to date using 16 observational studies, which included most of the articles examined by Onishi and colleagues[9] and Zhang and colleagues[14] as mentioned earlier. Compared with the general population, the relative risk (RR) of cancer in scleroderma was 1.75, with particularly strong associations between scleroderma and lung cancer (RR, 4.35) and hematologic neoplasms (RR, 2.24). Of the included studies assessing liver cancer or esophageal cancer, all showed an increased risk, with SIRs ranging from 3.30 to 7.35 and 2.86 to 35.0, respectively. Available data for the incidence of stomach, pancreas, skin, and oral cavity cancers were conflicting, and the investigators again did not find an increased risk of any sex-specific cancers.

The development of particular tumor types in scleroderma may in part depend on the severity and pattern of a given individual's end-organ involvement and/or the immunosuppressive medications they have received, although these associations have not been consistently characterized in the literature. These potential mechanisms linking cancer and scleroderma are discussed in more detail later.

Other demographic and phenotypic features of scleroderma that have been variably associated with an increased risk of cancer in early studies include older age of onset of scleroderma,[1,19–22] male sex,[6,8,9] smoking history,[23] and diffuse cutaneous involvement,[5] although these findings have not been consistently reproduced. Scleroderma autoantibody status, particularly anti-RNA polymerase III (anti-POLR3) positivity, has a dramatic effect on the overall risk and timing of cancer and may account for the discordant results from previous studies that did not control for this effect. This aspect of risk stratification is discussed in more detail elsewhere in this review.

POTENTIAL MECHANISMS LINKING CANCER AND SCLERODERMA

The relationship between cancer and scleroderma is likely complex and bidirectional. Cancers may emerge around the time of scleroderma onset or years after scleroderma diagnosis. These temporal relationships raise the question of whether malignancies or cancer treatments could trigger the development of scleroderma in some patients, whereas scleroderma or scleroderma therapies could increase the risk of subsequent cancer development in others. It is also possible that both diseases share a common inciting exposure or genetic predisposition.[24]

Data suggest that scleroderma disease activity and damage, particularly within individual organs, may predispose to malignant transformation within the same target tissues. For instance, patients with scleroderma may have a higher risk of esophageal cancer associated with severe reflux and Barrett esophagus, lung cancer in the context of known interstitial lung disease (ILD), liver cancer if there is overlap primary biliary cirrhosis, or thyroid cancer if there is autoimmune thyroiditis.[1,12,25,26] Data conflict as to whether scleroderma-ILD is a risk factor for lung cancer,[1,6,9,23,27] but the higher risk of lung cancers in patients with anti–topoisomerase 1 antibodies and reduced forced vital capacity is suggestive.[28] In a Japanese cohort of patients with scleroderma, risk factors for cancer were examined; all 10 lung cancer cases occurred in patients with ILD.[4] Interestingly, of the 4 patients who had autopsies in this study, the primary lung cancer was found in tissue affected by ILD in all cases.

Another possibility is that cytotoxic therapies used to treat scleroderma could increase the risk of subsequent cancer. Cyclophosphamide is an alkylating agent that has been used to treat severe scleroderma cutaneous and pulmonary disease. Data from vasculitis, scleroderma, and lupus suggest that the risk of hematologic and bladder cancers may be increased with exposure to cyclophosphamide, in particular with higher cumulative doses and in smokers.[29–33] Increasingly, mycophenolate mofetil is used to treat active cutaneous disease, ILD, and myositis in scleroderma. The data on cancer risk with mycophenolate in the rheumatic diseases are less clear, as most of the studies are from the transplant area, where patients are often treated with combinations of immunosuppressive drugs. Data in the transplantation literature conflict as to whether there is a higher risk of lymphoproliferative diseases and non-melanoma skin cancers,[34–37] with 1 recent report suggesting a higher risk of primary central nervous system lymphoma.[38] The data on cancer risk with immunosuppressive drugs in patients with scleroderma are limited. In our cohort, we have not observed an increased risk of cancer with immunosuppressive drug use, including cyclophosphamide and mycophenolate mofetil.[22] Whether these agents could directly promote malignant transformation is unclear. In the lupus literature, it has been postulated that immunosuppressive drugs may inhibit clearance of oncogenic viral infections, thereby increasing the risk of virus-associated cancers.[24,33] For discussion of other immunomodulatory agents commonly used in the rheumatic diseases and cancer risk, readers are referred to a recent review by Cappelli and colleagues.[39]

It is also important to note that patients with scleroderma may have a high cumulative exposure to ionizing radiation from medical tests over time, including plain radiographs, computed tomography (CT), and nuclear medicine studies.[40] This exposure could potentially increase the risk of cancer development.

A subset of patients develops scleroderma after cancer diagnosis and therapy. Cancer therapeutics, including chemotherapy, radiation therapy, and immunotherapy, may increase the risk of developing scleroderma. Case reports describe the development of scleroderma-like fibrosing syndromes and critical digital ischemia after exposure to bleomycin, gemcitabine, paclitaxel, and carboplatin.[41–46] Radiation therapy may trigger both cutaneous and pulmonary fibrosis; most reports describe localized scleroderma or exaggerated fibrosis developing in patients with known scleroderma.[1,47–49] It remains unclear whether de novo scleroderma could be a consequence of radiation exposure. A newer cancer therapeutic class, immune checkpoint inhibitors, works by blocking negative costimulatory receptors or ligands on T cells and antigen-presenting cells. These drugs can cause nonspecific T-cell activation and have resulted in several rheumatic immune-related adverse events. Recently, features resembling scleroderma have been reported after therapy with pembrolizumab or nivolumab (both PD-1 [programmed cell death protein 1] inhibitors).[50–53] Critical digital ischemia after immune checkpoint inhibitor therapy has also been reported.[54]

A close temporal relationship between the onset of cancer and scleroderma has been found in certain individuals, raising the question of whether scleroderma could be a paraneoplastic disease. This finding was initially observed in case reports and case series across a range of tumor types, although with particularly striking temporal clustering of breast cancer and scleroderma.[12,15–18] In 1 series, the breast cancer–scleroderma interval was 12 months or less in 27 of 44 individuals (61.4%), with simultaneous disease onset in 11 (25%).[17] Nearly half of this cohort was diagnosed with breast cancer before the onset of scleroderma. Further supporting the idea of scleroderma as a paraneoplastic phenomenon are reports of cancer treatment resulting in dramatic improvements in scleroderma.[55,56] Although it has been challenging to discern whether this improvement is due to cancer treatment or simply the use of potent immunosuppression, a recent report of a patient improving solely with resection of tumor suggests that cancer itself may be a driver of scleroderma.[57]

UNIQUE AUTOANTIBODIES IDENTIFY PATIENT SUBGROUPS WITH A HIGH RISK OF CANCER-ASSOCIATED SCLERODERMA

Given data suggesting that scleroderma could be a paraneoplastic disease, our group hypothesized that tumor antigen expression might be associated with scleroderma-specific autoantibody responses. In an initial study of 23 individuals with both cancer and scleroderma, we found that those with anti-POLR3 antibodies had a significantly shorter cancer-scleroderma interval compared with those with anti–topoisomerase 1 or anticentromere antibodies (medians of -1.2 years, $+13.4$ years, and $+11.1$ years, respectively).[58] Furthermore, participants who had anti-POLR3 antibodies had robust nucleolar expression of RNA polymerase III in their cancerous cells, which was not found in cancer cells from the other antibody groups or in healthy control tissues.

This association between anti-POLR3 antibodies and increased risk of concurrent cancer and scleroderma onset has since been reproduced in multiple international cohorts, including from Australia, Italy, Japan, and the United Kingdom.[20,21,59,60] Recently, this finding was validated in the European League Against Rheumatism Scleroderma Trials and Research group (EUSTAR) cohort.[19] A total of 4986 individuals with scleroderma from 13 participating EUSTAR centers were included, and 158 participants with anti-POLR3 antibodies were compared with 199 anti-POLR3–negative controls matched for sex, cutaneous phenotype, age of scleroderma onset, and disease duration. Cancer was significantly more common in the anti-POLR3–positive group (17.7% vs 9.0%), particularly with respect to cancers diagnosed within 2 years of scleroderma onset (9.0% vs 2.5%). Individuals with a synchronous onset of cancer and scleroderma in the setting of anti-POLR3 antibodies were significantly older at scleroderma onset and more likely to have diffuse cutaneous disease. The risk of concurrent-onset nonbreast cancers and scleroderma was also significantly higher in men than in women. These demographic and phenotypic risk factors are consistent with the findings from early epidemiologic studies as discussed earlier.

The findings in our pilot study have also been validated using a much larger cohort of 1044 individuals from the Johns Hopkins Scleroderma Center cohort.[22] Logistic regression analyses were used to evaluate the relationship of overall cancer risk and a shortened cancer-scleroderma interval with autoantibody status, demographic features, and scleroderma phenotypic features. Once again, anti-POLR3 positivity was associated with a significantly increased risk of cancer diagnosis within 2 years of scleroderma onset (odds ratio, 5.08). There was also an increased temporal clustering of cancer and scleroderma in the group of participants who were negative for anticentromere, anti–topoisomerase I, and anti-POLR3 antibodies (CTP negative).

A major limitation of these prior studies was that cancer risk was investigated in patients with scleroderma with a given autoantibody compared with patients with scleroderma who were negative for that specificity. This study design does not permit determination of the magnitude or types of cancer at high risk compared with the general population, information that is needed to inform cancer screening strategies in scleroderma. To address this limitation, the authors examined cancer incidence within 3 years of scleroderma onset (ie, cancer-associated scleroderma) in distinct serologic and phenotypic groups and compared this with the US Surveillance, Epidemiology, and End Results (SEER) cancer registry.[61] Of 2383 participants with scleroderma, 205 (~9%) had a history of cancer. Patients with anti-POLR3 antibodies and CTP-negative patients had a 2.8-fold and 1.8-fold increased risk of cancer within 3 years of scleroderma onset, respectively (**Fig. 1**). Within 3 years of scleroderma onset, patients with anti-POLR3 antibodies and diffuse cutaneous disease had a higher risk of breast cancer (SIR, 5.14), prostate cancer (SIR, 7.17), and tongue cancer (SIR, 43.9), whereas patients with anti-POLR3 antibodies and limited cutaneous disease had an increased risk of lung cancer (SIR, 10.4). Similarly, within 3 years of scleroderma onset, CTP-negative patients with limited scleroderma had a higher risk of

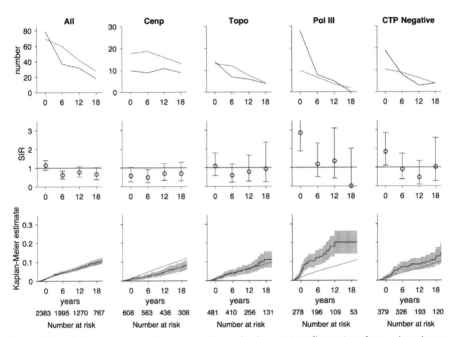

Fig. 1. Risk of all cancers over time. In each graph, the x-axis reflects time from scleroderma onset (defined as time zero). (*Top and middle rows*) Each time window represents a 6-year period (±3 years); for example, data plotted at time zero reflect cancer risk within plus or minus 3 years of scleroderma onset. The number at risk for each time window is denoted at the bottom of the graph. (*Top row*) The observed number of cancer cases (*blue*) is presented in comparison with the number of cancer cases that are expected based on SEER data (*red*). (*Middle row*) The ratio between the observed and expected cancer cases is presented as an SIR along with its 95% confidence interval. Values of 1 denote a cancer risk equivalent to that of the background population. (*Bottom row*) The cumulative incidence of cancer among patients with scleroderma (*solid blue line*) starting at 3 years before scleroderma onset is presented with 95% confidence intervals (*shaded blue region*). Red lines represent the expected cumulative incidence of cancer based on SEER data for the general population. Patients with scleroderma with anticentromere antibodies seem to have a decreased risk of cancer over time. Patients with scleroderma with anti-POLR3 antibodies and the CTP-negative group have an increased risk of cancer that is prominent at scleroderma onset. The cumulative incidence of cancer is significantly higher than that observed in the general population among patients with anti-POLR3 antibodies. Cenp, centromere; Topo, topoisomerase-1; Pol III, RNA polymerase III. (*From* Igusa T, Hummers LK, Visvanathan K, et al. Autoantibodies and scleroderma phenotype define subgroups at high-risk and low-risk for cancer. Ann Rheum Dis. 2018;77(8):1179-1186; with permission.)

breast cancer (SIR, 4.44) and melanoma (SIR, 7.10), and CTP-negative patients with diffuse scleroderma had an increased risk of tongue cancer (SIR, 40.5). When examining overall cancer risk, patients with anticentromere antibodies had a significantly lower risk of cancer than that expected in the general population (SIR, 0.59; see **Fig. 1**).

The CTP-negative subgroup in scleroderma is a heterogeneous population that likely consists of patients with many different scleroderma immune responses. It remains an important priority to identify the distinct subpopulations within CTP-negative patients, because this may guide risk stratification for cancer. Recently, our group has focused on autoantibody discovery in CTP-negative individuals in whom cancers were detected close to the time of scleroderma onset. In an initial investigation, phage immunoprecipitation sequencing was used for autoantibody discovery in participants who were either CTP negative with synchronous cancer and scleroderma, or had anti-POLR3 antibodies with or without cancer.[62] This method identified antibodies against the RNA binding region containing 3 (RNPC3), a component of the minor spliceosome complex, in 4 of 16 (25%) in the CTP-negative group and in none (0 of 32) in the anti-POLR3–positive group. These findings were subsequently reproduced in a larger population of 318 people with scleroderma and cancer.[63] Among them, a total of 12 (3.8%) had anti-RNPC3 antibodies. Compared with those with anticentromere antibodies, individuals with anti-RNPC3 or anti-POLR3 antibodies had a significantly higher risk of developing cancer within 2 years of scleroderma onset, with odds ratios of 4.3 and 4.5 respectively. Interestingly, 66.7% of the cancers in the anti-RNPC3 group were gynecologic tumors in women, with 50% having breast cancer, although this did not reach statistical significance across antibody subgroups because of small sample sizes.

The association between scleroderma-specific antibodies and cancer risk is likely limited to individuals who manifest clinical features of autoimmune disease and thus far does not seem to inform cancer risk in the general population. In a case control study of 50 women with breast cancer and 50 matched healthy controls (all without rheumatologic disease), all participants were negative for anti-POLR3 antibodies except for 1 control who was only borderline positive.[64] Similarly, anti-RNPC3 antibodies have not been detected in small comparison cohorts of healthy controls, patients with pancreatic cancer without rheumatic disease, and patients with lupus and cancer.[63]

EVIDENCE FOR A MODEL OF CANCER-INDUCED AUTOIMMUNITY

The striking co-occurrence of cancer and scleroderma onset in individuals with anti-POLR3 antibodies suggests a possible mechanistic link between the two disease processes and raised the question that cancer might be the trigger initiating autoimmunity in this subset of people. This possibility was investigated in a landmark study of tumors obtained from 16 patients with scleroderma, 8 of whom had anti-POLR3 antibodies, and 8 lacking these antibodies (they had antibodies against topoisomerase 1 or centromere, the two other prominent scleroderma antibody specificities).[65] In 6 of 8 (75%) cancers from the anti-POLR3–positive patients, alterations in the *POLR3A* gene locus were found. In contrast, none were detected in the tumors from the other 8 patients. Of the 6 patients with genetic abnormalities in *POLR3A*, 3 were somatic mutations; in each, this resulted in a single amino acid change (different in each patient). Furthermore, in 2 of these 3 patients, T cells that reacted with the mutated neoantigens were detected in peripheral blood. Given the rarity of POLR3A mutations in cancer, these findings are consistent with initiation of the anti-POLR3 immune response by such somatic mutations. A second kind of genetic alteration was found in this study: 5 out of 8 patients had loss of heterozygosity (LOH) at the *POLR3A* gene locus. Because LOH was not detected in the cancers from the 8 patients lacking anti-POLR3 antibodies, it is likely that the anti-POLR3 antibody response participates in shaping cancer evolution.

Anti-POLR3 antibodies in the patients with somatic mutations cross-reacted with both the mutated and wild-type RNA polymerase III protein.[65] These data suggest a model of cancer-induced autoimmunity in scleroderma, where the anti-POLR3 immune response is initiated against the mutated protein in the cancer (ie, an anti-tumor immune response), followed by subsequent spreading to the wild-type protein (**Fig. 2**).[66] In susceptible hosts, this cross-reactive immune response could damage target tissue and become self-sustaining, resulting in scleroderma propagation.

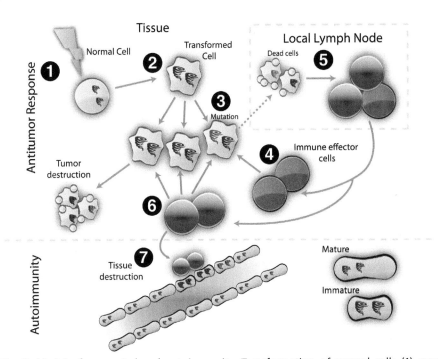

Fig. 2. Model of cancer-induced autoimmunity. Transformation of normal cells (1) may result in gene expression patterns that resemble immature cells involved in tissue healing (2). Occasionally, autoantigens become mutated (3); these are not driver mutations, and not all cancer cells have them. The first immune response is directed against the mutated form of the antigen (4), and may spread to the wild-type version (5). Immune effector cells directed against the mutant (*red*) delete exclusively cancer cells containing the mutation (6). Immune effector cells directed against the wild-type (*blue*) delete cancer cells without the mutation and also cross-react with the patient's own tissues (particularly immature cells expressing high levels of antigen, found in damaged/repairing tissue) (7). Once autoimmunity has been initiated, the disease is self-propagating. Immature cells (expressing high antigen levels) that repair the immune-mediated injury can themselves become the targets of the immune response, sustaining an ongoing cycle of damage/repair that provides the antigen source that fuels the autoimmune response. (*From* Shah AA, Casciola-Rosen L, Rosen A. Review: cancer-induced autoimmunity in the rheumatic diseases. Arthritis Rheumatol. 2015;67(2):317-326.; with permission.)

Additional studies are warranted to examine whether the mechanisms identified for RNA polymerase III apply more broadly to other subgroups with a high risk of cancer-associated scleroderma, such as patients with anti-RNPC3 antibodies.

CANCER PROTECTIVE IMMUNE RESPONSES MAY MODIFY CANCER RISK IN SCLERODERMA

Although the data suggesting a cancer-induced autoimmunity model in patients with scleroderma with anti-POLR3 antibodies are compelling, it is striking that 80% to 85% of these patients remain cancer free even over a prolonged period of follow-up. Could cancer be the initial trigger for scleroderma in patients with anti-POLR3 antibodies, with the subsequent antitumor response varying in its ability to eliminate the cancer or keep it in equilibrium without cancer emergence? Well-recognized features of the immune response include intramolecular and intermolecular spreading. That many scleroderma antibody specificities target multicomponent complexes, with multiple components being recognized by the antibody, is consistent with antigenic spreading. These features raised the question of whether targeting of additional autoantigens by the immune response could be cancer protective in anti-POLR3–positive patients with scleroderma.

To investigate this, our group identified 168 individuals with scleroderma and anti-POLR3 antibodies (based on clinically available assays and confirmed by enzyme-linked immunosorbent assay) with a roughly even mix of individuals with cancer or without cancer after at least 5 years of follow-up.[67] A comparison of the antibody profiles (generated by immunoprecipitation and visualized by fluorography) in these two subgroups showed clear enrichment of a 194-kDa protein targeted by antibodies in the cancer-negative group. This protein was subsequently identified as the catalytic subunit of RNA polymerase 1 (RPA194). When the full cohort was tested for antibodies against RPA194, anti-RPA194 was found to be significantly more common in the entire group without cancer (18.2%) compared with the group with cancer (3.8%), suggesting a potentially protective effect.

These findings raise the possibility that combinations of immune responses may have a previously unappreciated role in controlling cancer. They also highlight that knowledge of biomarkers that precisely define homogenous disease subgroups will enable improved precision in cancer prediction in relevant subsets. For instance, although patients with anti-POLR3 antibodies have a significantly increased risk of cancer-associated scleroderma that warrants intensive cancer detection strategies, patients with both anti-POLR3 and anti-RPA194 may not require additional cancer screening at scleroderma onset.

IMPLICATIONS FOR CANCER SCREENING

Given compelling data suggesting a model of cancer-induced autoimmunity in subsets of patients with scleroderma, important clinical questions arise. Do patients with new-onset scleroderma require intensive cancer detection strategies? If so, how do clinicians direct the right cancer screening tests to the appropriate patients, such that they maximize detection while minimizing the harms (ie, false-positive results and costs) of overscreening? If cancer is detected and treated early, could this effectively treat scleroderma and improve outcomes? Although there is not a strong evidence base to guide clinical decision making at this time, we share our current approach to cancer screening here.

Rheumatologists and primary care providers should ensure that all patients with scleroderma undergo comprehensive physical examination and age-based, sex-based, and risk factor–based cancer screening tests according to recommen-dations for the general population.[68,69] Additional cancer screening studies may be considered based on the presence of scleroderma-specific risk factors. For example, patients with severe reflux that is refractory to standard proton pump inhib-itor or H_2 blocker therapy should be referred for upper endoscopy to evaluate for Barrett esophagus, and serial endoscopies may be required if there is evidence of dysplasia or severe erosive esophagitis.[70] Patients with a persistent globus sensa-tion or unexplained dysphagia may need otolaryngology evaluation given the increased risk of head and neck cancers in scleroderma.[61,71] If cirrhosis has devel-oped, for instance because of primary biliary cirrhosis overlap, the American Asso-ciation for the Study of Liver Diseases has recommended cross-sectional imaging with or without alpha fetoprotein assessment at intervals of 6 to 12 months.[72] Hema-tology referral may be warranted in patients with new, unexplained cytopenias. There may be a role for serial chest CT or low-dose chest CT monitoring for the development of lung cancer in patients with scleroderma with ILD, but this requires further study. Exposure to immunosuppressive therapies may also be an important risk factor. Patients with prior cyclophosphamide exposure may benefit from annual urinalysis and urine cytology, whereas patients treated with mycophenolate mofetil should be advised to report any new or changing skin lesions. If there is a history of extensive sun exposure or prior skin cancers, serial full skin examinations to eval-uate for atypical lesions should be considered.

Although there are no published studies assessing cancer screening strategies in scleroderma, the data showing an increased risk of cancer around the time of sclero-derma onset in distinct autoantibody subsets raises the question of whether aggres-sive cancer detection strategies should be considered. In dermatomyositis, another rheumatic disease where a mechanism of cancer-induced autoimmunity has been postulated, aggressive cancer screening measures, including CT of the chest, abdomen, and pelvis, and whole body PET-CT, are often performed clinically. Whether a similar approach in high-risk patients with scleroderma, such as those with anti-POLR3 antibodies or CTP-negative patients, would add value beyond tradi-tional cancer screening tests requires further study. However, the data suggest that there may be a role for targeted cancer detection strategies based on autoantibody type and clinical phenotype.[61] For instance, anti-POLR3–positive patients with diffuse scleroderma have an increased risk of breast, prostate, and tongue cancer, suggest-ing a role for mammography, PSA assessment and prostate examination, and otolar-yngology examination in these patients. Similarly, anti-POLR3–positive patients with limited scleroderma have an increased risk of lung cancer, suggesting a role for chest CT examination. Additional studies are underway to define the optimal approach to cancer screening in these high-risk subsets that maximizes cancer detection while minimizing the harms of overscreening.[73]

SUMMARY

The increased risk of cancer in scleroderma may be caused by multiple mechanisms, with biological data suggesting the development of cancer-induced autoimmunity in some patients. Recent epidemiologic studies indicate that autoantibody status and clinical phenotype may be useful filters to identify patient subgroups at high risk or low risk for cancer in scleroderma. Further work is needed to test the value of targeted cancer detection strategies in scleroderma, and to define whether early cancer detec-tion and treatment improves scleroderma outcomes. It is also likely that careful inves-tigation at the scleroderma-cancer interface may provide insight into mechanisms of naturally occurring antitumor immunity and development of autoimmunity in the rheumatic diseases.

CLINICS CARE POINTS

- Scleroderma may be a paraneoplastic phenomenon in unique patient subgroups, including those with anti-RNA polymerase III antibodies or those who are negative for centromere, topoisomerase 1, or RNA polymerase III antibodies (CTP negative).
- All patients with new-onset scleroderma should undergo comprehensive physical examination and age-based, sex-based, and risk factor–based cancer screening tests.
- Recent data suggest that autoantibody and cutaneous subtype may define cancer risk, type, and timing in scleroderma. If validated, these findings may inform the development of targeted cancer screening guidelines.

DISCLOSURE

The authors have nothing to disclose.

REFERENCES

1. Abu-Shakra M, Guillemin F, Lee P. Cancer in systemic sclerosis. Arthritis Rheum 1993;36(4):460–4.
2. Bonifazi M, Tramacere I, Pomponio G, et al. Systemic sclerosis (scleroderma) and cancer risk: systematic review and meta-analysis of observational studies. Rheumatology (Oxford) 2013;52(1):143–54.
3. Derk CT, Rasheed M, Artlett CM, et al. A cohort study of cancer incidence in systemic sclerosis. J Rheumatol 2006;33(6):1113–6.
4. Hashimoto A, Arinuma Y, Nagai T, et al. Incidence and the risk factor of malignancy in Japanese patients with systemic sclerosis. Intern Med 2012;51(13): 1683–8.
5. Hill CL, Nguyen AM, Roder D, et al. Risk of cancer in patients with scleroderma: a population based cohort study. Ann Rheum Dis 2003;62(8):728–31.
6. Kang KY, Yim HW, Kim IJ, et al. Incidence of cancer among patients with systemic sclerosis in Korea: results from a single centre. Scand J Rheumatol 2009;38(4):299–303.
7. Kuo CF, Luo SF, Yu KH, et al. Cancer risk among patients with systemic sclerosis: a nationwide population study in Taiwan. Scand J Rheumatol 2012;41(1):44–9.
8. Olesen AB, Svaerke C, Farkas DK, et al. Systemic sclerosis and the risk of cancer: a nationwide population-based cohort study. Br J Dermatol 2010;163(4): 800–6.
9. Onishi A, Sugiyama D, Kumagai S, et al. Cancer incidence in systemic sclerosis: meta-analysis of population-based cohort studies. Arthritis Rheum 2013;65(7): 1913–21.
10. Rosenthal AK, McLaughlin JK, Linet MS, et al. Scleroderma and malignancy: an epidemiological study. Ann Rheum Dis 1993;52(7):531–3.
11. Rosenthal AK, McLaughlin JK, Gridley G, et al. Incidence of cancer among patients with systemic sclerosis. Cancer 1995;76(5):910–4.
12. Roumm AD, Medsger TA. Cancer and systemic sclerosis. An epidemiologic study. Arthritis Rheum 1985;28(12):1336–40.

13. Siau K, Laversuch CJ, Creamer P, et al. Malignancy in scleroderma patients from south west England: a population-based cohort study. Rheumatol Int 2011;31(5): 641–5.

14. Zhang J-Q, Wan Y-N, Peng W-J, et al. The risk of cancer development in systemic sclerosis: a meta-analysis. Cancer Epidemiol 2013;37(5):523–7.

15. Duncan SC, Winkelmann RK. Cancer and scleroderma. Arch Dermatol 1979; 115(8):950–5.

16. Forbes AM, Woodrow JC, Verbov JL, et al. Carcinoma of breast and scleroderma: four further cases and a literature review. Br J Rheumatol 1989;28(1):65–9.

17. Launay D, Le Berre R, Hatron P-Y, et al. Association between systemic sclerosis and breast cancer: eight new cases and review of the literature. Clin Rheumatol 2004;23(6):516–22.

18. Lee P, Alderdice C, Wilkinson S, et al. Malignancy in progressive systemic sclerosis–association with breast carcinoma. J Rheumatol 1983;10(4):665–6.

19. Lazzaroni M-G, Cavazzana I, Colombo E, et al. Malignancies in patients with Anti-RNA Polymerase III antibodies and systemic sclerosis: analysis of the EULAR scleroderma trials and research cohort and possible recommendations for screening. J Rheumatol 2017;44(5):639–47.

20. Moinzadeh P, Fonseca C, Hellmich M, et al. Association of anti-RNA polymerase III autoantibodies and cancer in scleroderma. Arthritis Res Ther 2014;16(1):R53.

21. Nikpour M, Hissaria P, Byron J, et al. Prevalence, correlates and clinical usefulness of antibodies to RNA polymerase III in systemic sclerosis: a cross-sectional analysis of data from an Australian cohort. Arthritis Res Ther 2011; 13(6):R211.

22. Shah AA, Hummers LK, Casciola-Rosen L, et al. Examination of autoantibody status and clinical features associated with cancer risk and cancer-associated scleroderma. Arthritis Rheumatol 2015;67(4):1053–61.

23. Pontifex EK, Hill CL, Roberts-Thomson P. Risk factors for lung cancer in patients with scleroderma: a nested case-control study. Ann Rheum Dis 2007;66(4): 551–3.

24. Egiziano G, Bernatsky S, Shah AA. Cancer and autoimmunity: harnessing longitudinal cohorts to probe the link. Best Pract Res Clin Rheumatol 2016;30(1): 53–62.

25. Trivedi PJ, Lammers WJ, van Buuren HR, et al. Stratification of hepatocellular carcinoma risk in primary biliary cirrhosis: a multicentre international study. Gut 2016;65(2):321–9.

26. Antonelli A, Ferri C, Ferrari SM, et al. Increased risk of papillary thyroid cancer in systemic sclerosis associated with autoimmune thyroiditis. Rheumatology (Oxford) 2016;55(3):480–4.

27. Peters-Golden M, Wise RA, Hochberg M, et al. Incidence of lung cancer in systemic sclerosis. J Rheumatol 1985;12(6):1136–9.

28. Colaci M, Giuggioli D, Sebastiani M, et al. Lung cancer in scleroderma: results from an Italian rheumatologic center and review of the literature. Autoimmun Rev 2013;12(3):374–9.

29. Faurschou M, Sorensen IJ, Mellemkjaer L, et al. Malignancies in Wegener's granulomatosis: incidence and relation to cyclophosphamide therapy in a cohort of 293 patients. J Rheumatol 2008;35(1):100–5.

30. Kasifoglu T, Yasar Bilge S, Yildiz F, et al. Risk factors for malignancy in systemic sclerosis patients. Clin Rheumatol 2016;35(6):1529–33.

31. Monach PA, Arnold LM, Merkel PA. Incidence and prevention of bladder toxicity from cyclophosphamide in the treatment of rheumatic diseases: a data-driven review. Arthritis Rheum 2010;62(1):9–21.

32. Bernatsky S, Ramsey-Goldman R, Joseph L, et al. Lymphoma risk in systemic lupus: effects of disease activity versus treatment. Ann Rheum Dis 2014;73(1): 138–42.

33. Dreyer L, Faurschou M, Mogensen M, et al. High incidence of potentially virus-induced malignancies in systemic lupus erythematosus: a long-term followup study in a Danish cohort. Arthritis Rheum 2011;63(10):3032–7.

34. Bichari W, Bartiromo M, Mohey H, et al. Significant risk factors for occurrence of cancer after renal transplantation: a single center cohort study of 1265 cases. Transplant Proc 2009;41(2):672–3.

35. Brewer JD, Colegio OR, Phillips PK, et al. Incidence of and risk factors for skin cancer after heart transplant. Arch Dermatol 2009;145(12):1391–6.

36. Marcen R, Galeano C, Fernandez-Rodriguez A, et al. Effects of the new immunosuppressive agents on the occurrence of malignancies after renal transplantation. Transplant Proc 2010;42(8):3055–7.

37. Wang K, Zhang H, Li Y, et al. Safety of mycophenolate mofetil versus azathioprine in renal transplantation: a systematic review. Transplant Proc 2004;36(7): 2068–70.

38. Crane GM, Powell H, Kostadinov R, et al. Primary CNS lymphoproliferative disease, mycophenolate and calcineurin inhibitor usage. Oncotarget 2015;6(32): 33849–66.

39. Cappelli LC, Shah AA. The relationships between cancer and autoimmune rheumatic diseases. Best Pract Res Clin Rheumatol 2020;101472. PMID: 32029389.

40. Picano E, Semelka R, Ravenel J, et al. Rheumatological diseases and cancer: the hidden variable of radiation exposure. Ann Rheum Dis 2014;73(12):2065–8.

41. Berger CC, Bokemeyer C, Schneider M, et al. Secondary Raynaud's phenomenon and other late vascular complications following chemotherapy for testicular cancer. Eur J Cancer 1995;31A(13–14):2229–38.

42. Bessis D, Guillot B, Legouffe E, et al. Gemcitabine-associated scleroderma-like changes of the lower extremities. J Am Acad Dermatol 2004;51(2 Suppl):S73–6.

43. Clowse ME, Wigley FM. Digital necrosis related to carboplatin and gemcitabine therapy in systemic sclerosis. J Rheumatol 2003;30(6):1341–3.

44. Cohen IS, Mosher MB, O'Keefe EJ, et al. Cutaneous toxicity of bleomycin therapy. Arch Dermatol 1973;107(4):553–5.

45. De Angelis R, Bugatti L, Cerioni A, et al. Diffuse scleroderma occurring after the use of paclitaxel for ovarian cancer. Clin Rheumatol 2003;22(1):49–52.

46. Finch WR, Rodnan GP, Buckingham RB, et al. Bleomycin-induced scleroderma. J Rheumatol 1980;7(5):651–9.

47. Colver GB, Rodger A, Mortimer PS, et al. Post-irradiation morphoea. Br J Dermatol 1989;120(6):831–5.

48. Shah DJ, Hirpara R, Poelman CL, et al. Impact of radiation therapy on scleroderma and cancer outcomes in scleroderma patients with breast cancer. Arthritis Care Res (Hoboken) 2018;70(10):1517–24.

49. Varga J, Haustein UF, Creech RH, et al. Exaggerated radiation-induced fibrosis in patients with systemic sclerosis. Jama 1991;265(24):3292–5.

50. Barbosa NS, Wetter DA, Wieland CN, et al. Scleroderma induced by pembrolizumab: a case series. Mayo Clin Proc 2017;92(7):1158–63.

51. Suárez-Díaz S, Coto-Hernández R, Yllera-Gutiérrez C, et al. Scleroderma-like syndrome associated with pembrolizumab. J Scleroderma Relat Disord 2020. Available at: https://journals.sagepub.com/doi/10.1177/2397198320905192.

52. Tjarks BJ, Kerkvliet AM, Jassim AD, et al. Scleroderma-like skin changes induced by checkpoint inhibitor therapy. J Cutan Pathol 2018;45(8):615–8.

53. Cho M, Nonomura Y, Kaku Y, et al. Scleroderma-like syndrome associated with nivolumab treatment in malignant melanoma. J Dermatol 2019;46(1):e43–4.

54. Khaddour K, Singh V, Shayuk M. Acral vascular necrosis associated with immune-check point inhibitors: case report with literature review. BMC Cancer 2019;19(1):449.

55. Hasegawa M, Sato S, Sakai H, et al. Systemic sclerosis revealing T-cell lymphoma. Dermatology 1999;198(1):75–8.

56. Juarez M, Marshall R, Denton C, et al. Paraneoplastic scleroderma secondary to hairy cell leukaemia successfully treated with cladribine. Rheumatology (Oxford) 2008;47(11):1734–5.

57. Bruni C, Lages A, Patel H, et al. Resolution of paraneoplastic PM/Scl-positive systemic sclerosis after curative resection of a pancreatic tumour. Rheumatology (Oxford) 2017;56(2):317–8.

58. Shah AA, Rosen A, Hummers L, et al. Close temporal relationship between onset of cancer and scleroderma in patients with RNA polymerase I/III antibodies. Arthritis Rheum 2010;62(9):2787–95.

59. Airo P, Ceribelli A, Cavazzana I, et al. Malignancies in Italian patients with systemic sclerosis positive for anti-RNA polymerase III antibodies. J Rheumatol 2011;38(7):1329–34.

60. Saigusa R, Asano Y, Nakamura K, et al. Association of anti-RNA polymerase III antibody and malignancy in Japanese patients with systemic sclerosis. J Dermatol 2015;42(5):524–7.

61. Igusa T, Hummers LK, Visvanathan K, et al. Autoantibodies and scleroderma phenotype define subgroups at high-risk and low-risk for cancer. Ann Rheum Dis 2018;77(8):1179–86.

62. Xu GJ, Shah AA, Li MZ, et al. Systematic autoantigen analysis identifies a distinct subtype of scleroderma with coincident cancer. Proc Natl Acad Sci U S A 2016; 113(47):E7526–34.

63. Shah AA, Xu G, Rosen A, et al. Brief report: anti-RNPC-3 antibodies as a marker of cancer-associated scleroderma. Arthritis Rheumatol 2017;69(6):1306–12.

64. Shah AA, Rosen A, Hummers LK, et al. Evaluation of cancer-associated myositis and scleroderma autoantibodies in breast cancer patients without rheumatic disease. Clin Exp Rheumatol 2017;35(Suppl 106 4):71–4.

65. Joseph CG, Darrah E, Shah AA, et al. Association of the autoimmune disease scleroderma with an immunologic response to cancer. Science 2014; 343(6167):152–7.

66. Shah AA, Casciola-Rosen L, Rosen A. Review: cancer-induced autoimmunity in the rheumatic diseases. Arthritis Rheumatol 2015;67(2):317–26.

67. Shah AA, Laiho M, Rosen A, et al. Protective effect against cancer of antibodies to the large subunits of both RNA polymerases I and III in scleroderma. Arthritis Rheumatol 2019;71(9):1571–9.

68. Shah AA, Casciola-Rosen L. Cancer and scleroderma: a paraneoplastic disease with implications for malignancy screening. Curr Opin Rheumatol 2015;27(6): 563–70.

69. Shah AA, Kuwana M. Cancer in systemic sclerosis. In: Varga J, Denton CP, Wigley FM, et al, editors. Scleroderma: from pathogenesis to comprehensive management. 2nd edition. New York: Springer; 2016. p. 525–32.

70. Shaheen NJ, Weinberg DS, Denberg TD, et al. Upper endoscopy for gastro-esophageal reflux disease: best practice advice from the clinical guidelines committee of the American College of Physicians. Ann Intern Med 2012;157(11): 808–16.

71. Derk CT, Rasheed M, Spiegel JR, et al. Increased incidence of carcinoma of the tongue in patients with systemic sclerosis. J Rheumatol 2005;32(4):637–41.

72. Lindor KD, Gershwin ME, Poupon R, et al. Primary biliary cirrhosis. Hepatology 2009;50(1):291–308.

73. Shah AA, Casciola-Rosen L. Mechanistic and clinical insights at the scleroderma-cancer interface. J Scleroderma Relat Disord 2017;2(3):153–9.

Risk Factors and Cancer Screening in Myositis

Siamak Moghadam-Kia, MD, MPH[a,b], Chester V. Oddis, MD[a,c],
Dana P. Ascherman, MD[d], Rohit Aggarwal, MD, MSc[a,c,*]

KEYWORDS

- Idiopathic inflammatory myopathies • Dermatomyositis • Cancer screening

KEY POINTS

- The idiopathic inflammatory myopathies, particularly dermatomyositis, are associated with an increased risk of cancer.
- Clinical risk factors for cancer-associated myositis include older age at disease onset, male gender, dysphagia, cutaneous necrosis, ulceration and vasculitis, rapid onset of myositis, and refractory myositis.
- Autoantibodies associated with greatest increase in the risk of cancer in myositis include anti–TIF1-gamma and antinuclear matrix protein-2.

INTRODUCTION

The idiopathic inflammatory myopathies (IIMs) are a group of heterogeneous, systemic autoimmune rheumatic diseases that include adult polymyositis (PM), adult dermatomyositis (DM), necrotizing myopathy (NM), myositis associated with another autoimmune disease, cancer-associated myositis, juvenile myositis (mostly juvenile DM [JDM]), and inclusion body myositis (IBM). The IIMs are multisystemic diseases that can affect many organs, including skeletal muscle, skin, lungs, joints, and the esophagus. An association between IIM and cancer is well-established by epidemiologic evidence from numerous large population studies.[1–5] The association is strong for patients with DM and less for PM, uncertain for NM or IBM, and not

No financial conflicts of interest or any funding source relevant to this article.
[a] Myositis Center, Division of Rheumatology and Clinical Immunology, Department of Medicine, University of Pittsburgh, 3601 5th Avenue, Suite 2B, Pittsburgh, PA 15261, USA; [b] VA Pittsburgh Healthcare System, Pittsburgh, 4100 Allequippa St, Pittsburgh, PA 15219, USA; [c] UPMC Arthritis and Autoimmunity Center, Falk Medical Building, 3601 Fifth Avenue, Suite 2B, Pittsburgh, PA 15213, USA; [d] Division of Rheumatology and Clinical Immunology, Department of Medicine, Myositis Center, University of Pittsburgh School of Medicine, 1218 Scaife Hall, 3550 Terrace Street, Pittsburgh, PA 15261, USA
* Corresponding author. Division of Rheumatology and Clinical Immunology, Department of Medicine, University of Pittsburgh, 3601 5th Avenue, Suite 2B, Pittsburgh, PA 15261.
E-mail address: aggarwalr@upmc.edu

present with JDM. The precise pathophysiologic links between cancer and myositis are not well-understood. In this review, we evaluate the risk stratification for cancer in myositis based on clinical and serologic features, including screening strategies.

DEFINITION AND TIMING OF CANCER-ASSOCIATED MYOSITIS

The association between inflammatory myopathy and cancer has led to the term cancer-associated myositis, generally referring to cancer that typically develops within 3 years of the diagnosis of myositis.[1–5] Although most cancers are diagnosed simultaneously with or during the first year after the diagnosis of myositis,[2,6] the cancer risk gradually decreases over 3 to 5 years and remains increased compared with the general population, particularly in DM.[6–10] Adenocarcinomas of the lung, ovaries, breast, cervix, bladder, pancreas, and upper and lower gastrointestinal tract, along with hematologic malignancies including Hodgkin lymphoma, are among the most commonly reported myositis-associated cancers.[2,5] However, the risk and distribution of malignancies may be influenced by genetic background and ethnicity. For example, southeast Asia has a higher frequency of nasopharyngeal, lung, and hematopoietic malignancies associated with DM.[6] Although the treatment of cancer may result in improvement or even resolution of myositis, a new myositis diagnosis or its recurrence has been reported with cancer relapse.[2,6]

Cancer Risk Based on Disease Subsets

Cancer risk is significantly higher in DM compared with PM, with reported standardized incidence ratios (SIRs) nearly double that of PM. In a meta-analysis of case control and cohort studies including 1078 myositis subjects (565 PM and 513 DM) with a comparable number of controls, the overall odds ratio (OR) for associated cancers with DM and PM was 4.4 and 2.1, respectively.[7] SIRs from large population-based studies in Denmark,[4] Australia,[3] Scotland,[2] and Taiwan[6] range from approximately 3.0 to 7.7 in DM and 1.3 to 2.1 in PM. In a Taiwan national health insurance database of 1012 DM and 643 PM patients from 1997 to 2007 with no prior malignancy history, there were 95 cancers (9.4%) in patients with DM and 33 cancers (4.4%) in patients with PM, resulting in SIRs of 5.11 (95% confidence interval [CI], 5.01–5.22) and 2.15 (95% CI, 2.08–2.22) in patients with DM and PM, respectively.[6] A recent meta-analysis of 5 studies with 4538 patients with DM or PM reported an overall relative risk (SIR) of cancer of 4.66 for patients with DM and 1.75 for patients with PM.[8] Clinically amyopathic DM has also been shown to have an association with cancer. In a systematic review of amyopathic dermatomyositis, 14% of 301 patients in the analysis had an associated malignancy.[11]

There is a paucity of studies assessing malignancy risk in IBM. In an Australian population-based cohort study, the SIR for IBM was 1.8,[3] whereas most epidemiologic studies report no increased risk of cancer in IBM.[12] Further, no association of cancer is reported in JDM, myositis associated with another autoimmune disease, the antisynthetase syndrome, or patients with anti- signal recognition particle (SRP)-positive NM.

Proposed risk stratification based on myositis clinical subtype

Based on published evidence as well as the authors' experiences, we propose the following cancer risk stratification.

- *High risk*: DM
- *Intermediate risk*: clinically amyopathic DM, PM

- *Low risk*: Juvenile myositis (including JDM), IBM, antisynthetase syndrome, NM (anti-SRP antibody positive), myositis in overlap with another autoimmune disease

CLINICAL AND SEROLOGIC RISK FACTORS FOR CANCER ASSOCIATED MYOSITIS

Although various studies report a greater cancer risk in patients with myositis with particular clinical features and serum autoantibodies, there also seem to be protective clinical features for cancer-associated myositis.[13–20]

Clinical Risk Factors

- *Older age at disease onset:* patients with myositis with disease onset after age 50 have a higher risk factor for cancer-associated myositis. A meta-analysis of 20 studies with 380 patients and 1575 controls reported that older age increases the risk of cancer.[13] In a review of 198 patients with IIM, patients with DM with cancer were more frequently older than 45 years of age, whereas those without cancer were younger than age 45.[14] Another study of malignancy among 251 patients with myositis found cancer-associated DM significantly more common in older patients.[15] A Japanese study of 145 patients diagnosed with either DM/PM or clinically amyopathic DM noted that patients with malignancy were older than their counterparts without cancer (61.5 years vs 51.1 years; $P<.005$).[16]
- *Male gender:* Males are at greater risk for cancer-associated myositis, even though myositis is more common in females[13,20] — and a recent meta-analysis of 31 studies confirmed this observation. Further, in the aforementioned study of 198 patients with IIM, patients with DM with cancer were more frequently male.[14]
- *Dysphagia:* Dysphagia owing to weakness of the striated muscle of the upper one-third of the esophagus is associated with more severe disease and a worse prognosis, but is also an independent risk factor for cancer (OR, 2.41; 95% CI, 1.50–3.86).[13] This risk has been confirmed in other studies.[15,16]
- *Cutaneous necrosis, ulceration and vasculitis:* Cutaneous ulcerations as well as necrosis of the skin and subcutaneous tissue are occasionally seen in severe DM, as well as amyopathic DM. Although it is generally associated with refractory disease and a poor prognosis, skin ulceration and more specifically skin necrosis has been associated with cancer associated DM (OR, 5.5; 95% CI, 3.5–8.7).[13] The association between cutaneous manifestations and cancer has been suggested in a few other studies as well.[20–22] Furthermore, leukocytoclastic vasculitis (histopathologically characterized by neutrophilic infiltration and fibrinoid necrosis within and around blood vessel walls) was significantly associated with cancer in a small retrospective review of 23 patients with DM.[17]
- *Rapid onset of myositis:* In a retrospective study of 33 patients with DM and 7 patients with PM, the rapid onset of myositis (defined by a diagnosis made within 2 months of initial signs and/or symptoms) was associated with malignancy ($P = .02$).[19]
- *Refractory myositis:* Severe and refractory disease, especially involving the skin, often suggests an occult malignancy.[15,20,21,23]
- *Laboratory features:* In addition to elevated inflammatory markers such as the erythrocyte sedimentation rate and C-reactive protein, higher total creatine kinase levels may also be associated with a higher cancer risk.[19,21,24]

Protective Factors

Features of IIM that may be associated with a lower risk of cancer include interstitial lung disease (ILD), inflammatory arthropathy, and Raynaud phenomenon,[6,13,16,19,20] but this risk reduction is only relative.

- *ILD:* In 147 patients with DM or PM from Taiwan, patients with ILD had a significantly lower frequency of malignancies compared with patients with IIM without ILD (P<.001).[6] In a more recent meta-analysis of 20 studies with 380 patients with DM and patients with PM and 1575 controls, ILD was protective against cancer (OR, 0.32; 95% CI, 0.20–0.51).[13]
- *Inflammatory arthropathy:* This meta-analysis also showed that arthritis was associated with a lower cancer risk in myositis (OR, 0.38; 95% CI, 0.24–0.61),[13] a conclusion supported by another independent study.[15]
- *Raynaud phenomenon:* In a study of 309 patients with myositis, Raynaud phenomenon was less frequent in the cancer-associated myositis group (11% vs 26%; P<.05).[20] In another retrospective study of 33 consecutive adult patients with DM and 7 patients with PM, the absence of Raynaud phenomenon was associated with cancer (P<.01).[16]

Proposed risk stratification based on myositis clinical factors

Based on the evidence presented elsewhere in this article, we propose the following risk stratification.

High risk: Multiple risk factors (generally ≥ 2), but no protective factors.
Intermediate risk: One risk factor or 2 risk factors with protective factors.
Low risk: No risk factors and 1 or more protective factors.

Red flags for cancer include unexplained weight loss, loss of appetite, unexplained pain, lymphadenopathy, mass, nonhealing ulcers, excessive fatigue, night sweats, pruritus.

SEROLOGIC RISK FACTORS FOR CANCER-ASSOCIATED MYOSITIS

Myositis autoantibodies are highly specific biomarkers associated with unique clinical phenotypes having prognostic significance. Several "cancer-associated" autoantibodies may help in the risk stratification for cancer in patients with myositis and guide cancer screening strategies.[25–29]

Myositis Autoantibodies

- *Anti–TIF1-gamma:* This myositis autoantibody, also identified as anti-p155 or anti-p155/140, targets a 155-kDa protein and has been linked to cancer in several studies.[9,30–32] A recent review on the relationship between anti–TIF1-gamma and cancer-associated myositis encompassed 312 adult patients with DM[33]; in this analysis, the pooled sensitivity of anti–TIF1-gamma for diagnosing cancer-associated DM was 78% (95% CI, 45%–94%), with a specificity of 89% (95% CI, 82%–93%). The diagnostic OR for anti–TIF1-gamma was 27.26 (95% CI, 6.59–112.82), with a positive likelihood ratio of 6.79 (95% CI, 4.11–11.23) and a negative likelihood ratio of 0.25 (95% CI, 0.08–0.76). No association between cancer and anti–TIF1-gamma was seen in juvenile myositis (despite the high frequency of this autoantibody in JDM). Of note, this autoantibody is not typically found in PM or NM. In 263 DM cases with 3252 person-years of follow-up for a median of 11 years, all of the detected malignancy cases in the TIF1-gamma–positive cohort occurred between 3 years before and 2.5 years after DM onset.[10]

- *Antinuclear matrix protein (NXP)-2*: Anti–NXP-2 (previously termed anti-MJ) recognizes a 140-kDa protein and is one of the myositis autoantibodies seen in JDM as well as adult DM. Similar to TIF1-gamma, this autoantibody is associated with cancer only in adult patients with DM. In 213 patients with DM, a total of 17% and 38% had antibodies against NXP-2 and anti–TIF1-gamma by immunoprecipitation, respectively,[34] and cancer was associated with anti–NXP-2 or TIF1-gamma autoantibodies (OR, 3.78; 95% CI, 1.33–10.8) using multivariate analysis. Stratification by gender noted an NXP-2 cancer association only in males (OR, 5.78; 95% CI, 1.35–24.70). In a Japanese study of 507 patients, only 1.6% of patients had NXP-2 autoantibodies, but one-third developed malignancy, mostly within 1 year of diagnosis.[35]
- *Anti–3-hydroxy-3-methylglutaryl-coenzyme A reductase (HMGCR)*: Anti-HMGCR is seen in patients with statin associated immune-mediated NM. In 207 Australian patients, there was a nonstatistically significant trend toward increased malignancy ($P = .15$) in anti–HMGCR-positive patients.[36] A recent study showed a higher (nonstatistically significant) prevalence of malignancy in patients with anti-HMGCR antibody,[27] whereas a French study demonstrated a higher incidence of cancer in anti–HMGCR-positive immune-mediated NM, but not with the anti-SRP antibody.[37] In a recent study in our center, there was no significant difference between the cancer frequency in the anti–HMGCR-positive NM group as compared with anti–HMGCR-NM ($P = .92$).[38]
- *Other myositis-associated autoantibodies*: In 627 patients with IIM, patients who were myositis-specific antibody-negative (SIR, 3.9; 95% CI, 1.9–7.1) or who possessed anti-SAE1 antibodies (SIR, 12.9; 95% CI, 3.2–32.9) were noted to have an increased risk of cancer compared with the general population.[30] Myositis-specific antibody negativity has been suggested to be associated with an increased risk of cancer in myositis in other studies as well.[34,39] Conversely, in another study of 231 patients with DM where 140 (61%) were antinuclear antigen (ANA) positive and 91 (39%) were ANA negative, there was a strong association between ANA positivity and a lower likelihood of malignancy (OR, 0.16; $P<.001$).[39] Similarly, having an antisynthetase antibody, especially anti–Jo-1, was associated with a lower risk of cancer-associated myositis.[24,30] As indicated elsewhere in this article, the risk of cancer has not been reported with anti–SRP-positive immune-mediated NM, compared with the general population.[40,41] There is no reported significant association of cancer with anti–Mi-2 or anti-MDA5 antibodies.

PROPOSED RISK STRATIFICATION BASED ON MYOSITIS AUTOANTIBODIES

Based on the studies discussed, the risk of cancer development in patients possessing specific autoantibodies can be stratified into high-, intermediate-, and low-risk groups.

- *High risk*: anti–TIF1-gamma, anti-NXP2
- *Intermediate risk*: Anti-SAE, anti-HMGCR, myositis autoantibody negative
- *Low risk*: Anti-synthetase, anti-SRP, anti–Mi-2, anti-MDA5 (melanoma differentiation antigen 5), ANA, antibodies associated with overlap myositis

SCREENING STRATEGIES
Basic or Age-Appropriate Screening

Over the years, myositis experts have recommended age- and sex-appropriate cancer screening, including basic laboratory testing at least at diagnosis as well as yearly for 3 years from initial diagnosis. This basic screening should be considered in all patients with myositis regardless of their risk stratification. This analysis includes a complete history and physical examination, complete blood count, serum chemistry panel, and cancer screening as per the national guidelines (**Box 1**).

Enhanced Screening

Enhanced screening would include basic screening as well as computed tomography (CT) scanning of the chest, abdomen, and pelvis, which could be performed in patients with increased risk for developing cancer. In addition, tumor markers as well as gynecologic/pelvic examination and/or ultrasound examination in women and testicular ultrasound examination in men should be considered.

In a study of 40 consecutive adult patients with DM (33 cases) or PM (7 cases), the yield of malignancy searches was increased with thoracic CT scans.[19] As indicated elsewhere in this article, all high-risk female patients with cancer red flags need to undergo a gynecologic/pelvic examination and pelvic/transvaginal ultrasound examination to screen for occult ovarian cancer.[42,43] In addition, males less than 50 years of age should undergo testicular ultrasound examination given the high risk of testicular cancer in at-risk male patients.

However, the use of tumor markers in myositis-associated cancer screening is controversial. In a single blinded, case-control study of 14 women with DM and 10

Box 1
Cancer screening in myositis

Basic screening
- Comprehensive history and physical examination; family history
- Routine blood tests: Complete blood count, liver function tests, urinalysis
- Chest radiograph
- Age-appropriate screening
  - Colonoscopy: The USPSTF recommends screening for colorectal cancer starting at age 50 years and continuing until age 75 years.
  - Mammography: The USPSTF recommends biennial screening mammography for women aged 50 to 74 years.
  - Screening for cervical cancer: The USPSTF recommends screening for cervical cancer every 3 years with cervical cytology alone in women aged 21 to 29 years. For women aged 30 to 65 years, the USPSTF recommends screening every 3 years with cervical cytology alone, every 5 years with hrHPV testing alone, or every 5 years with hrHPV testing in combination with cytology (cotesting).
  - Screening for prostate cancer: Per USPSTF, for men aged 55 to 69, the decision to undergo periodic prostate-specific antigen-based screening for prostate cancer should be an individual one.

Enhanced screening: Includes basic screening and consideration of one or more of the following evaluations.
- Computed tomography scanning of the chest/abdomen/pelvis
- Tumor markers
- Gynecologic/pelvic ultrasound examination in women, and testicular ultrasound examination in men (age <50 years)

Comprehensive screening: Includes basic or enhanced screening with consideration of the following evaluations.
- PET with computed tomography scanning of the chest/abdomen/pelvis

Abbreviations: hrHPV, high-risk human papillomavirus; USPSTF, US Preventive Service Task Force.

healthy controls, CA 125 was found to have a sensitivity of 50% and specificity of 100% for the detection of ovarian cancer.[44] A more recent study assessing the diagnostic values of CA 125, carcinoembryonic antigen, CA 19-9, and CA 15-3 for the detection of solid cancer in DM/PM patients also concluded that CA125 and CA19-9 assessment could be useful markers of cancer risk in patients with DM and PM.[45] For example, elevated CA125 and CA 19-9 at screening were higher in patients who developed cancer within 1 year or in patients without ILD. Based on these studies, a physician can consider CA 125 and CA 19-9 for the screening of patients at higher risk for cancer associated myositis. However, these findings have not been confirmed in other studies, and in a 21-year retrospective study, tumor markers did not predict occult tumors.[20] Furthermore, transient elevation of CA 15-3 was reported as a marker of ILD rather than underlying cancer in a patient with amyopathic DM.[46]

Comprehensive Screening

Comprehensive screening including basic or enhanced screening as well as PET with CT scanning of the chest, abdomen, and pelvis can be considered in patients with a particularly high risk for cancer. This advanced imaging approach (which combines [18F] fluorodeoxyglucose [FDG] labeling/PET and CT scanning) represents one of the most sensitive techniques available for the detection of occult malignancy and are increasingly being used in patients with myositis.[47,48] In a large prospective study of 55 consecutive patients with a recent diagnosis of myositis, whole body FDG-PET/CT scanning was compared with conventional cancer screening for the detection of malignancy.[47] The performance of a single FDG-PET/CT scan for diagnosing occult cancer in patients with myositis was comparable with that of a large number of conventional cancer screening techniques, including a complete physical examination, laboratory testing (complete blood count and serum chemistry panel), thoracoabdominal CT scanning, tumor markers (CA125, CA 19-9, carcinoembryonic antigen and prostate-specific antigen), and gynecologic examination in women, including ultrasound examination and mammography. The authors concluded that it is reasonable to perform PET/CT scans for high-risk patients rather than subjecting them to a many tests and procedures. Moreover, a cost analysis study showed that the expense of a whole body PET/CT scan was greater than conventional panels for insurance companies, but lower for patients in terms of out-of-pocket expenses.[49] These findings were supported by a Japanese study, where PET/CT scanning was able to effectively detect underlying cancer in patients with myositis.[50] However, a retrospective cohort study from Canada evaluating 100 FDG PET/CT studies in 63 unique patients (31 DM, 1 PM, 25 overlap myositis, 1 IBM, 1 orbital myositis, and 4 unspecified myositis) failed to show any additional benefit of FDG PET/CT scanning.[51] Unfortunately, all of these studies assessed the usefulness of the whole body FDG PET/CT in consecutive patients with myositis, irrespective of their cancer risk. Further studies are therefore necessary to determine the role and specificity of FDG-PET/CT scanning in risk-stratified cancer screening among patients with IIM.

APPROACH TO SCREENING

Despite an increasing number of studies examining the usefulness of various screening strategies, existing data do not permit consensus, evidence-based recommendations for cancer screening in myositis. However, based on these limited data and personal observation, we recommend that all newly diagnosed patients with myositis (duration of <3 years) undergo stratification of cancer risk. Age- and sex-appropriate screening, including history, physical examination, and basic laboratory testing, should be done on all patients with myositis regardless of their risk category. This comprehensive history and physical examination should include an assessment of clinical risk factors, protective factors, and any red flags for malignancy as discussed elsewhere in this article. Serum should also be assessed for myositis-specific autoantibodies in all newly diagnosed patients with IIM for the identification of high-risk patients. Patients can then be categorized into low-risk, intermediate-risk, and high-risk groups based on clinical characteristics and myositis autoantibody results (**Fig. 1**). Although not entirely evidence based, we further recommend that patients at low risk, intermediate risk, and high risk be considered for basic, enhanced, or comprehensive cancer screening, respectively. Finally, high-risk patients should likely undergo basic cancer screening annually for 3 years from diagnosis; **Fig. 1** provides further details.

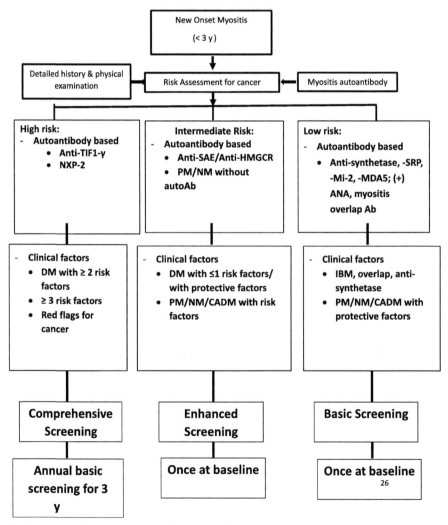

Fig. 1. Approach to cancer screening in myositis.

SUMMARY

Cancer screening is important in myositis, particularly at disease onset and within the first 3 years of disease. Risk stratification for cancer in patients with myositis can be completed based on a combination of clinical risk factors and protective factors, myositis clinical subtypes, and autoantibody profile. Despite a paucity of data- or consensus-driven recommendations, we have proposed a cancer screening strategy based on this paradigm of risk stratification. Large multicenter studies are needed to test our proposed recommendations as well as other strategies for early detection of cancer in myositis. High-risk patients should be monitored regularly and receive aggressive cancer screening to detect occult malignancy, although all patients should continue to obtain age- and gender-appropriate cancer screening as recommended for the general population.

CLINICS CARE POINTS

- Risk stratification for cancer in myositis can be completed based on a combination of myositis clinical subtypes, clinical risk factors, and autoantibodies.
- Cancer risk is significantly higher in DM as compared with other myositis clinical subtypes.
- Clinical risk factors for cancer in myositis include older age at disease onset, male sex, dysphagia, cutaneous ulceration, necrosis or vasculitis, rapid onset of myositis, refractory myositis and laboratory features including elevated inflammatory markers.
- The risk of cancer development in patients with myositis possessing anti–TIF1-gamma and anti-NXP2 is the highest among the myositis-associated and myositis-specific autoantibodies.
- Appropriate cancer screening strategies in IIMs are based on the risk level and include a comprehensive history and physical examination; routine blood tests; age-appropriate malignancy screening; CT scanning of the chest, abdomen, and pelvis; tumor markers; gynecologic/pelvic ultrasound examination in women; testicular ultrasound examination in men; and PET-CT scanning of the chest, abdomen, and pelvis.

REFERENCES

1. Yang Z, Lin F, Qin B, et al. Polymyositis/dermatomyositis and malignancy risk: a metaanalysis study. J Rheumatol 2015;42(2):282–91.
2. Stockton D, Doherty VR, Brewster DH. Risk of cancer in patients with dermatomyositis or polymyositis, and follow-up implications: a Scottish population-based cohort study. Br J Cancer 2001;85(1):41–5.
3. Buchbinder R, Forbes A, Hall S, et al. Incidence of malignant disease in biopsy-proven inflammatory myopathy. a population-based cohort study. Ann Intern Med 2001;134(12):1087–95.
4. Chow WH, Gridley G, Mellemkjaer L, et al. Cancer risk following polymyositis and dermatomyositis: a nationwide cohort study in Denmark. Cancer Causes Control 1995;6(1):9–13.
5. Sigurgeirsson B, Lindelöf B, Edhag O, et al. Risk of cancer in patients with dermatomyositis or polymyositis. A population-based study. N Engl J Med 1992; 326(6):363–7.
6. Chen YJ, Wu CY, Huang YL, et al. Cancer risks of dermatomyositis and polymyositis: a nationwide cohort study in Taiwan. Arthritis Res Ther 2010;12(2):R70.

7. Zantos D, Zhang Y, Felson D. The overall and temporal association of cancer with polymyositis and dermatomyositis. J Rheumatol 1994;21(10):1855–9.

8. Qiang JK, Kim WB, Baibergenova A, et al. Risk of malignancy in dermatomyositis and polymyositis. J Cutan Med Surg 2017;21(2):131–6.

9. Targoff IN, Mamyrova G, Trieu EP, et al, Childhood Myositis Heterogeneity Study Group; International Myositis Collaborative Study Group. A novel autoantibody to a 155-kd protein is associated with dermatomyositis. Arthritis Rheum 2006; 54(11):3682–9.

10. Oldroyd A, Sergeant JC, New P, et al. The temporal relationship between cancer and adult onset anti-transcriptional intermediary factor 1 antibody-positive dermatomyositis. Rheumatology (Oxford) 2019;58(4):650–5.

11. Gerami P, Walling HW, Lewis J, et al. A systematic review of juvenile-onset clinically amyopathic dermatomyositis. Br J Dermatol 2007;157(4):637–44.

12. Limaye V, Luke C, Tucker G, et al. The incidence and associations of malignancy in a large cohort of patients with biopsy-determined idiopathic inflammatory myositis. Rheumatol Int 2013;33(4):965–71.

13. Wang J, Guo G, Chen G, et al. Meta-analysis of the association of dermatomyositis and polymyositis with cancer. Br J Dermatol 2013;169(4):838–47.

14. Antiochos BB, Brown LA, Li Z, et al. Malignancy is associated with dermatomyositis but not polymyositis in Northern New England, USA. J Rheumatol 2009; 36(12):2704–10.

15. Ponyi A, Constantin T, Garami M, et al. Cancer-associated myositis: clinical features and prognostic signs. Ann N Y Acad Sci 2005;1051:64–71.

16. Azuma K, Yamada H, Ohkubo M, et al. Incidence and predictive factors for malignancies in 136 Japanese patients with dermatomyositis, polymyositis and clinically amyopathic dermatomyositis. Mod Rheumatol 2011;21(2):178–83.

17. Hunger RE, Dürr C, Brand CU. Cutaneous leukocytoclastic vasculitis in dermatomyositis suggests malignancy. Dermatology 2001;202(2):123–6.

18. Urbano-Márquez A, Casademont J, Grau JM. Polymyositis/dermatomyositis: the current position. Ann Rheum Dis 1991;50(3):191–5.

19. Sparsa A, Liozon E, Herrmann F, et al. Routine vs extensive malignancy search for adult dermatomyositis and polymyositis: a study of 40 patients. Arch Dermatol 2002;138(7):885–90.

20. András C, Ponyi A, Constantin T, et al. Dermatomyositis and polymyositis associated with malignancy: a 21-year retrospective study. J Rheumatol 2008;35(3): 438–44.

21. Gallais V, Crickx B, Belaich S. [Prognostic factors and predictive signs of malignancy in adult dermatomyositis]. Ann Dermatol Venereol 1996;123(11):722–6.

22. Prohic A, Kasumagic-Halilovic E, Simic D, et al. Clinical and biological factors predictive of malignancy in dermatomyositis. J Eur Acad Dermatol Venereol 2009;23(5):591–2.

23. Leow YH, Goh CL. Malignancy in adult dermatomyositis. Int J Dermatol 1997; 36(12):904–7.

24. Basset-Seguin N, Roujeau JC, Gherardi R, et al. Prognostic factors and predictive signs of malignancy in adult dermatomyositis. A study of 32 cases. Arch Dermatol 1990;126(5):633–7.

25. Dobloug GC, Garen T, Brunborg C, et al. Survival and cancer risk in an unselected and complete Norwegian idiopathic inflammatory myopathy cohort. Semin Arthritis Rheum 2015;45(3):301–8.

26. Ceribelli A, Isailovic N, De Santis M, et al. Myositis-specific autoantibodies and their association with malignancy in Italian patients with polymyositis and dermatomyositis. Clin Rheumatol 2017;36(2):469–75.
27. Tiniakou E, Mammen AL. Idiopathic inflammatory myopathies and malignancy: a comprehensive review. Clin Rev Allergy Immunol 2017;52(1):20–33.
28. Hervier B, Devilliers H, Stanciu R, et al. Hierarchical cluster and survival analyses of antisynthetase syndrome: phenotype and outcome are correlated with anti-tRNA synthetase antibody specificity. Autoimmun Rev 2012;12(2):210–7.
29. Udkoff J, Cohen PR. Amyopathic dermatomyositis: a concise review of clinical manifestations and associated malignancies. Am J Clin Dermatol 2016;17(5):509–18.
30. Chinoy H, Fertig N, Oddis CV, et al. The diagnostic utility of myositis autoantibody testing for predicting the risk of cancer-associated myositis. Ann Rheum Dis 2007;66(10):1345–9.
31. Kaji K, Fujimoto M, Hasegawa M, et al. Identification of a novel autoantibody reactive with 155 and 140 kDa nuclear proteins in patients with dermatomyositis: an association with malignancy. Rheumatology (Oxford) 2007;46(1):25–8.
32. Trallero-Araguás E, Labrador-Horrillo M, Selva-O'Callaghan A, et al. Cancer-associated myositis and anti-p155 autoantibody in a series of 85 patients with idiopathic inflammatory myopathy. Medicine (Baltimore) 2010;89(1):47–52.
33. Trallero-Araguás E, Rodrigo-Pendás JÁ, Selva-O'Callaghan A, et al. Usefulness of anti-p155 autoantibody for diagnosing cancer-associated dermatomyositis: a systematic review and meta-analysis. Arthritis Rheum 2012;64(2):523–32.
34. Fiorentino DF, Chung LS, Christopher-Stine L, et al. Most patients with cancer-associated dermatomyositis have antibodies to nuclear matrix protein NXP-2 or transcription intermediary factor 1γ. Arthritis Rheum 2013;65(11):2954–62.
35. Ichimura Y, Matsushita T, Hamaguchi Y, et al. Anti-NXP2 autoantibodies in adult patients with idiopathic inflammatory myopathies: possible association with malignancy. Ann Rheum Dis 2012;71(5):710–3.
36. Limaye V, Bundell C, Hollingsworth P, et al. Clinical and genetic associations of autoantibodies to 3-hydroxy-3-methyl-glutaryl-coenzyme a reductase in patients with immune-mediated myositis and necrotizing myopathy. Muscle Nerve 2015;52(2):196–203.
37. Allenbach Y, Keraen J, Bouvier AM, et al. High risk of cancer in autoimmune necrotizing myopathies: usefulness of myositis specific antibody. Brain 2016;139(Pt 8):2131–5.
38. Aggarwal R, Moghadam-Kia S, Lacomis D, et al. Anti-hydroxy-3-methylglutaryl-coenzyme A reductase (anti-HMGCR) antibody in necrotizing myopathy: treatment outcomes, cancer risk, and role of autoantibody level. Scand J Rheumatol 2019;5:1–7.
39. Yang H, Peng Q, Yin L, et al. Identification of multiple cancer-associated myositis-specific autoantibodies in idiopathic inflammatory myopathies: a large longitudinal cohort study. Arthritis Res Ther 2017;19(1):259.
40. Hoesly PM, Sluzevich JC, Jambusaria-Pahlajani A, et al. Association of antinuclear antibody status with clinical features and malignancy risk in adult-onset dermatomyositis. J Am Acad Dermatol 2019;80(5):1364–70.
41. Day JA, Limaye V. Immune-mediated necrotising myopathy: a critical review of current concepts. Semin Arthritis Rheum 2019;49(3):420–9.
42. Whitmore SE, Rosenshein NB, Provost TT. Ovarian cancer in patients with dermatomyositis. Medicine (Baltimore) 1994;73(3):153–60.

43. Cherin P, Piette JC, Herson S, et al. Dermatomyositis and ovarian cancer: a report of 7 cases and literature review. J Rheumatol 1993;20(11):1897–9.
44. Whitmore SE, Anhalt GJ, Provost TT, et al. Serum CA-125 screening for ovarian cancer in patients with dermatomyositis. Gynecol Oncol 1997;65(2):241–4.
45. Amoura Z, Duhaut P, Huong DL, et al. Tumor antigen markers for the detection of solid cancers in inflammatory myopathies. Cancer Epidemiol Biomarkers Prev 2005;14(5):1279–82.
46. Wong RC, Brown S, Clarke BE, et al. Transient elevation of the tumor markers CA 15-3 and CASA as markers of interstitial lung disease rather than underlying malignancy in dermatomyositis sine myositis. J Clin Rheumatol 2002;8(4):204–7.
47. Selva-O'Callaghan A, Grau JM, Gámez-Cenzano C, et al. Conventional cancer screening versus PET/CT in dermatomyositis/polymyositis. Am J Med 2010; 123(6):558–62.
48. Maliha PG, Hudson M, Abikhzer G, et al. 18F-FDG PET/CT versus conventional investigations for cancer screening in autoimmune inflammatory myopathy in the era of novel myopathy classifications. Nucl Med Commun 2019;40(4):377–82.
49. Kundrick A, Kirby J, Ba D, et al. Positron emission tomography costs less to patients than conventional screening for malignancy in dermatomyositis. Semin Arthritis Rheum 2019;49(1):140–4.
50. Owada T, Maezawa R, Kurasawa K, et al. Detection of inflammatory lesions by f-18 fluorodeoxyglucose positron emission tomography in patients with polymyositis and dermatomyositis. J Rheumatol 2012;39(8):1659–65.
51. Motegi SI, Fujiwara C, Sekiguchi A, et al. Clinical value of (18) F-fluorodeoxyglucose positron emission tomography/computed tomography for interstitial lung disease and myositis in patients with dermatomyositis. J Dermatol 2019;46(3): 213–8.

Paraneoplastic Musculoskeletal Syndromes

Fahad Khan, MD[1], Hilary Kleppel, BS[1], Alexa Meara, MD*

KEYWORDS

- Paraneoplastic • Rheumatologic • Cancer • Malignancy • Dermatomyositis

KEY POINTS

- Clinical changes that may represent paraneoplastic phenomena should cue physicians to be vigilant for a concomitant or impending underlying malignancy.
- Treatment of a culprit malignancy can result in the resolution or amelioration of the associated paraneoplastic phenomenon.
- Atypical presentations of clinical entities not often thought to be related to cancer, such as Raynaud phenomenon or polymyalgia rheumatica, may serve as clues to their manifestation as paraneoplastic phenomena.
- When a paraneoplastic phenomenon is encountered, physicians should strongly consider a focused work-up for associated cancers, especially with new diagnoses of dermatomyositis.

INTRODUCTION

Paraneoplastic syndromes are diseases caused by malignancies through means other than mass effect or metastasis.[1] Even though they occur in only about 10% of patients with cancer, physicians are wise to be vigilant for them for several reasons: a paraneoplastic phenomenon can be the first sign of cancer in an undiagnosed individual, and it can be severe enough to cause death.[2] Despite the tumor being distinctly separate from the area where the paraneoplastic syndrome manifests, it is important to realize that paraneoplastic phenomena are not caused by metastases of the neoplasm. For example, hypercalcemia caused by osteolysis caused by bony metastases does not count as a paraneoplastic disease, but hypercalcemia from production of parathyroid hormone–related protein by a tumor does. Paraneoplastic rheumatic syndromes can occur with hematologic cancers, lymphoproliferative diseases, and solid tumors.[3] Diseases that feature an advanced age at onset, significant constitutional upset, inadequate response to treatment, and otherwise atypical characteristics should increase the index of suspicion for a paraneoplastic syndrome.

Division of Rheumatology and Immunology, Department of Internal Medicine, Columbus, OH, USA
[1] Present address: 543 Taylor Avenue, Columbus, OH 43203.
* Corresponding author. 543 Taylor Avenue, Columbus, OH 43203.
E-mail address: alexa.meara@osumc.edu

Rheum Dis Clin N Am 46 (2020) 577–586
https://doi.org/10.1016/j.rdc.2020.04.002
0889-857X/20/© 2020 Elsevier Inc. All rights reserved.

SPECIFIC PARANEOPLASTIC SYNDROMES
Arthropathy

Carcinomatous polyarthritis (CP) is arthritis in the setting of malignancy that is not caused by the mass effect of a tumor or space-occupying effect of its metastases.[3] Solid tumors of the oropharynx, larynx, esophagus, stomach, colon, lung, breast, ovary, and pancreas, as well as lymphoproliferative diseases, have been associated with CP.[4] CP generally affects patients older than 50 years and is rapidly progressive on onset, which is often around the time of diagnosis of the responsible cancer. It is a diagnosis of exclusion that must be distinguished from other diseases, such as seronegative spondyloarthropathies (eg, reactive arthritis and enteric arthritis) and crystalline arthropathies. Distinguishing between CP and rheumatoid arthritis (RA) can pose a challenge, because both entities feature an increasing incidence with age and similar clinical presentations. In general, CP differs from RA in its asymmetric distribution, predilection for joints in the legs rather than wrists and hands, and seronegativity for the rheumatoid factor (RF) and anti–cyclic citrullinated peptide (CCP) antibodies.[5] However, there are reports of CP presenting with symmetric involvement of the wrists and hands as well as RF and anti-CCP antibody positivity.[5,6] The RF positivity may be explained by the malignancy. Although these features may render it difficult to exclude the possibility of RA, CP should eventually reveal a temporal association with a malignancy, whose treatment should resolve the arthritis symptoms.[7] For example, a 44-year-old woman who developed an aggressive polyarthritis was found to have medullary carcinoma of the breast and experienced resolution of her arthritis a week after mastectomy[8] without recurrence over a year of surveillance. Similarly, a 43-year-old man with CP associated with bronchogenic carcinoma experienced complete resolution of his arthritis following treatment with cisplatinum and etoposide.[6] In that case, it is not possible to say whether treatment of the underlying malignancy effected an enduring cure of the associated CP, because his health soon declined, and the patient died. However, the investigators conclude their report by stating that the treatment of CP is tantamount to treatment of the associated cancer, and that recurrence of arthritis should increase suspicion for recurrence of cancer.

Hypertrophic osteoarthropathy (HOA) causes proliferation of skin and bone associated with effusions in large joints.[9] Patients experience a progressive and bilateral periostosis at tubular bones, such as the tibia and fibula. Although HOA can be a primary disorder, it can also be secondary to numerous causes, among which are malignancies of the pulmonary and gastrointestinal systems. Symptomatic patients report leg pain and tenderness. The predominant physical examination finding in HOA is digital clubbing, which is a bulbous change of the distal part of the fingers associated with a convex deformity of the nails. In addition, there may be hypertrophy of the skin in the nailbeds or face. If a large joint effusion is aspirated, synovial fluid analysis reveals an increased viscosity and a paucity of white blood cells. A 1988 literature review of primary HOA found that synovial fluid analysis of joint effusions in 9 instances revealed thick, viscous fluid with low counts of white blood cells.[10] The synovial fluid was noninflammatory except for 1 case, which showed hemarthrosis. Plain films show periostosis as a thickened cortex of affected bones. HOA can be associated with lung malignancies,[11] especially non–small cell lung cancer.[12] Secondary causes of HOA are usually pulmonary but can also be pleural, mediastinal, or cardiovascular malignancies. Gastrointestinal tumors have also been linked to HOA. When it is associated with cancer, HOA can regress with treatment of the underlying malignancy.[13] Patients who have HOA in the setting of cystic fibrosis (CF) have been managed with nonsteroidal antiinflammatory drugs, physical therapy, and steroids. A 2002 case report describes a patient with CF who was treated with serial doses of pamidronate and experienced full resolution of symptoms with each.[14] Furthermore, a 2009 review of the use of pamidronate in various rheumatic conditions reports that it has been very effective for analgesia in primary as well as paraneoplastic HOA.[15]

Remitting seronegative symmetric synovitis with pitting edema (RS3PE) can exist as a primary disorder or occur secondary to malignancy.[13] In addition, patients with RS3PE have a higher incidence of malignancy.[16] RS3PE can occur with cancers of the stomach, colon, prostate, ovary, and endometrium, as well as malignant lymphoma, leukemia, and myelodyspasias.[13,16] When secondary to a malignancy, patients may have fever, weight loss, and an inadequate response to steroids. RS3PE has a predilection for the elderly and features bilateral synovitis and edema of the hands and feet.[17] Edema can lend a boxing-glove appearance to the hands.[13] Laboratory investigations reveal increase of erythrocyte sedimentation rate (ESR) and C-reactive protein (CRP) and absence of RF and anti-CCP antibodies.[17]

Polymyalgia rheumatica (PMR) is a disease of the elderly that causes pain and stiffness in the proximal muscles as well as fatigue.[3] Laboratory investigation typically shows anemia of chronic disease and increased ESR. One of the hallmarks of PMR is a dramatic response to a moderate dose of steroids; for example, 20 mg of prednisone daily. The following atypical features may be clues to an underlying cancer: onset before 50 years of age, asymmetric distribution, profound anemia, proteinuria, ESR greater than 100 mm/h or less than 40 mm/h, and an inadequate response to steroids.[3] Atypical PMR (aPMR) can precede a cancer diagnosis by up to about a year and has been associated with malignancies of the kidney, lung, and colon, and multiple myeloma.[3,13] Treatment of the underlying malignancy may alleviate symptoms of aPMR. A 2016 case report from Portugal describes an 82-year-old man with disabling pain and stiffness of his shoulders and hips associated with increased ESR and CRP level who was diagnosed with PMR and started on a steroid called deflazacort, 12 mg daily, but experienced inadequate relief despite increasing the dose to 18 mg daily. Further investigation of incidental macroscopic hematuria revealed diagnoses of bladder and prostate cancer, which were treated with radical cystectomy and prostatectomy; the patient was asymptomatic 1 month following discharge and showed improvement in inflammatory markers.[18,19]

Gout is a well-known inflammatory arthritis that can exist by itself, but it can also be secondary to the hyperuricemia that results from accelerated nucleic acid breakdown in patients with malignancy undergoing chemotherapy and radiation.[13] Hematologic malignancies such as leukemia, polycythemia vera, and lymphoma are associated with gout.[7] Liver involvement by the malignancy can affect the severity of gout. In addition, chemotherapy used to treat malignancy can lead to gout, because radiation or antiblastic therapies can cause hyperuricemia.[13]

Amyloidosis is the deposition of insoluble amyloid protein that can cause organ failure. Amyloidosis can also affect the synovium and periarticular space leading to joint pain, most commonly in the shoulders, wrists, and knees.[13] A low-grade but frank arthritis may be seen in an asymmetric pattern in multiple myeloma and Waldenström macroglobulinemia.

Myopathy

Inflammatory myopathy is an immune-mediated attack on skeletal muscle that manifests in weakness.[3] Dermatomyositis (DM) seems to have the strongest association with malignancy out of all the types of autoimmune myopathies, because 6% to 60% of patients with DM develop malignancy. The malignancy is usually diagnosed within a couple of years into the diagnosis of DM, and associated cancers include ovarian, lung, gastric, and nasopharyngeal types. Patients with polymyositis are also at increased risk for developing cancer, with up to 28% developing malignancy. Clinically amyopathic DM is also associated with cancer. Patients with inflammatory myopathy in whom to be especially vigilant about underlying malignancy include those with the following features: diagnosis at age greater than 50 years, male sex, rapidly progressive course, shawl sign, distal weakness, weakness of the pharynx and diaphragm, difficult-to-treat disease, leukocytoclastic vasculitis (LCV), skin ulceration/necrosis/vasculitis, lack of lung involvement, increased creatine kinase level, increased ESR, increased CRP level, anti–p155-140 (anti–transcriptional intermediary factor-1γ) antibody, and anti–nuclear matrix protein (NXP)-2 (anti-MJ) antibody. Treatment of the underlying malignancy can lead to improvement of the associated myopathy and cutaneous manifestations.[20] Cancer-associated myositis (CAM) and the malignancy of which it is a paraneoplastic phenomenon can have a parallel clinical course, and a relapse of malignancy can be accompanied by a similar resurgence of myositis. Patients with CAM rarely have myositis-specific and myositis-associated autoantibodies. The features of an inflammatory myopathy that are associated with a lower risk of cancer include the anti–Jo-1 antibody, anti-extractable nuclear antigens(includes Anti-SM, Anti-RNP, anti-RO/LA) antibodies, interstitial lung disease, joint involvement, and Raynaud phenomenon.[3] Age-appropriate cancer screening should be ensured in patients with inflammatory myopathy, and this vigilance for underlying cancer should be continued in case the malignancy develops years after the myopathy. Other means of discovering a malignancy in this setting include imaging the chest, abdomen, and pelvis and checking serum levels of tumor markers.

Vascular

Cancer-associated vasculitis affects about 8% of patients with malignancy,[3] complicates lymphoproliferative and myeloproliferative diseases more than solid tumors, and may antedate the discovery of cancer. It is generally a small vessel vasculitis that affects the skin rather than internal organs. Although cutaneous vasculitis and polyarteritis nodosa (PAN) are the most frequent paraneoplastic vasculitides,[21] the central nervous and cardiovascular systems can also be affected. Cutaneous vasculitis most commonly presents with palpable purpura of the legs but can also cause urticaria and erythema elevatum diutinum.

LCV is a small vessel vasculitis that presents with palpable purpura with a predilection for the legs, arthralgias, arthritis, myalgias, and fever.[13] LCV has connections with lymphoproliferative disorders such as acute and chronic leukemias, lymphomas, myelodysplasias, and solid tumors.

PAN is a systemic necrotizing vasculitis with a predilection for medium-sized vessels.[13] Patients are generally seronegative for antineutrophil cytoplasmic autoantibodies (ANCA) and do not experience glomerulonephritis or pulmonary capillaritis, which serves to distinguish PAN from microscopic polyangiitis, which is an ANCA-associated vasculitis (AAV) that can also target small and medium-sized vessels.[22] Inflamed arteries may occlude or rupture, causing ischemia or hemorrhage in various organs. Patients can experience fever; malaise; weight loss; pain in the abdomen, joints, and muscles; paresthesia; orchitis; and high blood pressure.[21] The most commonly affected areas are the peripheral nervous system and skin. The most frequent neurologic derangement is mononeuritis multiplex, whereas the skin examination may show palpable purpura, livedoid changes, nodules, and ulcers. Kidneys can be affected by infarctions or hematomas secondary to ruptured microaneurysms, and those infarcts can go on to cause hematuria and proteinuria. Hypertension can occur from vasculitis of intrarenal vasculature. About 10% of cases are mostly limited to skin involvement, and those have a better course. Systemic PAN may be associated with hepatitis B infection or hairy-cell leukemia.[23,24] PAN is associated with solid tumors of the liver, colon, bladder, lung, and hypopharynx, and hematologic diseases such as leukemia and myelodysplasia.[13] Granulomatosis with polyangiitis, an AAV, may be temporally linked to renal cell carcinoma.[25] Cryoglobulinemia is the presence of immunoglobulins in the serum that precipitates at less than 37°C.[13] Of the 3 types of cryoglobulinemia recognized, type I has an association with malignancy. Type I cryoglobulinemia consists of monoclonal immunoglobulin (Ig) M IgG and is associated with Waldenström macroglobulinemia and multiple myeloma. It can cause symptoms of hyperviscosity, such as vertigo, encephalopathy, cephalgia, and stroke.[26] Types II and III feature both IgM and IgG and are therefore called mixed cryoglobulinemia. Most cases of type II cryoglobulinemia are associated with hepatitis C infection, whereas type III cryoglobulinemia can result from infections and autoimmune disorders. Approximately 15% of patients with type II or type III cryoglobulinemia develop vasculitis, and almost all of those experience skin disease, such as palpable purpura.[21] About 6% of patients with cryoglobulinemic vasculitis have a lymphoproliferative disorder. Patients with mixed cryoglobulinemia have a high risk for developing non-Hodgkin lymphoma.[13] Treatment of paraneoplastic vasculitis begins with identifying and treating the underlying neoplasm, because that may help resolve the cutaneous rash. In addition, most patients should receive systemic steroids and, if need be, steroid-sparing agents such as cyclophosphamide, methotrexate, or azathioprine.

Erythromelalgia causes erythema and a sensation of burning and heat in the arms and legs, with a preference for the feet. The face and ears can also be involved, and there may be swelling in addition to redness and warmth.[21] The onset ranges from sudden to gradual, and aggravating factors include exercise, heat, and dependency of the affected limb.[3] Relieving factors include cold temperature and limb elevation. Although erythromelalgia may exist as a primary disorder, it can also be associated with myeloproliferative diseases such as polycythemia vera and essential thrombocytosis. The pathophysiology is thought to be thrombocythemia or arteriovenous shunting. Breakdown products and microthrombi of platelets are also implicated. Treatment with aspirin can palliate the symptoms of erythromelalgia. Despite palliation of symptoms with aspirin, patients should be monitored periodically with complete blood counts, because paraneoplastic erythromelalgia can precede the diagnosis of an associated cancer.[25]

Severe, asymmetric Raynaud phenomenon (RP) that occurs after age 50 years and leads to digital necrosis can be a paraneoplastic phenomenon that warrants a pursuit of an underlying malignancy.[3] In a 2014 retrospective cohort study from France, 15% of patients admitted for an initial occurrence of digital ischemia had an underlying cancer; those associated malignancies included adenocarcinoma, squamous cell carcinoma, and lymphoid neoplasia.[27] Other cancer associations include gastrointestinal, lung, ovarian, and renal carcinomas[7] and sarcomas.[13] RP can precede the cancer diagnosis by 7 to 9 months. The development of digital necrosis in the setting of DM should especially cue physicians to consider the possibility of an underlying cancer.

Cutaneous

Systemic sclerosis (SSc) can occur around the time of diagnosis of a malignancy. Also, cutaneous lesions similar to those seen in SSc can occur in several cancers and are called pseudoscleroderma or pseudosclerosis.[13] Associated cancers include metastatic melanoma; osteoclastic myeloma; plasmacytomas; carcinoids; and gastric, breast, and lung tumors.[7] In addition, the plasma cell dyscrasia POEMS (polyneuropathy, organomegaly, endocrinopathy, monoclonal protein, skin changes) syndrome can result in sclerodermoid skin changes. Although technically not a paraneoplastic phenomenon, sclerodermoid skin changes can also be seen in patients with hematologic malignancy who develop chronic graft-versus-host disease following bone marrow transplant.[25]

Fasciitis-panniculitis syndrome (FPS) causes swelling and hardening of the skin and subcutis and is accompanied by fibrosis and inflammation.[3] Patients may experience a monoarticular or polyarticular arthritis and subcutaneous nodules. FPS can exist as a primary disorder or be secondary to various causes such as infection or trauma. Rarely, FPS can be associated with cancer. Associated cancers include myelomonocytic leukemia, chronic lymphocytic leukemia, myeloproliferative disorder, Hodgkin disease, T-cell lymphoma, breast carcinoma, prostate carcinoma, gastric adenocarcinoma, and pancreatic carcinoma.[28] When FPS occurs as a paraneoplastic phenomenon, it has a female predilection and poor response to prednisone. Eosinophilic fasciitis (EF) is in the category of FPS and mostly affects the limbs, causing pain and swelling because of induration of the skin.[3,13] Laboratory investigations reveal hypereosinophilia, hypergammaglobulinemia, and increased ESR. Malignancies associated with EF include Hodgkin disease, lymphoproliferative disorder, angioimmunoblastic lymphadenopathy, and peripheral T-cell lymphoma.[29]

Multicentric reticulohistiocytosis (MRH) presents with papules located on the face, dorsal hands, and periungual areas.[3] It is associated with a symmetric and erosive polyarthritis that affects the interphalangeal joints, wrists, elbows, shoulders, hips, knees, ankles, and feet.[30] Patients can develop arthritis mutilans. In addition to skin and joint involvement, MRH can affect internal organs such as the thyroid, heart, lungs, liver, and lymph nodes.[13] Biopsy of affected areas characteristically shows infiltration by histiocytes and multinucleated giant cells. MRH can be associated with lung, stomach, breast, cervix, colon, and ovarian cancer. Treatment agents include prednisone, methotrexate, and etanercept.

Palmar fasciitis (PF) is a fibrosing condition of the palmar fascia associated with bilateral finger contractures and inflammatory polyarthritis.[3] The most common sites of arthritis are the metacarpophalangeal and proximal interphalangeal joints, but the wrists, elbows, knees, ankles, and feet can also be involved. PF is almost always associated with an underlying cancer, such as that of the ovaries, breast, uterus, lung, stomach, pancreas,[13] or endometrium.[7] Leukemia and Hodgkin disease may also play a role.

Miscellaneous

Antiphospholipid antibody (aPL) positivity has a known association with thrombotic disease in primary antiphospholipid syndrome as well as a condition secondary to autoimmune diseases such as systemic lupus erythematosus.[3] Recent work has also revealed an association of aPLs with cancer, but an association of aPLs in this patient population with thromboembolism is less clear. Although the prevalence of aPLs in the general population is 1% to 5%, it is higher in patients who have solid malignancies or lymphoproliferative diseases. For example, a 1995 study comparing 216 patients with cancer with 88 healthy controls found an approximately 22% prevalence of anticardiolipin antibodies in the cancer arm and only approximately 3% in the control arm.[31] Rates of thromboembolism were much higher in patients with cancer with anticardiolipin antibodies (28%) compared with rates of thromboembolism in patients with cancer without anticardiolipin antibodies (14%). In a more recent prospective cohort study from 2014, 74% of 95 patients with cancer admitted to an intensive care unit had aPL antibodies.[32] However, vascular complication rates in that cohort were similar in patients with and without aPL antibodies. aPL positivity is associated with multiple types of cancer, including carcinoma of the stomach, colon, prostate, ovary, lung, kidney, liver, and breast, and B-cell lymphoma, chronic myeloid lymphoma, non-Hodgkin lymphoma, lymphoblastic leukemia, monocytic leukemia, and myelomonocytic leukemia.[33,34]Thrombotic events in aPL-positive patients may herald an underlying malignancy.[34] In a patient with venous thromboembolism and ovarian endometrial adenocarcinoma, surgical excision of the tumor was followed by disappearance of lupus anticoagulant and anticardiolipin antibody, suggesting that the cancer possibly induced the aPL antibodies[35] and hematologic malignancies alike.

Reflex sympathetic dystrophy (RSD), also called complex regional pain syndrome (CRPS), entails local pain, edema, vasomotor changes, and osteoporosis confined to a particular extremity.[3] The pathogenesis is thought to be sympathetic dysfunction, and it can be caused by stroke, heart attack, injury, or various malignancies, such as apical lung tumors. Such Pancoast tumors may disrupt the brachial plexus or the stellate ganglion and cause RSD. CRPS has also been associated with occult neoplasms of the brain, breast, bowel, and ovaries.[36] In rare cases, CRPS can be associated with the peripheral musculoskeletal tumors osteoid osteoma and epithelioid sarcoma. RSD may improve as the associated cancer is treated.

Oncogenic osteomalacia, also known as tumor-induced osteomalacia, results in renal phosphate wasting and causes severe biochemical and skeletal changes.[37] It is a rare paraneoplastic phenomenon associated with cancers that evolve fibroblast growth factor-23.[3] Osteomalacia refers to soft bones from inadequate calcification caused by kidney disease or vitamin D deficiency. Patients develop chronic, progressive pain in muscles and bones, fatigue, weakness, and recurrent fractures. In children, it may mimic rickets with signs such as gait abnormality, stunted growth, and skeletal changes. Laboratory investigations reveal hypophosphatemia, phosphaturia, and low or normal serum calcitriol level. (Normally, calcitriol level should be increased in the setting of hypophosphatemia.) The serum phosphorus level can be severely low (eg, 0.7 mg/dL). Bone histomorphometry reveals osteomalacia. Plain films may show diffuse osteopenia, pseudofractures, and coarsening of trabeculae. The fractures result from inadequate calcitriol production and renal phosphate wasting. The culprit tumors may be small, indolent, and unusually located; for example, in the craniofacial regions and extremities. Oncogenic osteomalacia may result from malignant or benign tumors, such as those originating from mesenchymal cells.[7] Removing the responsible tumor can lead to quick normalization of the biochemical abnormalities and remineralization of bone. If resection is not possible because of inability to identify the occult malignancy responsible, then medical management with phosphorus and calcitriol is indicated.

Sarcoidosis is not the only condition that causes noncaseating granulomas, because similar-appearing granulomas can be identified in lymph nodes that drain areas with cancer involvement.[3] Solid tumors and lymphomas are both associated with granuloma formation. Therefore, patients with presumed sarcoidosis should be thoroughly evaluated for an underlying malignancy. An increased risk of lung cancer, bile duct cancer, colorectal cancers, and lymphoma has been reported in the presence of sarcoidosis.[38]

Lymphomatoid granulomatosis (LG) is a lymphoproliferative disease that features lymphocytic infiltration of blood vessels.[3] It is angiodestructive; can affect the lungs, skin, and central nervous system; and carries a poor prognosis. LG has historically been associated with T-cell lymphomas.[39] A quarter of affected patients go on to develop lymphoma. In addition to lymphoma, LG may be associated with leukemia. It mostly affects middle-aged patients and has a male predilection.[40] Patients present with fever and cough. Plain films may show numerous, bilateral, nodular pulmonary infiltrates. The skin and nervous system are the most frequently affected sites outside the lungs. Pathology shows vascular infiltration by mononuclear cells and necrosis, cluster of differentiation (CD)-20 positive B cells, CD-3–positive T cells, plasma cells, and histiocytes. LG carries a mortality as high as 71%, with most deaths occurring within 2 years.

SUMMARY

Although cancers can cause morbidity and mortality through mass effect of the primary tumor or its metastases, they are also capable of exerting distant effects through paraneoplastic phenomena. Many types of paraneoplastic phenomena exist, including those relevant to rheumatology and the musculoskeletal system that affect the joints, muscles, vasculature, skin, and bones.

Clinics Care Points

- Clinical changes that may represent paraneoplastic phenomena should cue the physician to be vigilant for a concomitant or impending underlying malignancy.
- Treatment of a culprit malignancy can result in the resolution or amelioration of the associated paraneoplastic phenomenon.
- Atypical presentations of clinical entities not often thought to be related to cancer, such as RP or PMR, may serve as clues to their manifestation as paraneoplastic phenomena.
- When a paraneoplastic phenomenon is encountered, physicians should strongly consider a focused work-up for associated cancers, especially with new diagnoses of DM.

DISCLOSURE

The authors have nothing to disclose.

REFERENCES

1. Jameson JL, Longo DL. Paraneoplastic syndromes: endocrinologic/hematologic. In: Jameson JL, Fauci AS, Kasper DL, et al, editors. Harrison's principles of internal medicine. 20th edition. New York: McGraw-Hill Education; 2018.
2. Schoen FJ, Mitchell RN. Neoplasia. In: Robbins & Cotran pathologic basis of disease. 9th edition. Philadelphia, PA: Saunders/Elsevier; 2015. p. 265–340.
3. Vaseer S, Chakravarty EF. Musculoskeletal syndromes in malignancy. In: Kelley and Firestein's textbook of rheumatology. 10th edition. Philadelphia, PA: Saunders/Elsevier; 2017. p. 2048–65, e2046.
4. Gamage KKK, Rifath MIM, Fernando H. Migratory polyarthritis as a paraneoplastic syndrome in a patient with diffuse large B cell lymphoma: a case report. J Med Case Rep 2018;12(1):189.
5. Watson GA, O'Neill L, Law R, et al. Migrating polyarthritis as a feature of occult malignancy: 2 case reports and a review of the literature. Case Rep Oncol Med 2015;2015:934039.
6. Zupancic M, Annamalai A, Brenneman J, et al. Migratory polyarthritis as a paraneoplastic syndrome. J Gen Intern Med 2008;23(12):2136–9.
7. Sendur OF. Paraneoplastic rheumatic disorders. Archives of Rheumatology 2012; 27(1):18–23.

8. Chan MK, Hendrickson CS, Taylor KE. Polyarthritis associated with breast carcinoma. West J Med 1982;137(2):132–3.
9. Mader R. Proliferative bone diseases. In: Kelley and Firestein's textbook of rheumatology. 10th edition. Philadelphia, PA: Saunders/Elsevier; 2017. p. 1751–63.e3.
10. Martínez-Lavín M, Pineda C, Valdez T, et al. Primary hypertrophic osteoarthropathy. Semin Arthritis Rheum 1988;17(3):156–62.
11. Bozzao F, Bernardi S, Dore F, et al. Hypertrophic osteoarthropathy mimicking a reactive arthritis: a case report and review of the literature. BMC Musculoskelet Disord 2018;19(1):1–6.
12. Yap FY, Skalski MR, Patel DB, et al. Hypertrophic osteoarthropathy: clinical and imaging features. Radiographics 2017;37(1):157–95.
13. Manzini CU, Colaci M, Ferri C, et al. Paraneoplastic rheumatic disorders: a narrative review. 2018. Available at: https://wwwreumatismoorg/indexphp/reuma.
14. Garske LA, Bell SC. Pamidronate results in symptom control of hypertrophic pulmonary osteoarthropathy in cystic fibrosis. Chest 2002;121(4):1363–4.
15. Slobodin G, Rosner I, Feld J, et al. Pamidronate treatment in rheumatology practice: a comprehensive review. Clin Rheumatol 2009;28(12):1359–64.
16. Sakamoto T, Ota S, Haruyama T, et al. A case of paraneoplastic remitting seronegative symmetrical synovitis with pitting edema syndrome improved by chemotherapy. Case Rep Oncol 2017;10:1131–7.
17. Parperis K, Constantinidou A, Panos G. Paraneoplastic arthritides: insights to pathogenesis, diagnostic approach, and treatment. J Clin Rheumatol 2019. https://doi.org/10.1097/RHU.0000000000001202.
18. Pereira J, Eugénio G, Calretas S, et al. More than just a case of polymyalgia rheumatica. Eur J Case Rep Intern Med 2016;3. Available at: https://www-ncbi-nlm-nih-gov.proxy.lib.ohio-state.edu/pmc/articles/PMC6346904/pdf/374-1-2612-1-10-20160223.pdf.
19. West SG. Idiopathic inflammatory myopathies. In: Rheumatology secrets. 4th edition. Philadelphia, PA: Elsevier Health Sciences; 2020. p. 177–84.
20. Ponyi A, Constantin T, Garami M, et al. Cancer-associated myositis: clinical features and prognostic signs. Ann N Y Acad Sci 2005;1051(1):64–71.
21. Buggiani G, Krysenka A, Grazzini M, et al. Paraneoplastic vasculitis and paraneoplastic vascular syndromes. Dermatol Ther 2010;23(6):597–605.
22. Hernandez-Rodriguez J, Alba MA, Prieto-Gonzalez S, et al. Diagnosis and classification of polyarteritis nodosa. J Autoimmun 2014;48-49:84–9.
23. Elkon KB, Hughes GRV, Catovsky D, et al. Hairy-cell leukæmia with polyarthritis nodosa. Lancet 1979;314(8137):280–2.
24. Vankalakunti M, Joshi K, Jain S, et al. Polyarteritis nodosa in hairy cell leukaemia: an autopsy report. J Clin Pathol 2007;60(10):1181–2.
25. Fam AG. Paraneoplastic rheumatic syndromes. Baillieres Best Pract Res Clin Rheumatol 2000;14(3):515–33.
26. Stone JH. Immune complex–mediated small-vessel vasculitis. In: Kelley and Firestein's textbook of rheumatology. 10th edition. Philadelphia, PA: Saunders/Elsevier; 2017. p. 1571–80.
27. Le Besnerais M, Miranda S, Cailleux N, et al. Digital ischemia associated with cancer: results from a cohort study. Medicine (Baltimore) 2014;93(10):e47.
28. Shah A, Jack A, Liu H, et al. Neoplastic/paraneoplastic dermatitis, fasciitis, and panniculitis. Rheum Dis Clin North Am 2011;37(4):573–92.
29. Khanna D, Verity A, Grossman J. Eosinophilic fasciitis with multiple myeloma: a new haematological association. Ann Rheum Dis 2002;61(12):1111–2.

30. Chauhan A, Mikulik Z, Hackshaw KV. Multicentric reticulohistiocytosis with positive anticyclic citrullinated antibodies. J Natl Med Assoc 2007;99(6):678–80.
31. Zuckerman E, Toubi E, Golan TD, et al. Increased thromboembolic incidence in anti-cardiolipin-positive patients with malignancy. Br J Cancer 1995;72(2):447–51.
32. Vassalo J, Spector N, de Meis E, et al. Antiphospholipid antibodies in critically ill patients with cancer: a prospective cohort study. J Crit Care 2014;29(4):533–8.
33. Gomez-Puerta JA, Cervera R, Espinosa G, et al. Antiphospholipid antibodies associated with malignancies: clinical and pathological characteristics of 120 patients. Semin Arthritis Rheum 2006;35(5):322–32.
34. Miesbach W. Antiphospholipid antibodies and antiphospholipid syndrome in patients with malignancies: features, incidence, identification, and treatment. Semin Thromb Hemost 2008;34(3):282–5.
35. Asherson RA. Antiphospholipid antibodies, malignancies and paraproteinemias. J Autoimmun 2000;15(2):117–22.
36. Lipton S, Schwab P. Neoplasm mimics of rheumatologic presentations: sialadenitis, ocular masquerade syndromes, retroperitoneal fibrosis, and regional pain syndromes. Rheum Dis Clin North Am 2011;37(4):623–37.
37. Jan de Beur SM. Tumor-induced osteomalacia. JAMA 2005;294(10):1260–7.
38. Herron M, Chong SG, Gleeson L, et al. Paraneoplastic sarcoidosis: a review. QJM 2020;113(1):17–9.
39. Alexandra G, Claudia G. Lymphomatoid granulomatosis mimicking cancer and sarcoidosis. Ann Hematol 2019;98:1309–11.
40. Katzenstein A-LA, Doxtader E, Narendra S. Lymphomatoid granulomatosis: insights gained over 4 decades. Am J Surg Pathol 2010;34(12):e35–48.

Immune Checkpoint Inhibition—Does It Cause Rheumatic Diseases? Mechanisms of Cancer-Associated Loss of Tolerance and Pathogenesis of Autoimmunity

Uma Thanarajasingam, MD, PhD[a],*,
Noha Abdel-Wahab, MD, PhD[b,c,d]

KEYWORDS

- Immune checkpoint inhibitors • Immune-related adverse events
- Rheumatic diseases • Tolerance • Autoimmunity

KEY POINTS

- Immune checkpoints transmit inhibitory signals, preventing excessive cellular responses and helping to maintain self-tolerance and limit tissue damage during immune responses.
- Immune checkpoint inhibitors (ICIs) are cancer treatment strategies directed at improving the host response to cancer and are associated with the development of immune-related adverse events (irAEs).
- Rheumatic irAEs (Rh-irAEs) arise from ICI therapy and have a broad clinical spectrum that mirrors many classic rheumatic diseases.
- A breakdown in self-tolerance contributes in part to irAEs and Rh-irAEs but cannot account entirely for their emergence.

INTRODUCTION

The treatment paradigm of cancer has been transformed fully with the innovation of various immunotherapeutic modalities, such as tumor-specific monoclonal antibodies (mAbs), recombinant cytokines (interleukin [IL]-2 and interferon α-2b), adoptive

[a] Mayo Clinic, 200 1st Street Southwest, Rochester, MN 55906, USA; [b] Division of Internal Medicine, Section of Rheumatology and Clinical Immunology, The University of Texas MD Anderson Cancer Center, 1400 Pressler Street, Unit 1465, Houston, TX, USA; [c] Department of Rheumatology and Rehabilitation, The University of Texas MD Anderson Cancer Center, 1400 Pressler Street, Unit 1465, Houston, TX, USA; [d] Faculty of Medicine, Assiut University Hospital, Assiut, Egypt
* Corresponding author.
E-mail address: Thanarajasingam.Uma@mayo.edu

Rheum Dis Clin N Am 46 (2020) 587–603
https://doi.org/10.1016/j.rdc.2020.04.003
0889-857X/20/© 2020 Elsevier Inc. All rights reserved.

rheumatic.theclinics.com

transfer of ex vivo–activated immune cells, cancer vaccine sipuleucel-T, and more recently mAbs against T-cell regulatory checkpoints molecules.[1] Immune checkpoints have proved attractive and efficacious targets for cancer immunotherapy across multiple malignancies.[2] Immune checkpoint inhibitors (ICIs) target immune checkpoints, which are mechanisms critical for regulating T-cell responses to antigen and subsequent activation and proliferation. By blocking these immune checkpoints, the brakes are taken off the host immune system, and the host antitumor response is augmented. To date, 7 ICIs have been approved by the Food and Drug Administration (FDA), targeting 2 main signaling pathways: cytotoxic T-lymphocyte–associated protein 4 (CTLA-4) and programmed death 1 (PD-1)/programmed death-ligand 1 (PD-L1) inhibitory pathways, significantly enhancing overall survival in various cancers, including in the adjuvant setting.[3–11]

Anti–cytotoxic T-Lymphocyte–Associated Protein 4 Blocking Agents

Ipilimumab, a fully human IgG1 mAb, was the first ICI agent to receive FDA approval, in 2011, for metastatic melanoma[12] and in 2015 as an adjuvant therapy for high-risk stage III melanoma after complete resection.[7] No other anti-CTLA-4 inhibitors currently are approved.

Anti–programmed Death 1 Blocking Agents

Pembrolizumab, a humanized IgG4 mAb, was the first anti–PD-1 inhibitor to receive FDA approval, in 2014, for metastatic melanoma.[13,14] Its approval currently is expanded to 13 other cancers, including non–small cell lung cancer (NSCLC), head and neck squamous cell cancer, classical Hodgkin lymphoma, primary mediastinal large B-cell lymphoma, urothelial carcinoma, microsatellite instability-high cancer, gastric cancer, esophageal cancer, cervical cancer, hepatocellular carcinoma, Merkel cell carcinoma, renal cell carcinoma (RCC), and endometrial carcinoma,[4] and also in the adjuvant setting for melanoma.[8] Nivolumab, a fully human IgG4 mAb, was the second anti–PD-1 approved, in 2014, for metastatic melanoma[15] and currently is approved for 6 other cancers, including NSCLC, small cell lung cancer (SCLC), RCC, Hodgkin lymphoma, head and neck squamous cell cancer, urothelial carcinoma, and hepatocellular carcinoma,[3] and as an adjuvant therapy for melanoma.[11] Cemiplimab is the newest human IgG4 mAb against PD-1, approved in 2018 for metastatic and locally advanced cutaneous squamous cell carcinoma.[9]

Anti–programmed Death-Ligand 1 Blocking Agents

Atezolizumab, a humanized IgG1 mAb against PD-L1, was the first anti–PD-L1 inhibitor to receive FDA approval in 2016 for urothelial carcinoma,[10] followed by its approval for SCLC, NSCLC, and triple-negative breast cancer.[5] Durvalumab, a fully human IgG1 mAb against PD-L1, received FDA approval in 2017 for urothelial carcinoma[16] and in 2018 for NSCLC.[6] Avelumab, another fully human IgG1 mAb against PDL-1, was approved in 2017 for metastatic Merkel cell carcinoma[17] and subsequently for locally advanced or metastatic urothelial carcinoma[18] and RCC.[19]

Combination Therapy

Certain ICIs used in combination have elicited high response rates in advanced disease. Ipilimumab plus nivolumab initially was approved in 2016 for metastatic melanoma[20] and then for RCC,[21] and colorectal cancer with high microsatellite instability/mismatch repair deficiency.[22] Another promising combination is nivolumab plus bempegaldesleukin (a PEGylated IL-2) that recently received FDA breakthrough therapy designation for metastatic and previously untreated unresectable melanoma.[23]

IMMUNE-RELATED ADVERSE EVENTS

The hallmarks of cancer immunotherapy are durable clinical responses that presumably are mediated by persistent activation of the immune system. Such responses could result, however, in off-target inflammatory responses and irAEs that can be severe and occasionally fatal. The phenotype of irAEs varies widely; many patients develop toxicity involving multiple organs, others develop toxicity limited to 1 organ, and some patients may not develop toxicity despite continued ICI therapy. Gastrointestinal, liver, skin, endocrine, and pulmonary irAEs were those reported most frequently across ICI clinical trials. Any-grade irAEs have been reported in up to 90% of patients receiving ICI monotherapy.[24–29] Grade 3/4 toxicity has been reported in 22% of patients receiving anti–PD-1 monotherapy and in up to 59% of those receiving combination ICIs.[20,30–33] A meta-analysis of 21 trials compared 6528 patients who have received ICI with 4926 patients who have not; higher risks of all-grade colitis (RR 7.66' $P<.001$), aspartate aminotransferase elevation (relative risk [RR] 1.80; $P = .020$), skin rash (RR 2.50; $P = .001$), hypothyroiditis (RR 6.81; $P<.001$), and pneumonitis (RR 4.14; $P = .012$) were observed in ICI-treated patients.[27] In regard to high-grade toxicity, higher risks of colitis (RR 5.85; $P<.001$) and aspartate aminotransferase elevation (RR 2.79; $P = .014$) also were observed in ICI-treated patients. Ipilimumab use was associated with a higher risk of all-grade rash ($P = .006$) and high-grade colitis ($P = .021$) compared with anti–PD-1/PD-L1 agents. A total of 613 fatal irAEs have been reported in the World Health Organization pharmacovigilance database between 2009 and 2018; 193 related to anti–CTLA-4 (70% from colitis), 333 to anti–PD-1/PD-L1 (35% from pneumonitis, 22% from hepatitis, and 15% from neurologic irAEs), and 87 to combination ICIs (37% from colitis and 25% from myocarditis). A meta-analysis of 112 trials (19,217 patients) reported death because of irAEs in 0.36% and 0.38% of patients treated with anti–PD-1 and anti–PD-L1, respectively. Fatality rate increased to 1.08% among patients treated with anti–CTLA-4 and 1.23% among those treated with combinations ICIs.[29]

Rheumatic irAEs (Rh-irAEs) increasingly have been reported over the past 3 years.[34] Limited mechanistic understanding of irAEs, including Rh-irAEs, exists to date, and it remains to be fully understood whether or not irAEs arise merely as a consequence of systemic, tumor-agnostic immune activation, a breakdown in self-tolerance induced by checkpoint inhibition, unmasked autoimmunity marked by antigen-specific T-cell responses in susceptible hosts, or an alternative process of autoimmunity altogether.

The spectrum of Rh-irAEs is reviewed. The functions of 2 immune checkpoints targeted most commonly for cancer immunotherapy, CTLA-4 and the PD-1/PD-L1 pathways, are summarized. Subsequently, the role of these immune checkpoints in autoimmunity, the mechanisms and implications of immune checkpoint blockade in the context of cancer therapy, and available mechanistic understanding of irAEs, with a focus on Rh-irAEs are discussed.

RHEUMATIC IMMUNE-RELATED ADVERSE EVENTS

Rh-irAEs have been reported in 5% to 10% of cancer patients treated with ICIs,[35] yet the true incidence rates remain imprecise because most of these adverse events are not typically perceived as severe or life threatening and, therefore, are underreported in oncology trials.[36] A broad spectrum of Rh-irAEs has been reported so far; arthritis, sicca, myositis, and polymyalgia rheumatica are most frequent. Other rheumatic syndromes also have been reported, however, including de novo onset of sarcoidosis, vasculitis, lupus, antiphospholipid syndrome, scleroderma-like syndromes, hemophagocytic lymphohistiocytosis, bone abnormalities, and flares of preexisting autoimmune diseases after initiation of ICI therapy.[35,37–39] Most of the reported cases occurred after initiation of anti–PD-1/PD-L1 agents or combination ICIs, and median time to onset of rheumatic manifestations was variable (they can develop early on but also several months after ICI initiation). Rh-irAEs may persist despite discontinuation of immunotherapy, as in some patients with arthritis.[40,41] Death attributable to Rh-irAEs has been reported in few patients with complicated myositis or vasculitis.[35] In the following sections, the most common Rh-irAEs are summarized, the most severe ones as critical for early recognition highlighted, and finally the general concepts for management of Rh-irAEs summarized.

COMMON RHEUMATIC IMMUNE-RELATED ADVERSE EVENTS
Arthritis

Two systematic reviews of ICI trials and few additional observational studies have provided data primarily on Rh-irAEs; arthralgia was the most frequent, ranging from 1% to 43%, and arthritis occurred in 1% to 7%.[38,42–46] Most of the reported cases occurred after the administration of anti–PD-1 agents or combination ICIs, and duration between ICI initiation and onset of arthritis was variable (0.1–24 months). Different patterns of inflammatory arthritis have been reported so far. Seronegative polyarthritis was the most frequent (patients had negative rheumatoid factor [RF] and anti-citrullinated peptide (CCP) antibodies, but some had positive antinuclear antibody (ANA)), followed by erosive rheumatoid arthritis (RA)-like (patients had positive RF, anti-CCP, and/or ANA). In addition, some patients presented with features similar to seronegative spondyloarthritis, such as conjunctivitis, urethritis, and skin psoriasis; only a few were tested for HLA-B27 and were found negative. Furthermore, cases of de novo onset of undifferentiated oligoarthritis and monoarthritis have been reported.[47] In a few of these patients, inflammatory arthritis persisted for up to 2 years after ICI discontinuation, requiring immunomodulatory agents and significantly limiting patients' function and quality of life.[48,49] Approximately half of the patients with ICI-induced arthritis reported in literature also had other nonrheumatic irAEs.[47] Arthritis flares have been reported in patients with preexisting inflammatory arthritis when treated with ICIs[39] as well as in a few other patients with degenerative osteoarthritis and gouty arthritis.[46,50]

Moreover, few additional cases of remitting seronegative symmetric synovitis with pitting edema, inflammatory tenosynovitis (hands and/or shoulders), enthesitis, and Jaccoud arthropathy have been reported after initiation of ICIs.[51–56]

Sicca Syndrome

Two systematic reviews of ICI trials have reported sicca symptoms as a treatment-related adverse event, with an estimated prevalence of 1.2% to 24.2%.[43,57] The French registry, Registre des Effets Indésirables Sévères des Anticorps Monoclonaux Immunomodulateurs en Cancérologie (REISAMIC), which included patients who had received anti-PD-1/PD-L1 agents, identified that the prevalence of sicca in patients receiving single agent anti–PD-1 was 0.3% and increased to 2.5% in patients receiving combination ICIs.[44] All patients reported in REISAMIC registry fulfilled the 2002 American-European Consensus Group and the 2017 American College of Rheumatology(ACR)/European League Against Rheumatism (EULAR) diagnostic criteria for true Sjögren syndrome. Few additional small series of patients with de novo onset of sicca after initiation of ICI have been published.[37,41,58–62] Time to onset of symptoms after ICI initiation ranged from 1 month to 10 months. All reported patients had salivary gland hypofunction, few had dry mouth without keratoconjunctivitis, and 1 patient had bilateral parotid gland enlargement. Few patients had other Rh-irAEs (such as arthritis, polymyalgia rheumatica, cryoglobulinemic vasculitis, and RA flare), and others also had nonrheumatic irAEs. Autoantibodies, including ANA, RF, anti-SSA, or anti-SSB, were found positive in few patients, and 1 patient each was reported to have antisyn-thetase and anti-Scl-70 antibodies. In a few patients, the diagnosis was confirmed by salivary gland ultrasonography and/or labial salivary gland biopsy.[62]

Polymyalgia Rheumatica

Few observational studies have documented the development of polymyalgia rheumatica as an adverse event in cancer patients receiving ICIs, with an estimated prevalence of 0.2% to 2.1%.[38,44,63] A few other cases reports and small series also have been published.[35,37,44,58,59,64–72] Some of these patients fulfilled the 2012 EULAR/ACR diagnostic criteria for polymyalgia rheumatica. Most of the cases occurred after the administration of anti–PD-1/PD-L1 agents, and duration between ICI initiation and symptoms onset ranged from 0.3 month to 16 months. One of the reported patients had impaired vision,[63] and a few others had associated Rh-irAEs and nonrheumatic irAEs.

LIFE-THREATENING RHEUMATIC IMMUNE-RELATED ADVERSE EVENTS
Myositis

Three systematic reviews of ICI trials have reported myalgia as the second most common Rh-irAEs, with a prevalence ranging from 2% to 21%, whereas myositis was diagnosed less frequently (0.4% to 6%).[43,57,73] Several observational studies[37,44,74–79] as well as case reports and small series[35,58–60,70,75,76,78,80–94] have documented de novo onset of myositis as an adverse event in patients receiving ICIs. Most of the reported cases occurred after the administration of anti–PD-1 agents or combination ICIs, and duration between ICI initiation and symptoms onset was relatively short compared with other Rh-irAEs (0.4–3 months). Different patterns of myositis have been reported, including polymyositis, necrotizing myositis with rhabdomyolysis, nonspecific myopathy, dermatomyositis, and antisynthetase syndrome. In more than one-third of the cases, myositis was associated with myasthenia gravis (MG) or myocarditis; a few patients had the triad of MG/myositis/myocarditis, and others had additional nonrheumatic irAEs. Marked elevation of creatine phosphokinase (up to 19,794 IU/L) has been reported as well as elevation of aldolase, transaminases, and lactate dehydrogenase. Elevation of anti-acetylcholine receptor antibodies and/or troponin also has been reported in patients with the triad of MG/myositis/myocarditis. In a few patients, diagnosis was confirmed by muscle biopsy. Death primarily due to myositis has been reported.

Vasculitis

A few studies and a systematic review of published cases have identified de novo onset of vasculitis induced by ICI therapy, fulfilling the 2012 revised International Chapel Hill Consensus Conference nomenclature for vasculitis.[35,37,63,95–101] Most of the reported cases occurred after the administration of anti–PD-1 agents, apart from temporal arteritis, which was reported more frequently in patients who received anti–CTLA-4. The time between ICI initiation and onset of vasculitis symptoms ranged from 0.25 month to 18 months. Different types of vasculitis have been reported, yet large vessels vasculitis followed by nervous system vasculitis remain the most predominant types. Antineutrophil cytoplasmic antibodies–associated, necrotizing, granulomatous, uterine lymphocytic, retinal, cryoglobulinemic, autoimmune, cutaneous small vessels, digital, and acral vasculitis also have been reported. The time between ICI initiation and onset of vasculitis symptoms ranged from 0.7 month to 5.5 months. Vision was impaired in 28% of patients with temporal arteritis. Vasculitis-related death has been reported in few patients.[63]

IMMUNE CHECKPOINTS—MECHANISM OF ACTION

CTLA-4 is a coinhibitory molecule expressed on both activated T cells and regulatory T cells (T-reg). CTLA-4 is up-regulated on T cells that have received signal 1 through engagement of the T-cell receptor (TCR) with the cognate antigen–major histocompatabiltiy complex presented by an antigen-presenting cell (APC). CTLA-4 competes with the costimulatory molecule, CD28, for their shared ligands CD80 and CD86, whereas CD28 binding to these ligands results in an activating signal, which amplifies T-cell signaling and proliferation,[102] CTLA-4 dampens T-cell activation and T-cell–mediated immune responses in myriad ways. CTLA-4 signaling decreases CD80/86 expression on APCs,[103] thus decreasing the ability of T cells to engage CD28 and receive the critical signal 2 needed for full activation. CTLA-4 binding decreases IL-2 and IL-2 receptor expression, critical for T-cell proliferation.[104] In addition, CTLA-4 can induce APCs to secrete indoleamine 2,3-dioxygenase (IDO), which catalyzes tryptophan degradation thereby depleting a key molecule necessary for T-cell proliferation.[105] Beyond its coinhibitory effects on early activated T cells, CTLA-4 is constitutively expressed on regulatory T cells (Tregs), promoting their proliferation and immunosuppressive activities through enchanted production of various mediators, such as transforming growth factor-β, IL-10, and IDO.[106] Thus overall, CTLA-4 acts to dampen down T-cell responses by decreasing early T-cell activation and proliferation and enhancing Treg function.

Programmed Death 1

Similarly, PD-1 and its ligands PD-L1 and PD-L2 exert inhibitory functions, although at different stages of immune activation and via different mechanisms compared with CTLA-4. PD-1 and PD-L1 are focused on because they currently are targets of ICI therapy. PD-1 and PD-L1 are expressed more broadly than CTLA-4 and are seen on B cells, Tregs, macrophages, and APCs[107] in addition to T cells. In particular, PD-1 expression is up-regulated on effector/peripheral T cells, and its engagement with its ligand results in disruption of the TCR signaling cascade (via recruitment of tyrosine phosphatases) leading to diminished cytokine production, T-cell cytolytic function, and survival.[108,109] The net impact is that of diminished effector T-cell functionality in the periphery. The PD-1 pathway is thought to have similar immunosuppressive activity on other cell types[110] and its ligation on Tregs also enhances their immunosuppressive function.[109,111]

PD-1 additionally plays a critical role in thymocyte development, regulating thresholds during positive selection, and inhibiting the proliferation of naive autoreactive T cells during negative selection.[107] PD-L1 expression also has been observed in so-called immune-privileged sites, supporting a role for its protecting the site from the immune response.[109] Thus, critical actions of PD-1 and PDL-1 include roles in the establishment of central tolerance and the maintenance of peripheral tolerance.[112] Some tumors have evolved to up-regulate the expression of PD-L1 on their cell surface, promoting T-cell exhaustion and inhibiting tumor-specific cytolytic T cells, thus harnessing the power of this immune checkpoint to evade detection by the host immune system.[113]

Cytotoxic T-Lymphocyte–Associated Protein 4 and Programmed Death 1: Murine Knockout Phenotype

The critical role of immune checkpoints in maintaining homeostasis of the immune system is illustrated by the phenotypes of their cognate knockouts in mouse models. Germline knockout of CTLA-4 leads to widespread autoimmunity in mice characterized by fulminant infiltration of activated lymphocytes into various organs (eg, spleen, lymph nodes, heart, lung, and liver) and elevated antibody levels and is fatal 3 weeks to 4 weeks after birth.[114] Conditional deletion of CTLA-4 in adult mice similarly results in spontaneous multiorgan lymphoproliferation and organ-specific antibodies but is not fatal, allowing the longer observation of the phenotype, which then was expanded to include the development of histologically evident pneumonitis, gastritis, insulitis, and marked expansion of Tregs.[115] Furthermore, the severity of collagen-induced arthritis is greater in adult mice with CTLA-4 deficiency compared with wild-type mice.[115]

PD-1–deficient mice, in a strain-specific manner, develop complement-mediated glomerulonephritis in a lupus-like pattern,[116] and a subset develops inflammatory arthritis. Compared with CTLA-4 knockouts, the restricted clinical phenotype and the delayed onset of autoimmunity (greater than 1 year) in PD-1–deficient mice likely result from the later stages of immune activation targeted by PD-1.[107]

In both CTLA-4 and PD-1 knockout mouse models, the phenotype varies based on mouse strain, underscoring the significant role of background genes in the development of autoimmunity in the context of ICI.

CYTOTOXIC T-LYMPHOCYTE–ASSOCIATED PROTEIN 4 AND PROGRAMMED DEATH 1 AND AUTOIMMUNITY

CTLA-4 has been implicated in several rheumatic diseases, including RA, systemic lupus erythematosus, and Sjögren syndrome. In RA, CTLA-4-Ig, or abatacept, is a useful treatment strategy attributable to a variety of mechanisms, including decreased Treg cell death, increased T-cell susceptibility to Treg functions, and down-regulation of proinflammatory cytokine production.[117]

The PD-1/PD-L1 pathway has been investigated in autoimmunity, primarily in experimental animal models, with limited study in humans. The putative role of PD-1 in systemic lupus erythematosus is highlighted by the phenotype of the PD-1 knockout mouse (discussed previously). In humans, the PD-1 pathway is down-regulated at various stages of RA disease progression and is reduced further with treatment of early RA,[118] implicating the PD-1 pathway in RA pathogenesis and as a potential treatment target. PD-1 single-nucleotide polymorphisms have been found associated with certain rheumatic diseases, such as RA and ankylosing spondylitis.[107] Although results varied considerably by sex and ethnic group, they are supportive for a strong role of this pathway in autoimmunity. Considering these observations, together with the mechanistic understanding of immune checkpoints, it is not surprising checkpoint inhibition is associated with irAEs that have been observed in almost every organ system.

Mechanisms of Immune Checkpoint Blockade in Cancer

Combination checkpoint blockade (CCB) with CTLA-4 and PD-1 inhibitors results in better antitumor responses but also more prevalent irAEs.[20] The exact mechanisms, however, underlying the antitumor efficacy of CTLA-4 and PD-1 blockade or the development of irAEs or whether these mechanisms are shared are not fully understood.

CTLA-4 blockade in cancer patients has been shown to overcome cancer-associated tolerance mechanisms and to augment antitumor efficacy by (1) impairing Treg effectiveness and longevity[119] and (2) reducing intratumoral Tregs[120] and possibly expanding and maintaining high-avidity T-cell clones with antitumor responses.[121] Furthermore, antibodies blocking CTLA-4 may lead to antibody-dependent cellular cytotoxicity of Tregs,[120] thus impeding peripheral tolerance and increasing the risk of autoimmunity. PD-1 blockade targets effector T cells in the periphery and thus preexisting antitumor T-cell responses. Clinically, this has translated into a more limited toxicity profile and increased therapeutic efficacy of the PD-1 inhibitors.[32]

It appears that shared and distinct cellular mechanisms underlie the antitumor efficacy related to CTLA-4 and PD-1 checkpoint blockade. Work by Wei and colleagues[122] demonstrated that anti–PDI-1 therapy induces the expansion of tumor-infiltrating CD8 T cells with an exhausted phenotype, whereas anti–CTLA-4 therapy induces the expansion of ICOS+TH1-like CD4 effector cells in addition to a subset of exhausted CD8 T cells. Further complicating matters are the observations that alternative inhibitory checkpoints are compensatory up-regulated after immune checkpoint blockade.[123] In the grand scheme of things, it is wise to view immune checkpoints as an intertwined and complex network that continually strives for immune homeostasis. Certainly, irAEs reflect a perturbation of such homeostasis. The putative mechanisms of irAEs are reviewed.

Mechanisms and Immunopathology of Immune-Related Adverse Events

Concurrent with CTLA-4 blockade has been observed the increase in circulating helper T cells type 17, which have been implicated in several autoimmune diseases, including colitis. PD-1 blockade is associated with the increased production of IL-6, IL-17, and enhanced Th1 responses, which could contribute as well to the development of autoimmunity.[124]

Greater diversification of the T-cell repertoire has been demonstrated in cancer patients treated with ICI who developed irAEs compared with those who did not.[15,125] In patients with prostate cancer receiving ipilimumab, an increased number of expanded CD8 T-cell clones in peripheral blood correlated with the presence of severe irAEs.[126,127] This TCR expansion could reflect overall immune activation in the context of ICI, which in turns leads to the mobilization and expansion of a diverse T-cell population, some of which may be autoreactive.

In 1 study, after CCB treatment in the setting of advanced melanoma, increases in the number of plasmablasts and markers of B-cell clonality were observed,[128] which correlated to higher rates of severe, delayed-onset irAEs. These observations support a role for B-cell autoreactivity, specifically in combined CCB, in the development of irAEs.

Despite data for a putative role for B cells in irAEs in general, autoantibody production is not associated strongly with Rh-irAEs in particular. Most patients with Rh-irAEs are seronegative.[34,41] Furthermore, in the limited studies available to date, only a minority of patients develop any positive autoantibodies after ICI therapy,[129] with anti-thyroid peroxidase antibodies the most common. The latter suggests that humoral immunity may feature more prominently in other, nonrheumatic irAEs.

In Rh-irAEs, the availability of immunopathologic studies supporting the diagnoses, although scant, suggest similar findings to those seen in some, but not all, of the classic rheumatic diseases.[130] For example, synovial fluid analyses from joints of patients who have developed inflammatory arthritis after ICI show increased cell counts with a neutrophil predominance, similar to findings that can be seen in, but are not specific for, RA. Furthermore, in a report of ICI-induced granulomatosis with polyangiitis, temporal artery biopsies echoed those seen in granulomatosis with polyangiitis and showed an inflammatory infiltrate of the adventitia and muscular layers with narrowing of the arterial lumen.[98]

In contrast, in ICI-induced myositis, the pathologic phenotype is varied and does not necessarily echo that seen in classical dermatomyositis (DM) or polymyositis (PM), with some biopsies showing features of inflammation, whereas others, predominantly muscle fiber atrophy or necrosis—suggesting distinct pathways of immune attack.[34] A series of patients with sicca syndrome had imaging findings of the parotid glands demonstrating hypoechoic lesions and lymphocytic aggregates as seen in Sjögren syndrome. None of these patients, however, was seropositive,[41] and, in other studies, minor salivary gland biopsies from patients with ICI-induced sicca tended to show a predominance of T-cell infiltration compared with the B-cell infiltrates seen in Sjögren syndrome.[62]

Cancer Immunity and Autoimmunity

Overall, there appears to be some shared but also distinct pathologic mechanisms that underlie Rh-irAEs compared with classical rheumatic disease. Furthermore, although CTLA-4 and PD-1 have been associated with autoimmune disease and their inhibition is associated with irAEs, whether their blockade directly causes autoimmunity and rheumatic disease remains unknown. In a landmark study of CTLA-4 function and antitumor immunity by Lute and colleagues,[131] anti-human CTLA-4 antibodies were studied in human *CTLA4* gene knockin mice for their ability to induce tumor rejection and autoimmunity. It was found that the antibody that induced the strongest protection against cancer induced the least autoimmune side effects—effectively uncoupling the autoimmune side effects and cancer therapeutic effects.

Cancer immunity and autoimmunity may overlap but are not one and the same. The effector arms of these immune responses vary, as do the tissues they target and the susceptibilities of those tissues to immune attack; additionally, the influence of host genetics and environmental factors cannot be underestimated. As such, although ICIs and Rh-irAEs provide novel and unique, in vivo opportunities to study autoimmunity, checkpoint inhibition cannot yet be pointed to as a direct causative factor for rheumatic disease. What is clear is that the most successful approaches moving forward, either antitumor or anti-irAEs, will be those that are able to selectively modulate the delicate balance between cancer immunity and autoimmunity.

SUMMARY

Immune checkpoints are critical for the immunomodulation of immune responses, and their absence or blockade has been associated with various manifestations of autoimmunity. ICI has proved an effective, largely tumor-agnostic cancer therapy but is associated with irAEs, including Rh-irAEs, which share variable clinical and pathologic similarities with classic rheumatic diseases. The mechanisms underlying ICI effectiveness and irAE occurrence, however, are far from fully understood. Disruption of self-tolerance and perturbations in T-cell clonality and Treg activity downstream of ICI seem to play prominent roles, but further study is crucial.

Clinics Care Points

ICIs have advanced the treatment of various cancers with remarkable survival benefits; however, their efficacy remains limited by the occurrence of irAEs.

- Rh-irAEs could have long-lasting effects and sequelae and sometimes are life threatening.
- Understanding the potential long-term adverse events of ICIs and how they could have an impact on patients' function and quality of life remains an unmet medical need.
- Identifying the specific immune correlates associated with the occurrence of irAEs could provide information on which targeted agents might be useful for irAEs management without hindering the antitumor immune response of ICI therapy.

DISCLOSURE

Dr. Thanarajasingam is supported by the "Catalyst" award for Advancing in Academics Program, funded by the Department of Medicine, Mayo Clinic, Rochester, MN.

REFERENCES

1. Papaioannou NE, Beniata OV, Vitsos P, et al. Harnessing the immune system to improve cancer therapy. Ann Transl Med 2016;4(14):261.
2. Topalian SL, Drake CG, Pardoll DM. Immune checkpoint blockade: a common denominator approach to cancer therapy. Cancer cell 2015;27(4):450–61.
3. Opdivo-nivolumab [package insert]. Princeton (NJ): NBMS; 2019. Available at: https://www.accessdata.fda.gov/drugsatfda_docs/label/2019/125554s075lbl.pdf.
4. KEYTRUDA- Pembrolizumab [package insert]. County Cork (Ireland): IM; 2019. Available at: https://www.accessdata.fda.gov/drugsatfda_docs/label/2020/125514s067lbl.pdf.
5. TECENTRIQ-atezolizumab [package insert]. South San Francisco CG. 2020. Available at: https://www.accessdata.fda.gov/drugsatfda_docs/label/2019/125377s104lbl.pdf. Accessed January, 2020.
6. Antonia SJ, Villegas A, Daniel D, et al. Durvalumab after chemoradiotherapy in stage III non-small-cell lung cancer. N Engl J Med 2017;377(20):1919–29.
7. Eggermont AM, Chiarion-Sileni V, Grob JJ, et al. Adjuvant ipilimumab versus placebo after complete resection of high-risk stage III melanoma (EORTC 18071): a randomised, double-blind, phase 3 trial. Lancet Oncol 2015;16(5):522–30.
8. Eggermont AMM, Blank CU, Mandala M, et al. Adjuvant pembrolizumab versus placebo in resected stage III melanoma. N Engl J Med 2018;378(19):1789–801.
9. Migden MR, Rischin D, Schmults CD, et al. PD-1 blockade with cemiplimab in advanced cutaneous squamous-cell carcinoma. N Engl J Med 2018;379(4):341–51.
10. Rosenberg JE, Hoffman-Censits J, Powles T, et al. Atezolizumab in patients with locally advanced and metastatic urothelial carcinoma who have progressed following treatment with platinum-based chemotherapy: a single-arm, multicentre, phase 2 trial. Lancet 2016;387(10031):1909–20.
11. Weber J, Mandala M, Del Vecchio M, et al. Adjuvant Nivolumab versus Ipilimumab in Resected Stage III or IV Melanoma. N Engl J Med 2017;377(19):1824–35.
12. Hodi FS, O'Day SJ, McDermott DF, et al. Improved survival with ipilimumab in patients with metastatic melanoma. N Engl J Med 2010;363(8):711–23.
13. Robert C, Ribas A, Wolchok JD, et al. Anti-programmed-death-receptor-1 treatment with pembrolizumab in ipilimumab-refractory advanced melanoma: a

randomised dose-comparison cohort of a phase 1 trial. Lancet 2014;384(9948): 1109–17.

14. Robert C, Schachter J, Long GV, et al. Pembrolizumab versus Ipilimumab in Advanced Melanoma. N Engl J Med 2015;372(26):2521–32.

15. Robert C, Long GV, Brady B, et al. Nivolumab in previously untreated melanoma without BRAF mutation. N Engl J Med 2015;372(4):320–30.

16. Massard C, Gordon MS, Sharma S, et al. Safety and efficacy of durvalumab (MEDI4736), an anti-programmed cell death ligand-1 immune checkpoint inhibitor, in patients with advanced urothelial bladder cancer. J Clin Oncol 2016; 34(26):3119–25.

17. Kaufman HL, Russell J, Hamid O, et al. Avelumab in patients with chemotherapy-refractory metastatic Merkel cell carcinoma: a multicentre, single-group, open-label, phase 2 trial. Lancet Oncol 2016;17(10):1374–85.

18. Patel MR, Ellerton J, Infante JR, et al. Avelumab in metastatic urothelial carcinoma after platinum failure (JAVELIN Solid Tumor): pooled results from two expansion cohorts of an open-label, phase 1 trial. Lancet Oncol 2018;19(1): 51–64.

19. Motzer RJ, Penkov K, Haanen J, et al. Avelumab plus Axitinib versus Sunitinib for Advanced Renal-Cell Carcinoma. N Engl J Med 2019;380(12):1103–15.

20. Larkin J, Chiarion-Sileni V, Gonzalez R, et al. Combined Nivolumab and Ipilimumab or Monotherapy in Untreated Melanoma. N Engl J Med 2015;373(1):23–34.

21. Motzer RJ, Rini BI, McDermott DF, et al. Nivolumab plus ipilimumab versus sunitinib in first-line treatment for advanced renal cell carcinoma: extended follow-up of efficacy and safety results from a randomised, controlled, phase 3 trial. Lancet Oncol 2019;20(10):1370–85.

22. Morse MA, Overman MJ, Hartman L, et al. Safety of Nivolumab plus Low-Dose Ipilimumab in Previously Treated Microsatellite Instability-High/Mismatch Repair-Deficient Metastatic Colorectal Cancer. Oncologist 2019;24(11):1453–61.

23. Hurwitz ME, Cho DC, Balar AV, et al. Baseline tumor-immune signatures associated with response to bempegaldesleukin (NKTR-214) and nivolumab. J Clin Oncol 2019;37(15_suppl):2623.

24. Khoja L, Day D, Wei-Wu Chen T, et al. Tumour- and class-specific patterns of immune-related adverse events of immune checkpoint inhibitors: a systematic review. Ann Oncol 2017;28(10):2377–85.

25. Bertrand A, Kostine M, Barnetche T, et al. Immune related adverse events associated with anti-CTLA-4 antibodies: systematic review and meta-analysis. BMC Med 2015;13:211.

26. El Osta B, Hu F, Sadek R, et al. Not all immune-checkpoint inhibitors are created equal: Meta-analysis and systematic review of immune-related adverse events in cancer trials. Crit Rev Oncol Hematol 2017;119:1–12.

27. De Velasco G, Je Y, Bosse D, et al. Comprehensive meta-analysis of key immune-related adverse events from CTLA-4 and PD-1/PD-L1 inhibitors in cancer patients. Cancer Immunol Res 2017;5(4):312–8.

28. Shoushtari AN, Friedman CF, Navid-Azarbaijani P, et al. Measuring toxic effects and time to treatment failure for nivolumab plus ipilimumab in melanoma. JAMA Oncol 2018;4(1):98–101.

29. Wang DY, Salem JE, Cohen JV, et al. Fatal toxic effects associated with immune checkpoint inhibitors: a systematic review and meta-analysis. JAMA Oncol 2018;4(12):1721–8.

30. Schachter J, Ribas A, Long GV, et al. Pembrolizumab versus ipilimumab for advanced melanoma: final overall survival results of a multicentre, randomised, open-label phase 3 study (KEYNOTE-006). Lancet 2017;390(10105):1853–62.

31. Hodi FS, Chiarion-Sileni V, Gonzalez R, et al. Nivolumab plus ipilimumab or nivolumab alone versus ipilimumab alone in advanced melanoma (CheckMate 067): 4-year outcomes of a multicentre, randomised, phase 3 trial. Lancet Oncol 2018;19(11):1480–92.

32. Weber JS, Hodi FS, Wolchok JD, et al. Safety profile of nivolumab monotherapy: a pooled analysis of patients with advanced melanoma. J Clin Oncol 2017; 35(7):785–92.

33. Eggermont AM, Chiarion-Sileni V, Grob JJ, et al. Prolonged survival in stage III melanoma with ipilimumab adjuvant therapy. N Engl J Med 2016;375(19): 1845–55.

34. Richter MD, Crowson C, Kottschade LA, et al. Rheumatic Syndromes Associated With Immune Checkpoint Inhibitors: A Single-Center Cohort of Sixty-One Patients. Arthritis Rheumatol 2019;71(3):468–75. https://doi.org/10.1002/art. 40745.

35. Abdel-Wahab N, Suarez-Almazor ME. Frequency and distribution of various rheumatic disorders associated with checkpoint inhibitor therapy. Rheumatology (Oxford) 2019;58(Supplement_7):vii40–8.

36. Cappelli LC, Shah AA, Bingham CO. Immune-related adverse effects of cancer immunotherapy- implications for rheumatology. Rheum Dis Clin North Am 2017; 43(1):65–78.

37. Richter MD, Crowson C, Kottschade LA, et al. Rheumatic syndromes associated with immune checkpoint inhibitors: a single-center cohort of sixty-one patients. Arthritis Rheumatol 2019;71(3):468–75.

38. Kostine M, Rouxel L, Barnetche T, et al. Rheumatic disorders associated with immune checkpoint inhibitors in patients with cancer-clinical aspects and relationship with tumour response: a single-centre prospective cohort study. Ann Rheum Dis 2018;77(3):393–8.

39. Abdel-Wahab N, Shah M, Lopez-Olivo MA, et al. Use of immune checkpoint inhibitors in the treatment of patients with cancer and preexisting autoimmune disease a systematic review. Ann Intern Med 2018;168(2):121.

40. Cappelli LC, Brahmer JR, Forde PM, et al. Clinical presentation of immune checkpoint inhibitor-induced inflammatory arthritis differs by immunotherapy regimen. Semin Arthritis Rheum 2018;48(3):553–7.

41. Cappelli LC, Gutierrez AK, Baer AN, et al. Inflammatory arthritis and sicca syndrome induced by nivolumab and ipilimumab. Ann Rheum Dis 2017;76(1): 43–50.

42. Abdel-Rahman O, Eltobgy M, Oweira H, et al. Immune-related musculoskeletal toxicities among cancer patients treated with immune checkpoint inhibitors: a systematic review. Immunotherapy 2017;9(14):1175–83.

43. Cappelli LC, Gutierrez AK, Bingham CO, et al. Rheumatic and musculoskeletal immune-related adverse events due to immune checkpoint inhibitors: a systematic review of the literature. Arthritis Care Res 2017;69(11):1751–63.

44. Le Burel S, Champiat S, Mateus C, et al. Prevalence of immune-related systemic adverse events in patients treated with anti-Programmed cell Death 1/anti-Programmed cell Death-Ligand 1 agents: A single-centre pharmacovigilance database analysis. Eur J Cancer 2017;82:34–44.

45. Lidar M, Giat E, Garelick D, et al. Rheumatic manifestations among cancer patients treated with immune checkpoint inhibitors. Autoimmun Rev 2018;17(3): 284–9.

46. Buder-Bakhaya K, Benesova K, Schulz C, et al. Characterization of arthralgia induced by PD-1 antibody treatment in patients with metastasized cutaneous malignancies. Cancer Immunol Immunother 2018;67(2):175–82.

47. Pundole X, Abdel-Wahab N, Suarez-Almazor ME. Arthritis risk with immune checkpoint inhibitor therapy for cancer. Curr Opin Rheumatol 2019;31(3):293–9.

48. Braaten TJ, Brahmer JR, Forde PM, et al. Immune checkpoint inhibitor-induced inflammatory arthritis persists after immunotherapy cessation. Ann Rheum Dis 2019;79(3):332–8.

49. Calabrese L, Velcheti V. Checkpoint immunotherapy: good for cancer therapy, bad for rheumatic diseases. Ann Rheum Dis 2017;76(1):1–3.

50. Kim ST, Bittar M, Kim HJ, et al. Recurrent pseudogout after therapy with immune checkpoint inhibitors: a case report with immunoprofiling of synovial fluid at each flare. J Immunother Cancer 2019;7(1):126.

51. Gauci ML, Baroudjian B, Laly P, et al. Remitting seronegative symmetrical synovitis with pitting edema (RS3PE) syndrome induced by nivolumab. Semin Arthritis Rheum 2017;47(2):281–7.

52. Ngo L, Miller E, Valen P, et al. Nivolumab induced remitting seronegative symmetrical synovitis with pitting edema in a patient with melanoma: A case report. J Med Case Rep 2018;12(1):48.

53. Wada N, Uchi H, Furue M. Case of remitting seronegative symmetrical synovitis with pitting edema (RS3PE) syndrome induced by nivolumab in a patient with advanced malignant melanoma. J Dermatol 2017;44(8):e196–7.

54. de Velasco G, Bermas B, Choueiri TK. Autoimmune arthropathy and uveitis as complications of programmed death 1 inhibitor treatment. Arthritis Rheumatol 2016;68(2):556–7.

55. Inamo J, Kaneko Y, Takeuchi T. Inflammatory tenosynovitis and enthesitis induced by immune checkpoint inhibitor treatment. Clin Rheumatol 2018; 37(4):1107–10.

56. Smith MH, Bass AR. Arthritis after cancer immunotherapy: symptom duration and treatment response. Arthritis Care Res (Hoboken) 2019;71(3):362–6.

57. Abdel-Rahman O, Oweira H, Petrausch U, et al. Immune-related ocular toxicities in solid tumor patients treated with immune checkpoint inhibitors: a systematic review. Expert Rev Anticancer Ther 2017;17(4):387–94.

58. Calabrese C, Kirchner E, Kontzias K, et al. Rheumatic immune-related adverse events of checkpoint therapy for cancer: case series of a new nosological entity. RMD Open 2017;3(1):e000412.

59. Narvaez J, Juarez-Lopez P, J.L.L., et al. Rheumatic immune-related adverse events in patients on anti-PD-1 inhibitors: Fasciitis with myositis syndrome as a new complication of immunotherapy. Autoimmun Rev 2018;17(10):1040–5.

60. Leipe J, Christ LA, Arnoldi AP, et al. Characteristics and treatment of new-onset arthritis after checkpoint inhibitor therapy. RMD Open 2018;4(2):e000714.

61. Teyssonneau D, Cousin S, Italiano A. Gougerot-Sjogren-like syndrome under PD-1 inhibitor treatment. Ann Oncol 2017;28(12):3108.

62. Warner BM, Baer AN, Lipson EJ, et al. Sicca Syndrome Associated with Immune Checkpoint Inhibitor Therapy. Oncologist 2019;24(9):1259–69.

63. Salem JE, Manouchehri A, Moey M, et al. Cardiovascular toxicities associated with immune checkpoint inhibitors: an observational, retrospective, pharmacovigilance study. Lancet Oncol 2018;19(12):1579–89.

64. Belkhir R, Burel SL, Dunogeant L, et al. Rheumatoid arthritis and polymyalgia rheumatica occurring after immune checkpoint inhibitor treatment. Ann Rheum Dis 2017;76(10):1747–50.
65. Chan KK, Bass AR. Checkpoint inhibitor-induced polymyalgia rheumatica controlled by cobimetinib, a MEK 1/2 inhibitor. Ann Rheum Dis 2019;78(7):e70.
66. Garel B, Kramkimel N, Trouvin AP, et al. Pembrolizumab-induced polymyalgia rheumatica in two patients with metastatic melanoma. Joint Bone Spine 2017; 84(2):233–4.
67. Imai Y, Tanaka M, Fujii R, et al. [Effectiveness of a Low-dose Corticosteroid in a Patient with Polymyalgia Rheumatica Associated with Nivolumab Treatment]. Yakugaku zasshi 2019;139(3):491–5.
68. Iskandar A, Hwang A, Dasanu CA. Polymyalgia rheumatica due to pembrolizumab therapy. J Oncol Pharm Pract 2018;25(5):1282–4.
69. Kuswanto WF, MacFarlane LA, Gedmintas L, et al. Rheumatologic symptoms in oncologic patients on PD-1 inhibitors. Semin Arthritis Rheum 2018;47(6): 907–10.
70. Mitchell EL, Lau PKH, Khoo C, et al. Rheumatic immune-related adverse events secondary to anti-programmed death-1 antibodies and preliminary analysis on the impact of corticosteroids on anti-tumour response: A case series. Eur J Cancer 2018;105:88–102.
71. Bernier M, Guillaume C, Leon N, et al. Nivolumab causing a polymyalgia rheumatica in a patient with a squamous non-small cell lung cancer. J Immunother 2017. https://doi.org/10.1097/CJI.0000000000000163.
72. Nakamagoe K, Moriyama T, Maruyama H, et al. Polymyalgia rheumatica in a melanoma patient due to nivolumab treatment. J Cancer Res Clin Oncol 2017; 143(7):1357–8.
73. Baxi S, Yang A, Gennarelli RL, et al. Immune-related adverse events for anti-PD-1 and anti-PD-L1 drugs: systematic review and meta-analysis. BMJ 2018;360: k793.
74. Anquetil C, Salem JE, Lebrun-Vignes B, et al. Immune checkpoint inhibitor-associated myositis. Circulation 2018;138(7):743–5.
75. Pundole X, Shah M, Abdel-Wahab N, et al. Immune checkpoint inhibitors and inflammatory myopathies: data from the US food and drug administration adverse event reporting system. Arthritis Rheumatol 2017;69(10):1192–3.
76. Liewluck T, Kao JC, Mauermann ML. PD-1 Inhibitor-associated Myopathies: Emerging Immune-mediated Myopathies. J Immunother 2018;41(4):208–11.
77. Touat M, Maisonobe T, Knauss S, et al. Immune checkpoint inhibitor-related myositis and myocarditis in patients with cancer. Neurology 2018;91(10): e985–94.
78. Moreira A, Loquai C, Pfohler C, et al. Myositis and neuromuscular side-effects induced by immune checkpoint inhibitors. Eur J Cancer 2019;106:12–23.
79. Safa H, Johnson DH, Trinh VA, et al. Immune checkpoint inhibitor related myasthenia gravis: single center experience and systematic review of the literature. J Immunother Cancer 2019;7(1):319.
80. Chen YH, Liu FC, Hsu CH, et al. Nivolumab-induced myasthenia gravis in a patient with squamous cell lung carcinoma: Case report. Medicine 2017;96(27): e7350.
81. Delyon J, Brunet-Possenti F, Leonard-Louis S, et al. Immune checkpoint inhibitor rechallenge in patients with immune-related myositis. Ann Rheum Dis 2019; 78(11):e129.

82. Fellner A, Makranz C, Lotem M, et al. Neurologic complications of immune checkpoint inhibitors. J Neurooncol 2018;137(3):601–9.
83. Kadota H, Gono T, Shirai Y, et al. Immune checkpoint inhibitor-induced myositis: a case report and literature review. Curr Rheumatol Rep 2019;21(4):10.
84. John S, Antonia SJ, Rose TA, et al. Progressive hypoventilation due to mixed CD8(+) and CD4(+) lymphocytic polymyositis following tremelimumab - durvalumab treatment. J Immunother Cancer 2017;5(1):54.
85. Kang KH, Grubb W, Sawlani K, et al. Immune checkpoint-mediated myositis and myasthenia gravis: A case report and review of evaluation and management. Am J Otolaryngol 2018;39(5):642–5.
86. Mohn N, Suhs KW, Gingele S, et al. Acute progressive neuropathy-myositis-myasthenia-like syndrome associated with immune-checkpoint inhibitor therapy in patients with metastatic melanoma. Melanoma Res 2019;29(4):435–44.
87. Monge C, Maeng H, Brofferio A, et al. Myocarditis in a patient treated with Nivolumab and PROSTVAC: a case report. J Immunother Cancer 2018;6(1):150.
88. Reynolds KL, Guidon AC. Diagnosis and management of immune checkpoint inhibitor-associated neurologic toxicity: illustrative case and review of the literature. Oncologist 2018;24(4):435–44.
89. Roberts JH, Smylie M, Oswald A, et al. Hepatitis is the new myositis: immune checkpoint inhibitor-induced myositis. Melanoma Res 2018;28(5):484–5.
90. Suzuki S, Ishikawa N, Konoeda F, et al. Nivolumab-related myasthenia gravis with myositis and myocarditis in Japan. Neurology 2017;89(11):1127–34.
91. Pushkarevskaya A, Neuberger U, Dimitrakopoulou-Strauss A, et al. Severe ocular myositis after ipilimumab treatment for melanoma: a report of 2 cases. J Immunother 2017;40(7):282–5.
92. Shah M, Tayar JH, Abdel-Wahab N, et al. Myositis as an adverse event of immune checkpoint blockade for cancer therapy. Semin Arthritis Rheum 2018; 48(4):736–40.
93. Sheik Ali S, Goddard AL, Luke JJ, et al. Drug-associated dermatomyositis following ipilimumab therapy: a novel immune-mediated adverse event associated with cytotoxic T-lymphocyte antigen 4 blockade. JAMA Dermatol 2015; 151(2):195–9.
94. Kudo F, Watanabe Y, Iwai Y, et al. Advanced lung adenocarcinoma with nivolumab-associated dermatomyositis. Intern Med 2018;57(15):2217–21.
95. Daxini A, Cronin K, Sreih AG. Vasculitis associated with immune checkpoint inhibitors-a systematic review. Clin Rheumatol 2018;37(9):2579–84.
96. Perez-De-Lis M, Retamozo S, Flores-Chavez A, et al. Autoimmune diseases induced by biological agents. A review of 12,731 cases (BIOGEAS Registry). Expert Opin Drug Saf 2017;16(11):1255–71.
97. Mamlouk O, Selamet U, Machado S, et al. Nephrotoxicity of immune checkpoint inhibitors beyond tubulointerstitial nephritis: single-center experience. J Immunother Cancer 2019;7(1):2.
98. Goldstein BL, Gedmintas L, Todd DJ. Drug-associated polymyalgia rheumatica/giant cell arteritis occurring in two patients after treatment with ipilimumab, an antagonist of ctla-4. Arthritis Rheumatol 2014;66(3):768–9.
99. Roger A, Groh M, Lorillon G, et al. Eosinophilic granulomatosis with polyangiitis (Churg-Strauss) induced by immune checkpoint inhibitors. Ann Rheum Dis 2018;78(8):e82.
100. Castillo B, Gibbs J, Brohl AS, et al. Checkpoint inhibitor-associated cutaneous small vessel vasculitis. JAAD Case Rep 2018;4(7):675–7.

101. Comont T, Sibaud V, Mourey L, et al. Immune checkpoint inhibitor-related acral vasculitis. J Immunother Cancer 2018;6(1):120.
102. Ravetch JV, Lanier LL. Immune inhibitory receptors. Science 2000; 290(5489):84–9.
103. Qureshi OS, Zheng Y, Nakamura K, et al. Trans-endocytosis of CD80 and CD86: a molecular basis for the cell-extrinsic function of CTLA-4. Science 2011; 332(6029):600–3.
104. Phan GQ, Yang JC, Sherry RM, et al. Cancer regression and autoimmunity induced by cytotoxic T lymphocyte-associated antigen 4 blockade in patients with metastatic melanoma. Proc Natl Acad Sci U S A 2003;100(14):8372–7.
105. Uyttenhove C, Pilotte L, Theate I, et al. Evidence for a tumoral immune resistance mechanism based on tryptophan degradation by indoleamine 2,3-dioxygenase. Nat Med 2003;9(10):1269–74.
106. Fallarino F, Grohmann U, Hwang KW, et al. Modulation of tryptophan catabolism by regulatory T cells. Nat Immunol 2003;4(12):1206–12.
107. Gianchecchi E, Delfino DV, Fierabracci A. Recent insights into the role of the PD-1/PD-L1 pathway in immunological tolerance and autoimmunity. Autoimmun Rev 2013;12(11):1091–100.
108. Riley JL. PD-1 signaling in primary T cells. Immunol Rev 2009;229(1):114–25.
109. Francisco LM, Sage PT, Sharpe AH. The PD-1 pathway in tolerance and autoimmunity. Immunol Rev 2010;236:219–42.
110. Pardoll DM. The blockade of immune checkpoints in cancer immunotherapy. Nat Rev Cancer 2012;12(4):252–64.
111. Francisco LM, Salinas VH, Brown KE, et al. PD-L1 regulates the development, maintenance, and function of induced regulatory T cells. J Exp Med 2009; 206(13):3015–29.
112. Okazaki T, Honjo T. PD-1 and PD-1 ligands: from discovery to clinical application. Int Immunol 2007;19(7):813–24.
113. Weinmann SC, Pisetsky DS. Mechanisms of immune-related adverse events during the treatment of cancer with immune checkpoint inhibitors. Rheumatology (Oxford) 2019;58(Supplement_7):vii59–67.
114. Waterhouse P, Penninger JM, Timms E, et al. Lymphoproliferative disorders with early lethality in mice deficient in Ctla-4. Science 1995;270(5238):985–8.
115. Klocke K, Sakaguchi S, Holmdahl R, et al. Induction of autoimmune disease by deletion of CTLA-4 in mice in adulthood. Proc Natl Acad Sci U S A 2016;113(17): E2383–92.
116. Nishimura H, Nose M, Hiai H, et al. Development of lupus-like autoimmune diseases by disruption of the PD-1 gene encoding an ITIM motif-carrying immunoreceptor. Immunity 1999;11(2):141–51.
117. Hosseini A, Gharibi T, Marofi F, et al. CTLA-4: From mechanism to autoimmune therapy. Int Immunopharmacol 2020;80:106221.
118. Guo Y, Walsh AM, Canavan M, et al. Immune checkpoint inhibitor PD-1 pathway is down-regulated in synovium at various stages of rheumatoid arthritis disease progression. PLoS One 2018;13(2):e0192704.
119. Selby MJ, Engelhardt JJ, Quigley M, et al. Anti-CTLA-4 antibodies of IgG2a isotype enhance antitumor activity through reduction of intratumoral regulatory T cells. Cancer Immunol Res 2013;1(1):32–42.
120. Simpson TR, Li F, Montalvo-Ortiz W, et al. Fc-dependent depletion of tumor-infiltrating regulatory T cells co-defines the efficacy of anti-CTLA-4 therapy against melanoma. J Exp Med 2013;210(9):1695–710.

121. Cha E, Klinger M, Hou Y, et al. Improved survival with T cell clonotype stability after anti-CTLA-4 treatment in cancer patients. Sci Transl Med 2014;6(238): 238ra270.

122. Wei SC, Levine JH, Cogdill AP, et al. Distinct Cellular Mechanisms Underlie Anti-CTLA-4 and Anti-PD-1 Checkpoint Blockade. Cell 2017;170(6):1120–33.e7.

123. Koyama S, Akbay EA, Li YY, et al. Adaptive resistance to therapeutic PD-1 blockade is associated with upregulation of alternative immune checkpoints. Nat Commun 2016;7:10501.

124. June CH, Warshauer JT, Bluestone JA. Is autoimmunity the Achilles' heel of cancer immunotherapy? Nat Med 2017;23(5):540–7.

125. Oh DY, Cham J, Zhang L, et al. Immune Toxicities Elicted by CTLA-4 Blockade in Cancer Patients Are Associated with Early Diversification of the T-cell Repertoire. Cancer Res 2017;77(6):1322–30.

126. Armand P, Shipp MA, Ribrag V, et al. Programmed death-1 blockade with pembrolizumab in patients with classical hodgkin lymphoma after brentuximab vedotin failure. J Clin Oncol 2016;34(31):3733–9.

127. Subudhi SK, Aparicio A, Gao J, et al. Clonal expansion of CD8 T cells in the systemic circulation precedes development of ipilimumab-induced toxicities. Proc Natl Acad Sci U S A 2016;113(42):11919–24.

128. Das R, Bar N, Ferreira M, et al. Early B cell changes predict autoimmunity following combination immune checkpoint blockade. J Clin Invest 2018; 128(2):715–20.

129. de Moel EC, Rozeman EA, Kapiteijn EH, et al. Autoantibody Development under Treatment with Immune-Checkpoint Inhibitors. Cancer Immunol Res 2019; 7(1):6–11.

130. Ibraheim H, Perucha E, Powell N. Pathology of immune-mediated tissue lesions following treatment with immune checkpoint inhibitors. Rheumatology (Oxford) 2019;58(Supplement_7):vii17–28.

131. Lute KD, May KF Jr, Lu P, et al. Human CTLA4 knock-in mice unravel the quantitative link between tumor immunity and autoimmunity induced by anti-CTLA-4 antibodies. Blood 2005;106(9):3127–33.

Moving?

Make sure your subscription moves with you!

To notify us of your new address, find your **Clinics Account Number** (located on your mailing label above your name), and contact customer service at:

Email: journalscustomerservice-usa@elsevier.com

800-654-2452 (subscribers in the U.S. & Canada)
314-447-8871 (subscribers outside of the U.S. & Canada)

Fax number: 314-447-8029

Elsevier Health Sciences Division
Subscription Customer Service
3251 Riverport Lane
Maryland Heights, MO 63043

*To ensure uninterrupted delivery of your subscription,
please notify us at least 4 weeks in advance of move.

Printed and bound by CPI Group (UK) Ltd, Croydon, CR0 4YY

08/05/2025

01864694-0008